Principles of M

Laboratory Practice

Principles of IVF Laboratory Practice

Edited by

Markus Montag
ilabcomm GmbH, St Augustin, Germany

Dean Morbeck
Scientific Director, Fertility Associates, New Zealand

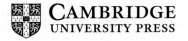
CAMBRIDGE
UNIVERSITY PRESS

CAMBRIDGE
UNIVERSITY PRESS

University Printing House, Cambridge CB2 8BS, United Kingdom

One Liberty Plaza, 20th Floor, New York, NY 10006, USA

477 Williamstown Road, Port Melbourne, VIC 3207, Australia

4843/24, 2nd Floor, Ansari Road, Daryaganj, Delhi - 110002, India

79 Anson Road, #06-04/06, Singapore 079906

Cambridge University Press is part of the University of Cambridge.

It furthers the University's mission by disseminating knowledge in the
pursuit of education, learning, and research at the highest international levels
of excellence.

www.cambridge.org
Information on this title: www.cambridge.org/9781316603512
10.1017/9781316569238

© Cambridge University Press 2017

First published 2017

Printed in the United Kingdom by TJ International Ltd. Padstow Cornwall
in April 2017.

A catalogue record for this publication is available from the British Library.

Library of Congress Cataloging-in-Publication Data
Names: Montag, Markus, editor. | Morbeck, Dean (Dean E.), editor.
Title: Principles of IVF laboratory practice / edited by Markus Montag,
Dean Morbeck.
Description: Cambridge ; New York, NY : University Printing House, 2017. |
Includes bibliographical references and index.
Identifiers: LCCN 2016047633 | ISBN 9781316603512 (pbk. : alk. paper)
Subjects: | MESH: Fertilization in Vitro–methods |
Clinical Laboratory Techniques | Laboratory Manuals
Classification: LCC RG135 | NLM WQ 25 | DDC 618.1/780599–dc23 LC
record available at https://lccn.loc.gov/2016047633

ISBN 978-1-316-60351-2 Paperback

Contents

Section 8 Embryo Biopsy

Section 9 Embryo Transfer

Section 10 Quality Management

The color plates appear between pages 144 and 145

Contributors

Mina Alikani
Reproductive Science Center of New Jersey, Eatontown, NJ, USA

Basak Balaban
Assisted Reproduction Unit, VKF American Hospital, Nisantasi-Istanbul, Turkey

C. Brent Barrett
Boston IVF, Boston, MA, USA

Dara S. Berger
UNC Fertility, Department of Obstetrics and Gynecology, Division of Reproductive Endocrinology and Infertility, Raleigh, NC, USA

Kathrin Berrisford
CARE Fertility, Nottingham, UK

Marcela Calonge
IVI Santiago de Chile, Chile

Alison Campbell
CARE Fertility, Nottingham, UK

Tiencheng Arthur Chang
University of Texas Health Science Center, San Antonio, TX, USA

Greg L. Christensen
University of Louisville, KY, USA

Melicia Clarke-Williams
New York University Langone Medical Center, New York, NY, USA

Tyler Cozzubbo
Weill Cornell Medical College, Ronald O. Perelman and Claudia Cohen Center for Reproductive Medicine, New York, NY, USA

Michael Crowe
Fertility Lab Sciences, Lone Tree, CO, USA

Nina Desai
Cleveland Clinic Fertility Center, Cleveland, OH, USA

Anick De Vos
Center for Reproductive Medicine, Brussels, Belgium

Andrew D. Dorfmann
Genetics & IVF Institute, Fairfax EggBank

Caroline Drew
CARE Fertility, Nottingham, UK

Thomas Ebner
Kinderwunsch Zentrum Linz and Johannes Kepler University Linz, Faculty of Medicine, Linz, Austria

Kara A. Ehlers
University of Louisville, KY, USA

Courtney Failor
University of Texas Health Science Center, San Antonio, TX, USA

Aisaku Fukuda
IVF Osaka Clinic, Japan

Giannoula Karagouga
Dept. of Biomarker Discovery, Center of Individualized Medicine, Mayo Clinic, Rochester, MN, USA

Kathryn J. Go
IVF New England, a Boston IVF partner, Lexington, MA, USA

Cristina Hickman
IVF Hammersmith, Ltd., Boston Place Clinic, London, UK

Heather S. Hoff
UNC Fertility, Department of Obstetrics and Gynecology, Division of Reproductive Endocrinology and Infertility, University of North Carolina, Raleigh, NC, USA

Rebecca Holmes
Boston IVF, Boston, MA, USA

Romain Imber
Centre Hospitalier Inter Régional Cavell
(CHIREC), Braine l'Alleud – Bruxelles,
Belgium

Benedetta Iussig
GENERA Centres for Reproductive
Medicine, Rome, Marostica, Umbertide,
Napoli, Italy

David Jareno
Centre Hospitalier Inter Régional Cavell
(CHIREC), Braine l'Alleud – Bruxelles,
Belgium

Sangita K Jindal
Montefiore's Institute for Reproductive
Medicine and Health, Department
Obstetrics, Gynecology and Women's
Health, Albert Einstein College of
Medicine, Bronx, NY, USA

Dawn A. Kelk
Yale University School of Medicine, Yale
Fertility Center, New Haven, CT, USA

Sabine Kliesch
Centre of Reproductive Medicine and
Andrology, University Hospital of
Münster, Germany

María José de los Santos
IVF Laboratory Director of IVI,
Valencia, Italy

Patty Ann Labella
NYU Fertility Center, New York University
Langone Medical Center, New York,
NY, USA

Alex Lagunov
Fertility Lab Sciences, Lone Tree, CO, USA

Georgios Liperis
Westmead Fertility Centre and Institute of
Reproduction, University of Sydney,
Westmead, Australia

Jonathan Lo
Yale Fertility Center, Yale University
School of Medicine, New Haven, CT, USA

Caroline McCaffrey
NYU Fertility Center, New York University
Langone Medical Center, New York,
NY, USA

David H. McCulloh
NYU Fertility Center, New York University
Langone Medical Center, New York,
NY, USA

Marius Meintjes
Frisco Institute for Reproductive Medicine,
Austin, TX, USA

Satoshi Mizuno
IVF Osaka Clinic, Japan

Maximilian Murtinger
IVF Centers Prof Zech, Bregenz, Austria

Queenie V. Neri
Weill Cornell Medical College, Ronald
O. Perelman and Claudia Cohen Center for
Reproductive Medicine, New York,
NY, USA

Verena Nordhoff
Centre of Reproductive Medicine and
Andrology, University Hospital of
Münster, Germany

Oriol Oliana
IVF Hammersmith, Ltd., Boston Place
Clinic, London, UK

Gianpiero D. Palermo
Weill Cornell Medical College,
Reproductive Medicine,
Ithaca, NY, USA

Thomas B. Pool
Fertility San Antonio, TX, USA

Nicolas Prados
IVF Laboratory Director of IVI,
Valencia, Italy

Pooja Rambhia
Case Western Reserve University School of
Medicine, Cleveland, OH, USA

Michael L. Reed
Center for Reproductive Medicine of New
Mexico, Albuquerque, NM, USA

Laura Rienzi
GENERA Centers for Reproductive
Medicine, Napoli, Italy

Mitchel C. Schiewe
Ovagen Fertility, Newport Beach,
CA, USA

Karen Schnauffer
Hewitt Fertility Centres, Liverpool
Women's Hospital, Liverpool, UK

Cecilia Sjöblom
Westmead Fertility Centre and Institute of
Reproduction, University of Sydney,
Westmead, Australia

Amy E.T. Sparks
University of Iowa Carver College of
Medicine, Department of Obstetrics and
Gynecology, Iowa City, IA, USA

Jason E. Swain
Fertility Lab Sciences,
Lone Tree, CO, USA

Jun Tao
Fertility Treatment Center, Tempe,
AZ, USA

Stephen Troup
Hewitt Fertility Centres, Liverpool
Women's Hospital, Liverpool, UK

Filippo M. Ubaldi
GENERA Centres for Reproductive
Medicine, Rome, Marostica, Umbertide,
Napoli, Italy

Pierre Vanderzwalmen
Centre Hospitalier Inter Régional Cavell
(CHIREC), Braine l'Alleud – Bruxelles,
Belgium

Sabine Vanderzwalmen
IVF Centers Prof Zech, Bregenz, Austria
Centre Hospitalier Inter Régional Cavell
(CHIREC), Braine l'Alleud – Bruxelles,
Belgium

Shunping Wang
Brown University, Providence, RI, USA

Klaus E. Wiemer
Poma Fertility, Kirkland, AZ, USA

Barbara Wirleitner
IVF Centers Prof Zech, Bregenz, Austria

Foreword

Soon we shall reach the 40th anniversary of the birth of Louise Brown, the world's first 'test-tube' baby, born in a small town in the north of England, thanks to the tireless work of Robert Edwards and Patrick Steptoe. During the intervening years, it has been wonderful to see how the technologies associated with the treatment of human infertility have developed and how widely they have been adopted around the world. It is estimated that around six million in vitro fertilization (IVF) children have now been born worldwide, a number that continues to increase steadily.

The IVF laboratory has changed dramatically over the intervening four decades and is consequently far more sophisticated with regards to the technologies used routinely to treat infertile couples, which now include intra-cytoplasmic sperm injection (ICSI), embryo biopsy, pre-implantation genetic screening, blastocyst culture, vitrification and time-lapse analysis. In parallel, there has been a rapid increase in the number of clinics worldwide. Consequently, this has created a pressing need for the standardization of training and education for embryologists.

In this book, Montag and Morbeck have assembled contributions from several experts around the world, who have penned detailed procedures for each component of IVF – from the very inception of a laboratory through to the very conception of a pregnancy. This book therefore represents a veritable gold mine of procedures which will be invaluable not only to new laboratories but also to all those clinics that strive to make our patients' dreams of having a family fulfilled, and hence a copy should be located in every clinic worldwide.

Professor David K. Gardner
School of BioSciences
The University of Melbourne
Parkville, Victoria
Australia

Preface

Since the first successful human in vitro fertilization (IVF) treatment in 1978, IVF has transformed from an experimental procedure to an established standard of care that is practiced throughout the world, every year helping thousands of infertile patients realize their dream of parenthood. We can deliver this incredible care only by standing on the shoulders of the pioneers of our field, who through trial, error and determination developed the foundation for how we practice today. We are fortunate to work in a field that rapidly advances, and the IVF laboratory, at the core of this advancement, has become increasingly complex. This complexity is not limited to the procedures themselves but starts during the planning and construction of an IVF laboratory and continues with the training of young embryologists. Operation of an IVF laboratory comprises a portfolio of techniques that cover basic as well as advanced practices. Capturing and transforming this breadth of material into a practical, cookbook-like manual seemed to be obvious, and we, the editors, were encouraged that perhaps this is a gap that needs filling.

Today's embryology world is rapidly changing, and with it come new challenges as new generations of embryologists begin their careers. As the pioneers of IVF transition to retirement, all the knowledge they acquired through learning by doing has yielded what we consider to be the *Principles in IVF Practice* – sound procedures that will work in almost every laboratory. It is our aim to capture these principles for all those who enter our expanding and fast-growing field and do not have the chance or the freedom to learn by trial and error. Many embryologists in laboratories around the globe use the basics that are described in this book. One can consider these methods as a foundation of good working practice for new embryologists.

One theme of this book is the mix of contributing authors that come from different parts of the world with very different points of view. Thus, experienced practitioners in the world of IVF can compare their own and established concepts with those of others and perhaps learn something new as well. We sincerely hope that this book will contribute to and stimulate discussions in many laboratories on how to perform or adapt procedures. We, too, learned much during the editing process and are eager to place the printed version on our laboratory bench.

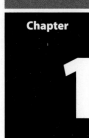

Chapter

Establishing and Equipping a New IVF Laboratory

Alex Lagunov, Michael Crowe and Jason E. Swain

Introduction

Attention to detail and robust quality control systems are essential components for a successful in vitro fertilization (IVF) laboratory, necessary to maintain high success rates. This not only pertains to daily laboratory operations, such as adequate staff training, monitoring of equipment function and weekly/monthly success rates, but also entails proper laboratory design and construction. A highly successful IVF laboratory requires careful consideration of layout and workflow and use of appropriate materials to avoid introducing potentially embryotoxic factors into the laboratory environment.

1.1 Background

The design and equipping of a new IVF laboratory can be a daunting and tedious endeavour. Numerous factors must be considered, including space requirements to accommodate staff and equipment as well as layout for optimal workflow. Proximity to other rooms, such as medical gas storage, operating/procedure rooms and transfer rooms, as well as IVF storage is also relevant. The potential for future laboratory expansion is also often desirable. Thus, initial planning of space requirements should consider these items. Each facility will have its own unique demands that will affect the ultimate size and layout of the laboratory space. However, commonalities exist between highly successful laboratories in terms of how the laboratory is built and equipped. Furthermore, key steps are often taken prior to clinical use to ensure proper functioning of the built space.

The following are abbreviated procedures addressing key components to ensure proper establishment and equipment of a modern IVF laboratory. Many key components focus on use of appropriate materials and systems to ensure proper air quality and growth conditions. Of paramount importance is constant oversight during the construction process to ensure that key details are met. Once these requirements have been met, diligence and a thorough quality management programme are required to ensure that optimal laboratory conditions remain intact.

1.2 Supplies and Equipment

- A professional team of architects and a general contracting firm experienced in medical facility build-out
- A penthouse suite or stand-alone building, allowing for proper laboratory layout
- A functional laboratory/clinic design plan that is approved by the laboratory director and architectural and construction teams

- Careful attention to required workflow, equipment, electrical and information technology (IT) needs

- Appropriately chosen construction materials
    - Low or no volatile organic compounds (VOCs)
        - Flooring /adhesives – sheet vinyl with welded seems, low-VOC adhesive
        - Insulation – avoid around perimeter of laboratory; formaldehyde free product or mineral wool if required
        - Paint – no-VOC latex paint product for all laboratory spaces
        - Cabinetry – powder-coated/painted-metal cabinetry, no particle board or laminate
        - Countertops – Corian, Trespa or some other low-VOC hard material without adhesives
        - Furniture – medical- or laboratory-grade furniture with vinyl covering and low-VOC materials
        - Avoid use of printers, corkboards, xylene markers inside the laboratory space
        - Copper piping for gas lines with brazed connection; stainless steel piping also appropriate
        - Tyvek wrap around lab perimeter behind drywall to help maintain positive pressure

    - Minimum 36-inch doors for equipment installation - with gaskets and sweeps
    - Security system on entry doors (lockable)
    - Gas manifold system – gas regulators, Tygon tubing
        - Automatic tank switchers may be used but are not required.
        - Regulators to measure tank pressures are needed at the gas source.
        - Low-pressure regulators at the gas outlet are recommended to meet varying pressure requirements of different incubator models.

    - Required laboratory equipment/vendor list
        - Microscopes, micromanipulators, centrifuges, laminar flow hoods, incubators, refrigerators, alarm system, computers, consumables, etc.

    - Backup generator allowing for all equipment to be supplied with uninterrupted power
        - Natural gas or diesel – may be dictated by code or building requirements. A minimum of eight-hour backup is recommended, and fuel tank size should be appropriate. Battery backups may be used for some equipment, but must be adequate to supply several hours of power.

    - Appropriate, dedicated heating, ventilation and air-conditioning (HVAC) system
        - VOC filtration (various systems exist that use combinations of UV light, carbon filters and potassium permanganate)
        - High-efficiency particulate air (HEPA) filtration
        - properly sized and designed unit to maintain positive pressure inside the laboratory
        - proper placement of air vents to avoid being directly over critical equipment

- Cleaning products
  - 3% Hydrogen peroxide solution or commercially available low-VOC, embryo-safe cleaning solutions
- Required laboratory manuals
  - Quality management programme, protocols and policies, equipment maintenance, safety (Material Safety Data Sheets), etc.

1.3 Quality Control

- Keep a record of meeting minutes and plan revisions with construction company and contractors to track discussions.
- Continue to monitor the construction process on a daily/weekly basis to ensure that design and specifications are followed.
  - Ensure the use of low-VOC products in full range of materials used to construct the laboratory (and procedure room if in proximity to the laboratory).
- Air quality testing prior to and after construction is recommended to achieve appropriate laboratory air quality (measurement of VOCs in ppb levels is recommended).
- Perform a mouse embryo assay (MEA) or approved bioassay prior to clinical cases.

1.4 Procedure

1.4.1 Initial Project Planning

1. Identify a location that suits the needs of the clinic/laboratory.
   a. Proximity to an existing clinic is recommended.
   b. Must be adjacent to procedure room/operating room (OR) and embryo transfer room.
   c. Adequate laboratory space for offices, storage, equipment, specimen collection, medical gasses, etc.

2. Locate and interview several construction and architectural companies based on previous experience in medical facility design and build-out in order to ensure that quality standards are clearly understood and met.

3. Prepare a laboratory floor plan considering workflow, including all laboratory equipment, maintaining close proximity between intracytoplasmic sperm injection (ICSI) stations and other IVF workstations to all incubators.
   a. Compile equipment list and plan locations.
   b. Plan placement of lights, air vents and electrical and IT outlets appropriately.
   c. Design a separate dedicated medical gas/liquid nitrogen storage room. It is recommended to be a sound proof, well-ventilated room located in close proximity to a freight elevator or delivery area, if possible. If feasible, locating this room near IVF liquid nitrogen or vapour tank storage area with vacuum jacketed lines for filling is recommended.
      i. Ensure that building regulations allow for use and transport of high-pressure medical gasses and liquid nitrogen.
   d. Design a separate room for consumables storage and off-gassing.

4. Once plans are approved and construction is initiated, ensure that HVAC is designed based on the required square footage and filtering capacity and meets requested standards (discussed further in HVAC).

5. Ensure that a natural gas or diesel backup power generator is included in the laboratory design and is sufficient to support more than eight hours of backup power supply. Set up generator service schedule to include initial two-hour load bank test, as well as semi-annual maintenance/inspections and yearly load tests.

   a. If a generator is not feasible, uninterruptible power supply (UPS) units are required on all crucial equipment with supply long enough to permit corrective action in case of power failure.

6. Fill out and submit required laboratory applications and paperwork to the relevant governing agencies.

1.4.2 Build-Out Process

1. Verify that all materials used are low or no VOCs (verify during onsite inspections).

   a. Insulation: Insulation is often used in construction. However, chemicals such as formaldehyde are often present. Presence of insulation on the direct periphery of the IVF laboratory should be avoided if possible. If unable to avoid due to the presence of an outside wall, use of a formaldehyde-free product is recommended. Alternatives for sound dampening include mineral wool.

   b. Flooring: Welded instead of glued seems of sheet vinyl flooring are recommended for sanitary reasons as well as minimal VOC release. Prior to clinical use, floors need to be cleaned with appropriate cleaners, such as hydrogen peroxide, along with simple regular sweeping, vacuuming or steam mopping. Avoid the use of any potentially harmful cleaners or waxes inside the laboratory.

   c. Paints: Latex-based no-VOC paints should be used on all painted surfaces.

   d. Cabinetry: Powder-coated metal cabinetry or stainless steel is suggested to avoid concerns with laminate and particle board, which would likely contain adhesives with high levels of VOCs.

   e. Furniture: Purchase all medical- or laboratory-grade chairs with vinyl-coated seating surfaces that are easily cleaned of any contamination. Tables and countertop should be made of either Trespa, Corian, stainless steel or some other hard material devoid of adhesives (laminate).

   f. Cleaners: Alcohol is discouraged due to VOCs. 3% Hydrogen peroxide–based cleaning solutions are recommended.

2. Ensure that HVAC ductwork uses cleaned steel instead of plastic or other materials.

   a. Ductwork should be cleaned onsite by the installation crew using alcohol. Swabs can be taken to verify cleanliness and absence of oil and dust, etc.

   b. Verify that ductwork is sealed during the construction process to avoid dust and contaminants..

3. Ensure that sufficient gas supply is provided for all planned equipment inside the IVF laborator.

   a. Verify that gas piping is in the correct location.

   b. Verify that proper manifold system and regulators are present and functional.

4. Ensure proper placement and functioning of various items.

   a. Confirm placement of light switches and outlets and all necessary equipment for performing daily operations.
   b. Confirm the placement and swing of doors, proper locks, seals, sweeps, etc.

5. Verify function of the generator. If a power outage creates a lag prior to generator power surge, ensure that all equipment is plugged into the UPS.
6. If windows are present, ensure that blackout blinds are available to help regulate light/ heat within the laboratory. Incubators and ICSI workstations should be protected from direct sunlight to avoid potential issues with light and/or temperature regulation.
7. Confirm the absence of cork boards, printers/toners or unapproved markers containing xylene within the confines of the laboratory during move-in. These items may be kept in a separate laboratory office area away from embryo culture and handling locations.

1.4.3 HVAC

1. Select an HVAC company.

   a. Decide on a commercially available 'plug-and-play' filtration system or have HVAC company built from scratch based on required IVF laboratory air quality demands. System should be dedicated to the IVF laboratory.

      i. Filtration should include pre-filters (MERV) and HEPA filtration to remove particulates. Importantly, filtration should also reduce VOC content and can include use of ultraviolet (UV) light for photo-catalytic oxidation or use of chemical filter beds with carbon and potassium permanganate mixtures.
      ii. Placement of filtration system is important; it should be as close to the outlet air ducts in the laboratory as possible to avoid risk for introduction of contaminants in-line after the filters.
      iii. Ensure that air supply duct placement is not directly above/near ICSI stations or incubators, as this will affect temperature regulation of the stage warming units.

   b. Ensure that only metal ductwork is used. This should be pre-cleaned and sealed during construction to avoid introduction of contamination.
   c. Achieve positive pressure in the laboratory.

      i. Request Tyvek wrapping of the laboratory, hard deck ceiling, gasketted lights and doors and door sweeps.

   d. Use proper air exchange rates and ratio of outside-to-inside air to achieve desired air quality.

      i. Recommendations vary and will depend on the HVAC system and beginning air quality.

   e. Ensure a proper water supply drawn to the HVAC unit to allow for constant humidity control.
   f. Ensure that a pressure display panel is installed inside the laboratory to monitor and record positive pressure for proper system functionality as per daily laboratory quality control.

g. Set up a regular maintenance contract with an appropriate company for servicing the belts and other items of the HVAC unit as well as all necessary filter changes to allow for initially targeted air quality standards.

1.4.4 Equipment

1. Determine volume estimates for the laboratory, and obtain quotes for selected equipment.

   a. Quotes and equipment specs (size, electrical requirements, heat output) should be obtained early on in the design process.

      i. Backup units of critical equipment should be considered (ICSI microscopes, incubators, fridges, freezers, etc.).

   b. Low-oxygen incubators are mandatory.

      i. Mix of bench-top units and box-type incubators is recommended.
      ii. Low oxygen may be supplied via premixed tanks or through use of separate nitrogen and carbon dioxide sources depending on type of incubator.
         (1) Nitrogen may be supplied through gas cylinders, high-pressure liquid nitrogen tanks or via a nitrogen generator. Cost, ease of delivery and usage are all factors to consider.
      iii. Use in-line VOC gas filters between gas supply and incubators – change out every four to six months.

2. Attempt to purchase equipment from vendors that are able to service the items within a short amount of time if equipment failures arise.
3. Set up a regular laboratory equipment maintenance system with local service providers (hoods, centrifuges, pipette calibration/validation).
4. Ensure that all incubators and cryo-storage vessels are monitored by an alarm with the ability to e-mail and/or call in case of an emergency.

   a. Wireless systems are now available to help with equipment movement and location and are recommended.

1.4.5 Burn-In

1. After construction, the laboratory should be wiped down with an approved disinfectant/cleaner.

   a. Walls, floors, cabinets and other surfaces should be wiped several times over the course of the burn-in period.

2. Equipment should be moved into the laboratory and cleaned/tested prior to clinical use.

   a. Of critical importance is burn-in of laboratory incubators. Incubators should be cleaned according to manufacturer's instructions and temperature raised to greater than 45°C for several days or up to two weeks to promote off-gassing, cleaned and tested.[1]
   b. Laboratory temperature can be raised to help with off-gassing of other laboratory items.
   c. Verify correct temperature, gas and functioning of all equipment for several days after burn-in on quality control sheets to verify proper environmental conditions and functioning.

3. Perform pH testing of culture media used for embryos and gametes with the aim of achieving desired pH based on incubator carbon dioxide concentration.[1-3]

4. Perform air quality testing measuring VOCs and particle counts before and after burn-in, and record the differences in the readings for quality control records.

   a. This can be performed by a professional company or by laboratory personnel if hand-held particle counters and VOC meters have been purchased by the laboratory or can be obtained from vendors. Sensitivity of these units should be considered (parts per billion recommended for VOC assessment).

5. Perform a MEA to ensure proper incubator conditions.

   a. All culture supplies should also be pre-tested with an appropriate bioassay prior to clinical use.

1.5 Notes

A. Rationale behind using low-VOC materials and a dedicate HVAC system is based on various publications suggesting the cytotoxicity of VOCs.[4-7] VOCs include various types of alkanes, aldehydes, ketones and alcohols commonly concentrated at high levels in paints, glues and flooring.

B. After laboratory commissioning, ongoing maintenance and quality control are required to ensure optimal function and culture conditions.

   i. Schedule for HVAC filter changes, routine cleaning and disinfecting of the laboratory, daily monitoring of incubator gas and temperature, testing of generator and alarm systems, etc.

   ii. Monitoring of key performance indicators (KPIs) to identify possible issues

   (1) Fertilization rates, embryo development rates, clinical pregnancy, etc.

References

1. Swain, J. and Lagunov, A. IVF incubator handling, in *Standard Operational Procedures in Reproductive Medicine Laboratory and Clinical Practice*, ed. B. Rizk and M. Montag. (Boca Raton, FL: CRC Press, in press).

2. Swain, J. E. Optimizing the culture environment in the IVF laboratory: impact of pH and buffer capacity on gamete and embryo quality. *Reprod Biomed Online* 2010; 21(1):6–16.

3. Swain, J. E. Is there an optimal pH for culture media used in clinical IVF? *Hum Reprod Update* 2012; 18(3):333–9.

4. Hall, J., et al. The origin, effects and control of air pollution in laboratories used for human embryo culture. *Hum Reprod* 1998; 13(Suppl. 4):146–55.

5. Schimmel, T., et al. Removal of volatile organic compounds from incubators used for gamete and embryo culture. *Fertil Steril* 1997; 68(Suppl. 1):S165.

6. Morbeck, D. E. Air quality in the assisted reproduction laboratory: a mini-review. *J Assist Reprod Genet* 2015; 32(7):1019–24.

7. Heitmann, R. J., et al. Live births achieved via IVF are increased by improvements in air quality and laboratory environment. *Reprod Biomed Online*, 2015.

Chapter 2

Basic Embryology Skills in the IVF Laboratory

Stephen Troup and Karen Schnauffer

Introduction

Before aspiring embryologists can even begin to perform the procedures that will comprise the majority of their routine workload, there are a number of essential basic skills that underpin their day-to-day work. Failure to acquire these basic skills at the outset can lead to an inability to perform even the simplest of tasks appropriately, an inability to troubleshoot problems and even the potential to place gametes, embryos and patients at risk. As such, considerable time and effort should be dedicated to the acquisition of these basic skills, and this is often reflected in the formally recognised embryology training schemes which now exist (e.g. European Society of Human Reproduction and Embryology (ESHRE) Embryology Certification). A competent embryologist will also equip himself or herself with an appropriate level of theoretical knowledge to allow an understanding of the rationale for processes and procedures. The fundamental nature of the work that an embryologist performs requires that all aspects of training be completed to the highest possible standard, and attention to detail must persist throughout. The importance and relevance of the basic skills described in this chapter should not be underestimated.

2.1 Confidentiality

It is a fundamental rule in medical ethics that information given by, or relating to, a patient remains private and that it should only be shared with a third party under certain agreed circumstances and more often than not with the permission of the patients themselves. In many countries, regulation determines the extent of patient confidentiality.[1] In the absence of such guidance, it remains the responsibility of the embryologist to give due consideration to the often extremely private and personal information that is made available to him or her during a patient's treatment in order to perform his or her tasks and, in particular, with whom this information should be shared. Assumptions should not be made that any third party to whom information is given will respect the confidential nature of the information, and involving the patient in any such disclosure is always advisable.

2.2 Record Keeping

It goes without saying that accurate record keeping within an embryology laboratory is of paramount importance – but it is all too often overlooked. The following set of basic rules, which seek to minimise risk associated with record keeping, should be adopted by embryologists in all areas of their work.

1. Any records pertaining to a patient should be identified using three identifiers, such as forename(s) and surname(s), the patient's date of birth and address and, importantly, a unique identifier such as the hospital/clinic number.
2. All written records should be made in black ink.
3. All entries in the patient record should be signed by the embryologist making the record, together with the date and time of the entry and the designation of the embryologist.
4. All written records should be clearly legible, and where a record needs to be corrected, this should be done by a single line through the incorrect entry (so as not to completely obscure the original entry), which then should be signed and dated as described in rule 3. Correction fluid should not be used.
5. Electronic patient records (EPRs) should be backed up regularly and securely.
6. Paper documents should be scanned into an EPR in such a way that the original document can be reconstituted.

2.3 Traceability

Traceability of gametes, embryos and everything else that comes into contact with them (i.e. consumables, culture media and equipment) for the duration of the treatment is essential and relies on robust recording keeping, as described earlier, to ensure that the correct identity of patients, gametes and embryos is maintained at all times. This enables gametes and embryos to be accurately tracked throughout treatment from procurement to replacement, storage or being discarded. In the event of a commercial product being withdrawn, the traceability system would identify which patients had been affected by the faulty product and enable a full investigation to be carried out. Below is a list of traceability points that should be included in a traceability system:

1. Centres should ensure that patients and partner(s)/donor(s) can be uniquely and accurately identified.
2. The treatment type and date should be clearly documented.
3. Any container used for culture of embryos or preparation of gametes should be fully labelled with the patient's details.
4. All equipment and materials coming into contact with a patient's gametes or embryos should be identified with a product description, source and batch numbers of the product used.
5. The centre from which the gametes or embryos have been created should be recorded.

2.3.1 Aseptic Technique

Successful culture of gametes and embryos *in vitro* depends on keeping the cultures free from contamination by micro-organisms such as fungi, bacteria and viruses. Within an assisted-conception laboratory, many potential sources of biological contamination exist, including the air within the laboratory, non-sterile supplies, unclean surfaces, equipment and clothing and also the individuals who work within the laboratory! In some countries, regulations exist specifying the 'quality' of air required within laboratories where gametes and embryos are handled.[2]

'Aseptic technique' is a set of procedures designed to create a 'barrier' between micro-organisms in the environment to reduce the probability of contamination from these sources. There are four basic elements of aseptic technique, namely, a sterile work area, good personal hygiene, sterile reagents and sterile handling techniques.

2.3.1.1 Sterile Work Area

The simplest and most effective way to reduce contamination from airborne particles and aerosols (i.e. dust, spores, sneezing, shed skin, etc.) is to use a safety cabinet. A number of sizes and designs are commercially available depending on the needs of the user, with some being specifically designed for assisted-conception use (ACU). Listed below are some important general considerations regarding their use:

1. The safety cabinet should be professionally installed and commissioned and be dedicated for ACU.
2. The safety cabinet should be located in an area that is free from drafts from doors, windows and other equipment and with minimal through traffic.
3. The safety cabinet should be left running at all times and only switched off when it will not be used for extended periods of time.
4. The work surface should be uncluttered and contain only items required for the procedure being undertaken.
5. The safety cabinet should not be used to process gametes or embryos from more than one patient at a time.
6. A Bunsen burner (or any naked flame) should not be used within an assisted-conception laboratory.
7. Before and after use and in-between patients, the surfaces of the cabinet should be disinfected using a suitable cleaning agent. Human gametes and embryos are particularly susceptible to damage by cleaning agents and by volatile organic compounds (VOCs)[3] often released by commonly used disinfecting agents. As such, it is advisable to use products which are known to be safe within the IVF laboratory.

2.3.1.2 Good Personal Hygiene

Wash your hands using a suitable proprietary hand cleaner regularly. This ideally should be on entering and leaving the laboratory and also between patients. If the latter is not feasible, then the use of alcohol hand gels is an acceptable alternative.

Wearing personal protective equipment (e.g. theatre scrubs which are regularly laundered) reduces the probability of contamination from shed skin as well as dirt and dust from your clothes. A theatre cap and dedicated clean laboratory footwear are also essential.

2.3.1.3 Aseptic Liquid Handling

The following general guidance will minimize the risk of contamination when handling the various culture media used within the embryology laboratory:

1. Ensure that your hands and the work area are clean.
2. Avoid pouring directly from bottles or flasks.
3. Use sterile glass or disposable plastic pipettes and a pipettor to work with liquids, and use each pipette only once to avoid cross-contamination. Do not unwrap sterile pipettes until they are to be used. Keep your pipettes within your work area.
4. Always cap bottles and flasks immediately after use.
5. Do not uncover a sterile flask, bottle, Petri dish and so forth until immediately prior to use, and do not leave any containers open to the environment. Return the cover/lid as soon as you are finished.
6. If you remove a cap or cover and have to put it down on the work surface, place the cap with its opening facing down.

Appendix 2A contains a list of suggestions and procedures regarding aseptic technique. Completion of this should help you to achieve effective aseptic technique.

2.4 Microscopy

Human gametes and embryos are not visible to the human eye, necessitating the use of a microscope for a very large proportion of the work performed by an embryologist. Embryologists use a variety of microscopes in their day-to-day work, including low-magnification stereomicroscopes for the observation and handling of eggs and embryos, higher-magnification compound microscopes to observe and assess sperm and very-high-magnification inverted compound microscopes with micro-manipulators attached to allow gametes and embryos to be handled with extremely fine control. In addition, a number of different illumination systems will be encountered to enable usually unstained, live gametes and embryos to be observed using the microscope (e.g. dark-field, phase-contrast, Hoffmann, etc.).

All microscopes are basically the same and comprise a light source, something to 'hold' the sample, a magnifying lens and an eyepiece(s) to focus the observer's eyes on the image. Whilst it would be impossible to describe how to correctly set up every different microscope, we have listed some basic tips which will help to achieve optimal performance from all microscopes:

1. Follow the manufacturer's instructions very carefully.
2. Familiarise yourself with the individual components of each microscope and how each piece fits together.
3. Keep all lenses and eyepieces clean by using an appropriate lens tissue. Avoid using tissue paper to clean lenses.
4. Ensure that no components of the microscope are loose.
5. Do not interchange lenses between microscopes.
6. Most microscopes have two eyepieces, at least one of which will be adjustable. Take time to adjust the eyepieces to suit your own eyes – this will significantly improve the image you see and avoid eye strain.
7. Keep a supply of spare bulbs and fuses for each microscope.
8. Ensure that the laboratory has ready access to any tools required to dismantle and reassemble the microscope.
9. Do not panic if the microscope appears to not be working – a properly set up microscope will always work!

2.5 Handling Gametes and Embryos

An embryologist will spend a significant amount of time handling gametes and embryos, more often than not using various forms of pipettes. These skills require a high degree of manual dexterity, and the ability to move gametes and embryos efficiently and safely is the key to being a successful embryologist. Although many different pipetting devices are available, the following basic rules apply throughout:

1. Always use a sterile pipette.
2. Never use the same pipette for more than one patient.
3. Ensure that the pipette is the correct size, particularly that its internal diameter is not too small.

4. If using a pipetting device, ensure that it is working properly before starting to use it.
5. Bubbles are the embryologist's nightmare as eggs and embryos will stick to them. As such, careful, controlled pipetting must be used at all times to avoid the generation of bubbles.
6. Ensure that the embryos are out of the incubator for the shortest time possible.

2.6 Risk Reduction and Witnessing

In every field where tasks are performed by humans, occasional mistakes will be made, and unfortunately, the embryology laboratory is not immune to the possibility of 'human error'. Although 'mix-ups' in the embryology laboratory are exceptionally rare, the consequences of such mistakes are devastating to all involved and can also attract a high level of public interest. One such unfortunate incident in a UK assisted-conception laboratory in the late 1990s led to the publication of a number of recommendations[4] which now form the basis of the way in which the chance of embryology mix-ups can be minimised.

Much of the risk reduction can be achieved by cross-checking and witnessing either manually, using bar-code or radio-frequency identification systems or both. The recommendations are summarised as follows:

1. Every sample of gametes or embryos should be identifiable at all stages of treatment.
2. Witnessing protocols should be employed when any of the following procedures take place:
   a. Collecting eggs.
   b. Collecting sperm.
   c. Preparing sperm.
   d. Mixing sperm and eggs or injecting sperm into eggs.
   e. Moving gametes or embryos between tubes or dishes.
   f. Transferring embryos into a woman.
   g. Inseminating a woman.
   h. Placing gametes or embryos into cryostorage.
   i. Removing gametes or embryos from cryostorage.
   j. Disposing of gametes or embryos.
   k. Transporting gametes or embryos.

3. Each witnessing stage should check the patient's full name and identifying code, and a formal record (including signatures) should be made of each stage (including the person performing the task, the person witnessing the task and the date and time the witnessing stage took place).
4. Consideration should be given to which members of staff are appropriate to perform witnessing and to provide them with specific witnessing training – it is not appropriate to ask someone who happens to be passing to 'quickly watch what you're doing'. Also, bear in mind that the risk of mistakes occurring is higher when staff are asked to perform procedures repetitively.[5]
5. Distractions in the laboratory should be kept to a minimum, and the use of mobile phones and entertainment systems is discouraged.
6. When developing witnessing procedures, consideration should be given to the disruption they may cause, as being interrupted and returning to a task are a common cause of mistakes.

References

1. Human Fertilisation and Embryology Authority (HFEA). *Code of Practice*, 8th edn. (London: HFEA, 2009, revised 2015).

2. Commission Directive 2006/17/EC of 8 February 2006 Implementing Directive 2004/23/EC of the European Parliament and of the Council as Regards Certain Technical Requirements for the Donation, Procurement and Testing of Human Tissues and Cells.

3. Khoudja, R. Y., Xu, Y., Li, T. and Zhou, C. Better IVF outcomes following improvements in laboratory air quality. *J Assist Reprod Genet* 2013; 30(1):69–76.

4. Toft, B. *Independent Review of the Circumstances Surrounding Four Adverse Events That Occurred in the Reproductive Medicine Units at The Leeds Teaching Hospitals NHS Trust, West Yorkshire,* Department of Health 40216 1P 0.4k Jun 4 (CWP).

5. Toft, B. and Mascie-Taylor, H. Involuntary automaticity: a work-system induced risk to safe health care. *Health Services Manage Res* 2005; 18(4):211–16.

Appendix 2A Questionnaire to Help Achieve Effective Aseptic Technique

Question	Date Completed	Signature

Work area

Is the safety cabinet properly installed and commissioned?

Is the safety cabinet in an area free from drafts and through traffic?

Is the work surface uncluttered, and does it contain only items required for your procedure?

Have the inner surfaces of the safety cabinet been decontaminated?

Are you routinely cleaning (and sterilising where possible) your safety cabinets, incubators, refrigerators and other laboratory equipment?

Personal hygiene

Did you wash your hands?

Are you wearing suitable laboratory clothing?

Are you changing your shoes when you enter and leave the 'clean area'?

If you have long hair, is it tied in the back?

Are you using a pipettor to work with liquids?

Reagents and media

Are all your bottles, flasks and other containers capped when not in use?

Do any of your reagents look cloudy? Contaminated? Do they contain floating particles?

Handling

Are you working slowly and deliberately, mindful of aseptic technique?

Are you placing the caps or lids face down on the work area?

Are you using sterile glass pipettes or sterile disposable plastic pipettes to manipulate all liquids?

Are you using a sterile pipette only once to avoid cross-contamination?

Are you careful not to touch the pipette tip to anything non-sterile, including the outside edge of the bottle threads or the work surface?

Chapter

3

Sperm Preparation for IVF
Training Protocol

Kara A. Ehlers and Greg L. Christensen

Introduction

The preparation of a clean, highly motile sperm sample is an important part of a successful in vitro fertilization (IVF) programme. Preparing sperm samples for IVF is also one of the first skills taught to junior embryologists and can help set both the tone and standard for how the remainder of their embryology training will occur. In addition to training junior embryologists on how to manipulate and process a sperm sample, it is also crucial that they are taught the importance of good quality control, correct labeling and sample identification, proper documentation and problem-solving skills. [1] The purpose of this brief chapter is to help identify how to help train a junior embryologist to prepare sperm for IVF rather than simply provide protocols for sperm preparation.

3.1 Background

Regardless of the industry, common sense teaches us that untrained or poorly trained staff will not perform efficiently, be able to provide high-quality service or have satisfaction in their work. Add to this the sensitive nature of assisted reproductive technology (ART), the high emotional investment of the patients and the serious consequences that an error could have and it becomes clear why having a good training programme and well-trained staff is so important.

The Clinical Laboratory Improvement Amendments (CLIA) of 1988 establish standards for the staff of high-complexity laboratories. These standards range from required education levels to ongoing assessment of competency. They also include requirements for the minimum levels of training required but do not specify how the training should occur. In this respect, it is the responsibility of the laboratory director or designee to develop a training programme that will give trainees the skill set to perform the required tasks independently, correctly and with confidence.

3.2 Trainees

In most cases, individuals selected for training in IVF sperm preparation have already been trained on performing semen analysis. Before advanced training on sperm preparation occurs, it is important that trainees have mastered the elements of the semen analysis, including assessment of concentration, motility and morphology.

Sperm preparation for insemination and IVF can be considered a therapeutic procedure rather than diagnostic, and some argue that it technically can be performed by individuals who do not meet high-complexity testing requirements. Regardless, it is our opinion that since many of the elements of sperm preparation are the same as for semen analysis, trainees should meet the same CLIA requirements in programmes where the CLIA are applicable. Per CLIA requirements, all high-complexity testing personnel must hold at minimum an associate's degree in laboratory science or the defined equivalent. Additionally, they must be evaluated and demonstrate competency to perform their assigned tasks semi-annually during the first year and annually thereafter.[2]

3.3 Training

The field of embryology is unique as it is largely an apprenticeship with more senior embryologists training junior embryologists. As a result, it is important for an ART laboratory to develop a training protocol with a mechanism to determine when proficiency has been reached for a specific task before allowing it to be performed independently. While there is no specific 'right' way to train someone on how to do sperm preparations for IVF, the following points are helpful in teaching this and other new skills:

1. *Designate the individual or individuals responsible for training.* In busy programmes with a lot of staff, this is especially important so that trainees know who to listen to and trainers know they have been given the assignment. The people selected to train should be knowledgeable, capable of explaining complex ideas and, ideally, patient.

2. *Maintain detailed written protocols as a reference.* Protocols should be clearly written and simple to follow. They should include a brief overview of the protocol, a list of supplies, instructions for preparing reagents and a clear list of steps to be followed. The designated trainers should be instructed to teach trainees how to prepare sperm samples according to the written protocol rather than their own personal versions. Trainees should be encouraged to reference the protocol as needed when they have questions. An example of a written protocol for preparing sperm for ART via density gradient separation is included at the end of this chapter.

3. *Train using the see-do-teach method.* Allow trainees to watch some sperm preparations until they are comfortable that they understand the process. The observation or 'see' phase of training is an excellent time to discuss how to handle outliers such as semen samples with high viscosity, low volume or very low concentration. Next, allow trainees to practice and perform sperm preparations under supervision, preferably using non-patient samples initially. Once they are confident that they understand and can perform the steps, have them teach the procedure to someone else, such as an administrative staff member.

It is important at the beginning of the training that the expectations are very clear. Trainees should be informed of what they will need to learn and be able to do before they are cleared to work unsupervised. This will vary from programme to programme but should include correct labelling and documentation of samples, slides and paperwork; the ability to perform the steps of the sperm preparation correctly; and demonstration of the knowledge needed to work independently. Trainees should be encouraged to ask questions, and trainers should give feedback wherever possible. For complex processes such as sperm preparation, it may be helpful to break the training process into sections.

Documentation of training, including how and when it was performed, and the status of an individual's ability to perform independently should be maintained in that person's personnel record.[2]

3.4 Competency Assessment

All staff within the laboratory should be evaluated periodically to document that they are competent to perform their job descriptions. When staff are trained on a new skill, such as sperm preparation, this competency assessment can be documented at the completion of the training process. For programmes regulated by the CLIA, a competency assessment must be completed for each test or procedure that personnel are approved to perform within the first six months of employment and yearly thereafter.

The six required elements of a CLIA competency assessment include the following[2]:

1. Direct observation of routine patient test performance, including patient preparation (if applicable) and specimen handling, processing and testing
2. Monitoring the recording and reporting of test results
3. Review of intermediate test results or worksheets, quality control records, proficiency testing results and preventive maintenance records
4. Direct observations of performance of instrument maintenance and function checks
5. Assessment of test performance by testing previously analyzed specimens, internal blind testing of samples or external proficiency testing of samples
6. Assessment of problem-solving skills

Inasmuch as these apply to sperm preparation for IVF, they should be incorporated into both the initial training programme and routine competency assessments.

3.5 Density Gradient Sperm Preparation for IVF: Sample Protocol

All programmes should incorporate protocols that have been first validated in their own facility, and the following protocol is intended only as an example. The notes following the protocol are intended to draw attention to a few specific points regarding some differences about preparing sperm for IVF on which technicians should be trained.

3.5.1 Protocol Overview

Sperm preparations used for inseminating oocytes or intracytoplasmic sperm injection (ICSI) must be very clean and highly motile. The density gradient produces such a sample by filtering out seminal fluids, debris and non-motile sperm or other cell types from the final samples. In brief, layers of density gradient medium, containing silane-coated silica particles, are placed in a centrifuge tube, and semen is layered on top. The sample is centrifuged, and the most motile sperm move through the density gradient medium during centrifugation to collect in a soft pellet at the bottom. The layers above the pellet are removed, leaving the pellet, which is washed free of the density gradient medium and re-suspended to an appropriate concentration for insemination or ICSI.

3.5.1.1 Supplies

- 15-ml centrifuge tubes
- 5-ml pipette
- Counting chamber
- Transfer pipettes
- Pre-stained morphology slides
- Centrifuge

- Phase-contrast microscope
- Personal protective equipment
- Pipette and pipette tips (1–20 μl)

3.5.1.2 Media

- 90% Gradient layer (see following table)
- 45% Gradient layer (see following table)
- 5 ml of fertilization medium in a medium tube (protein added and equilibrated overnight in a CO_2 incubator)

	90% Gradient medium	45% Gradient medium
100% Stock gradient solution	9 ml	4.5 ml
Human tubal fluid (HTF) + 5% protein	1 ml	5.5 ml

Once prepared, the gradient medium can be stored for up to two weeks at between 2 and 8°C.

3.5.1.3 Protocol

1. Label all materials including paperwork, specimen containers and centrifuge tubes with the patient's name, IVF case number and the date.
2. Prepare a density gradient column by placing 1 ml of 90% sperm gradient medium in the bottom of a sterile centrifuge tube. Gently layer an additional 1 ml of 45% sperm gradient medium on top of the 90% layer by running it down the side of the centrifuge tube. Maintain the column at 37°C until ready for use.
3. Once the semen sample has been checked into the laboratory, record the time of receipt on the sperm preparation form, and allow the sperm sample to liquefy at 37°C (liquefaction will take ~15 to 20 minutes). Once liquefied, gently swirl the container several times to mix the sample. Place a 5-μl drop of the semen on a counting chamber, and perform an analysis of motility and concentration. Place another 5-μl drop of semen on a pre-stained slide for morphology analysis, and place a coverslip over it. Record all the results for the initial analysis on the patient's worksheet along with any unusual observations. Refer to the semen analysis protocol for any questions regarding the semen analysis.
4. Measure the volume by aspirating the sample into a 5-ml pipette, and gently layer the semen on top of the prepared gradient column by running the sample down the side of the tube (Note A).
5. Centrifuge the sample at 300×g for 15 minutes, making sure that the centrifuge is correctly balanced.
6. Gently aspirate the supernatant (top layer of seminal fluid), the 45% layer and the upper half of the 90% layer, and set aside in the patient's specimen container. Be careful not to disturb the soft pellet at the bottom.
7. Dilute the remaining 90% layer with approximately 3 ml of CO_2 equilibrated fertilization medium. Gently invert the centrifuge tube to mix the sample (Note B).
8. Centrifuge the sample for 10 minutes at 300×g.
9. Gently decant the supernatant into the patient's specimen container and set it aside (Note C).

10. Using a clean syringe, add fresh fertilization medium to bring the final volume up to 1 ml, and re-suspend the sample by gently drawing it up and down with the syringe or by using a vortex.
11. Place a small aliquot of the sample on a counting chamber to evaluate the final motility and concentration. Record the results on the patient's worksheet, including the time the sample preparation was completed (Note D).
12. Maintain the sample at 37°C in an equilibrated incubator for a minimum of one hour before insemination (Note E).

3.5.1.4 Notes

A. Less sperm is needed for IVF preparations than for intrauterine insemination (IUI). Therefore, if the sample is being prepared for conventional insemination and has a normal concentration and motility, no more than 1 ml typically needs to be processed. The same principle applies for samples being prepared for ICSI when reasonable sperm numbers are present.

B. Whereas sperm samples prepared for IUI are routinely given a final wash in a HEPES-buffered medium or similar, sperm samples prepared for IVF insemination should receive a final wash in the same medium in which the oocytes are incubated at the time of insemination.

C. No portion of the gradient layers or other media used in processing the IVF sperm sample should be disposed of until the final analysis is complete and preferably not until the insemination is performed. If needed, extra sperm can be recovered from these layers as needed.

D. Typical insemination protocols call for concentrations of motile sperm ranging from 25,000 to 500,000 being added to insemination dishes. Trainees should be instructed on how to calculate the correct volume or dilution needed to achieve the right concentration for insemination.

E. Allowing the sample to incubate for a period of time prior to insemination can facilitate capacitation. If a cryopreserved specimen is going to be used, it can be prepared just prior to insemination, as cryopreserved specimens undergo capacitation spontaneously and do not maintain their progressive motility as long as fresh samples.

References

1. ASRM Practice Committee. Recommended practices for the management of embryology, andrology, and endocrinology laboratories: a committee opinion. American Society for Reproductive Medicine, Birmingham, AL, 2014.

2. Centers for Medical and Medicaid Services. What do I need to do to assess personnel competency? Available at www.cms.gov/Regulations-and-Guidance/Legislation/CLIA/Downloads/CLIA_CompBrochure_508.pdf (accessed 30 September, 2015).

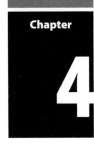

Chapter

4

Oocyte Pickup for IVF
Training Protocol

Alison Campbell, Caroline Drew and Kathryn Berrisford

Introduction

Oocyte pick-up is the process whereby oocytes are microscopically identified and pipetted from follicular fluid aspirates and placed into a culture environment prior to in vitro fertilization (IVF). This chapter sets out the laboratory operating procedure for oocyte pickup and considers practical training methods and competency assessment.

From the outset, it is important for embryologists or technicians to be aware that changes in the wider environment of a gamete or embryo can affect its immediate culture environment. The external environment includes not only the space in which the pickup is performed – the flow hood, which requires stable temperature and pH maintenance – but also the consumables and culture media used.

Task-based training leading to competency should follow a robust pathway. Oocyte pickup is a critical process and, as such, should be performed effectively and reproducibly by the embryologists on the team.

4.1 Equipment, Media and Consumables

Numerous equipment setups, culture media and consumables are available for oocyte pickup. Basic essentials are presented below.

4.1.1 Equipment
- Workstation providing grade A air quality with integrated microscope
- Mini incubator (if non-buffered medium is used)
- Electronic witnessing system (recommended)
- Tube warmer
- Microscope

4.1.2 Media
- IVF medium
- Mineral oil
- Flushing medium

4.1.3 Consumables
- 40-mm culture dish
- Centre-well dish
- Pasteur pipettes

- Rubber bung/teat
- Round-bottom tubes

4.2 Oocyte Pickup Procedure

4.2.1 Pre-Procedure Checks

In advance of the oocyte pickup, the laboratory may prepare by considering the number of follicles observed on an ultrasound scan. This can help in ensuring that an appropriate number of dishes are available. Blood test screening results and any special procedures to be undertaken that deviate from a standard treatment cycle, for example, use of pre-implantation genetic screening (PGS)/pre-implantation genetic diagnosis (PGD)/specialized media, should also be noted.

4.2.2 The Oocyte Pickup: Preparation on Day −1

4.2.2.1 Media Preparation Using Aseptic Technique

All media and culture dish preparation should be carried out in a suitable location away from biological fluids and under laminar airflow. Media expiry dates should be checked prior to use. Records of media and consumable lot numbers and date and time of first use should be maintained to ensure that all products used are traceable.

Hands should be washed thoroughly and dried before commencing any media preparation or dish handling. The laminar flow hood should be clear and be switched on at least 10 minutes before commencing the procedure (refer to the operating manual for precise requirements). Prior to commencing, the work area should be wiped with a non-embryo-toxic cleaning agent and allowed to dry thoroughly.

4.2.2.2 Labelling

All consumables should be labelled with at least two identifiers. Patient's name, date of birth, clinic identification number and a unique barcode or radiofrequency identification (RFID) tag are recommended.

4.2.2.3 Dish Preparation

Several dishes are required to wash the oocyte cumulus complexes at the point of identification, particularly if there is blood contamination. Some embryologists advocate reserving a clear follicular fluid aspirate for rinsing consecutive oocytes.

Following washing, oocytes should be placed into culture dishes for incubation prior to insemination. Commonly, 20- to 50-μl microdrops of medium, under mineral oil, are used (see Table 4.1).

4.2.2.4 Microdrop Preparation

Glass Pasteur pipettes or liquid-handling pipetters set to a fixed volume are used to make microdrops, and serological pipettes are used to dispense larger volumes of medium or oil overlay into dishes.

The advantage of pipetters with tips, as opposed to Pasteur pipettes, is that the volume of each microdrop will be consistent and standardized. It may also be quicker, especially if a multi-dispensing pipetter is used. Pasteur pipettes, unless purchased already rounded at the

Table 4.1 Schematic Table Depicting Example Dish Types, Media Volumes and Holding Conditions

Dish	Minimum number required for pickup	Day of preparation (day 0 = pickup day)	Medium
Oocyte collection/wash dish	2	Day −1	3 ml of IVF medium overlaid with 2 ml of mineral oil
Oocyte holding dish	1 per 5 follicles (for IVF) 1 per 10 follicles (for ICSI)	Day −1	1 ml of IVF medium overlaid with 1 ml of mineral oil
Standard culture	1 per 12 oocytes (ICSI) /1 per 12 follicles (IVF)	ICSI: Day −1 IVF: Day 0	25-µl microdrops of IVF medium overlaid with 4 ml of mineral oil

Photographs courtesy of Vitrolife Sweden AB.

tip, can also scratch the surface of the culture dish, damaging the tissue culture–coated surface of some plastic-ware.

Oil must be overlaid immediately after microdrop dispensing, and it must cover the entire surface of the drops. This will minimize evaporation and osmolarity changes. The osmolarity of most commercially available culture media is between 275 and 290 mosmol/kg.

Bubbles can form on the surface of or within culture drops or wells. These can obscure the oocyte/embryos and adhere to them, making visualizing and pipetting problematic. All bubbles should be removed.

4.2.2.5 Preparation of Flushing Medium

Flushing medium is commonly used by the clinical staff to rinse the pickup needle and to flush oocytes from the follicles. If required, this medium should be warmed thoroughly to 37°C prior to use. Flushing medium is kept at this temperature during the pickup using a tube or syringe warmer. Several flushing media are commercially available.

4.2.3 The Oocyte Pickup: Procedure on Day 0

4.2.3.1 Identification Check

Prior to the surgical procedure, the name of the patient should be checked in the procedure room by asking the patient to state her name and date of birth in the presence of the clinician and a nurse. The details are confirmed against the patient's notes, and the identity check section of the embryology notes should be signed by the clinician and the nurse. Electronic witnessing should be used where possible.

4.2.3.2 Preparation of Equipment

Oocyte pickup is carried out under ultrasound guidance by clinical staff in a procedure room adjacent to the embryology laboratory. According to the European Union Tissues and Cells Directive (EUTCD), oocyte processing must be performed in a Good Manufacturing Practice (GMP) Grade A environment (provided by the workstation) with a background of at least GMP Grade D.

Temperature must be maintained throughout the procedure using tube warmers and heated stages. Regular temperature checks using calibrated and certificated devices and validation ensure that optimal temperature is maintained in the dishes and tubes.

pH must be maintained by using appropriately buffered media or a workstation-based mini incubator or gas jar and overlaying dishes with oil. The pH working ranges advised by the manufacturers should be adhered to and based on carbon dioxide upper and lower limits.

Particularly important when a non-buffered system is used is rapid identification of oocytes within the aspirates to ensure that oocytes are not exposed to ambient gaseous partial pressures that may affect pH, which is generally between 7.2 and 7.4 (see below for further information on buffering of media).

- Ensure that Class II hood airflow is on and is ready for use – clear of used dishes, pipettes and tubes.
- Use a sterile pipette, and ensure that clean, warm (equilibrated if necessary) dishes are ready.

- Ensure that heated stages and tube warmer are on and at the correct temperature. If using a gas funnel, ensure that gas is flowing. A holding incubator may also be used if the holding and washing media are not buffered.
- *Mobile incubator.* If the laboratory is not located adjacent to the operating room, a mobile incubator should be prepared at this point to ensure that temperature and pH changes are controlled during movement of the gametes to the embryology laboratory.

4.2.4 Oocyte Pickup: Standard Operating Procedure

- Record the start time in the embryology notes or database. Aim to work quickly in order to maintain a physiological environment for the oocytes and to minimize light exposure.
- Immediately prior to commencing the oocyte pickup procedure, remove the wash dish from the main incubator, check the labelling against the patient identification and place the dish in the CO_2 holding incubator or under a flow of 5% CO_2 on a heated stage, unless a suitable buffer is being used, which does not necessitate this. If reduced O_2 is used for incubation, the same partial pressure of O_2 is also recommended during oocyte pickup where a non-buffered system is in place.
- Pour the contents of each tube into two to three collecting dishes and examine macroscopically and microscopically (ranging commonly from 8× to 60×) for the presence of the cumulus mass identifiable as a white pearlescent body.
- Once located, move to the washing dish or rinse in clear follicular fluid and aspirate in and out of the pipette to remove blood cells from the cumulus. Oocytes collected in the wash dish must be kept in the gassed/warm environment during collection unless a suitable buffer is used, which does not necessitate this measure.
- Constant communication is essential between laboratory and operating procedure room to keep the clinician informed of the following:
  - When an oocyte is retrieved and the total number of eggs collected in the procedure so far.
  - The presence and condition of granulosa cells.
  - The number of tubes waiting to be examined. (This should not exceed one tube waiting – the effect of blood contaminants, which may cause oxidative stress, is detrimental.)
- Checked follicular aspirate should be placed into a discard pot and a gel sachet added to solidify the discarded fluid.
- Once the collection is complete, there will be notification from the clinical staff of the last aspirate to be passed. A visual check of the tube warming block should be made at the end of the procedure to ensure that aspirates do not remain.
- The pre-equilibrated dish for holding the oocytes, prior to insemination/ICSI, should be removed from the incubator and appropriate witnessing procedures employed. The oocytes should be carefully pipetted into the fresh medium; up to five per dish is recommended. A separate pre-equilibrated wash dish may be employed at this point if there is excessive blood/cellular debris.
- Care should be taken not to move all the oocytes in one manoeuvre.
- Scratch or mark the number of oocytes present on the dish or label. Replace in the incubator.

- Record details of the number of oocytes collected in the patient record along with any other relevant details, such as the duration of the procedure and staff involved.
- The patient's name should be recorded on the outside of the incubator for ease of identification.
- The discard pot should be closed and placed into a clinical waste bag for incineration.
- If a spillage has occurred, wipe over with sterile water or approved cleaning solution when no cultures are out of the incubator.
- The entire workspace should be cleared of all used dishes and pipettes and cleaned thoroughly before commencement of the next case.

4.3 Additional Considerations

4.3.1 Witnessing

Throughout the process of oocyte pickup, manual or electronic witnessing of all steps should be adhered to. This is initiated by patient identification checks and culminates with the cohort of oocytes being pipetted into a culture dish labelled with at least two patient-unique identifiers. Clear, documented evidence of all witnessing steps should be undertaken.

4.3.2 Traceability and Quality Control

- There should be fully documented traceability of equipment, media and consumables used in the process of oocyte pickup.
- All equipment should be fully serviced and validated for use.
- All media should be mouse embryo assay (MEA) tested and Communauté Européenne (CE) marked specifically for IVF use (where available) and the process validated. MEA testing uses one- or two-cell mouse embryos to test the efficiency of media to culture embryos to the blastocyst stage. This is usually denoted by manufacturers as being 80% or more. CE marking is obtained by manufacturers for products providing certification for quality and safety. In Europe, the media used in IVF are usually defined as Class III medical devices because they contain medicinal products or substances acting in an ancillary manner. Other products intended for IVF, such as plastic ware, may have a different medical device classification.

4.4 Choice of Buffered Medium for Washing and Holding Oocytes

Two main media options exist for oocyte pickup.

4.4.1 Media for Use in Ambient Air

To provide flexibility in handling oocytes during pickup by allowing time for washing and manipulating oocytes, media buffered to maintain physiological pH in air at 37°C is available. The most common types of buffered media for IVF use either HEPES or MOPS buffering or a combination of both. HEPES can maintain the pH for approximately 15 minutes at 37°C; MOPS can maintain it for longer periods and is not affected by temperature changes.

4.4.2 Media for Use in Culture-Modified Conditions

Sodium bicarbonate buffers are used in many standard IVF media and maintain a pH between 7.2 and 7.4 (physiological) in an atmosphere of 5% to 6% CO_2 at 37°C, although subtle variations exist between media types and batches. To avoid the use of additional media and buffering methods, standard IVF medium may be used at oocyte pickup provided that an appropriate mixed gas source is available for maintaining the oocytes in incubation-similar conditions during the procedure. This typically involves a small, temporary incubator within the workstation or a simple integrated funnel of piped mixed gas.

4.5 Quality Assurance

As part of an ongoing quality assurance programme within the laboratory, performance audits of all staff should be carried out once they have been deemed to be competent in a procedure. In terms of oocyte retrieval, audits to highlight the differences in the average number of oocytes collected per embryologist and the subsequent maturity and fertilization rate of oocytes should be monitored. If statistical values fall outside the expected range, then additional training may be required.

4.6 Laboratory Training and Competency Assessment in Oocyte Pickup

4.6.1 Training
4.6.1.1 Knowledge

Practical training should be preceded by an understanding of the scientific theory behind the oocyte pickup procedure. Understanding the requirements for constant temperature throughout the process should be paramount. Cooling of the oocytes below 37°C has been demonstrated to induce microtubule disassembly and can cause irreversible disruption of the meiotic spindle.

Understanding the importance of observing the colour of the media is important. Most IVF media contain a concentration of phenol red, which is used as a pH indicator. When the pH of the medium is stable at its physiological level, the medium will be a pale pink colour. If the medium becomes a bright pink or orange, this is indicative of a pH change. Reasons for this include

- If the medium is in the incubator, the level of CO_2 in the incubator has changed.
- The drop of medium is not completely covered with oil and therefore has started to evaporate, and the osmolality has changed.
- There is an infection in the medium.

4.6.1.2 Practical Aspects

Practical training should begin with observation of an expert carrying out the procedure. Before the handling of patients' gametes can occur, trainees must exhibit skills in fine manipulation using a stereomicroscope. Hand-eye coordination can be encouraged and refined by the manipulation of granulosa cells left in the dishes after removal of the oocytes. Key skills to acquire include manipulation of cellular material within a small volume and speed of movement. The temperature of the medium within a dish may change by up to 3°C

Table 4.2 Task-Based Competency Assessment Form for Oocyte Pickup

Task description	Oocyte pickup	
	Embryologist	**Evaluator**
Demonstrates effective oral, written and non-verbal communication skills with colleagues and patients.		
Maintains documentation and records.		
Demonstrate critical judgement in professional practice.		
Evaluates and addresses issues surrounding equipment application and/or operation. Participates in equipment preventive maintenance programmes.		
Performs oocyte recovery procedure according to laboratory protocol.		
Demonstrates that procedures are witnessed either manually or electronically at the appropriate steps in the procedure.		
Is able to clean and disinfect equipment and apply infection prevention and control precautions.		
Is able to handle and dispose of biohazardous waste.		
Demonstrates use of personal protective equipment.		
Is able to discuss treatment plan with patient following oocyte pickup.		

Specific knowledge requirement for oocyte recovery	Evidence	Embryologist	Evaluator
Laboratory protocol: oocyte pickup	Read receipt		
Individual clinical data review: key performance indicator limits met	Completed proforma and report		

Embryologist and evaluator should initial the preceding boxes to confirm compliance with the description and knowledge requirements.

It is my opinion that _____ may undertake independent work on this task as he or she has demonstrated the appropriate knowledge and experience for competency.

This competency must be reviewed if there is a substantial change to protocols or task knowledge requirements.

Evaluator's name:

Signature:

Date:

Position:

during five minutes out of the incubator, and the temperature within a glass pipette may decrease by over 10°C in 10 seconds. Care should also be taken to minimize the time period that oocytes are exposed to light. Manipulation of the oocytes should also be kept to a minimum to avoid any physical damage; the diameter of the pipette should also be large enough to avoid squeezing.

Once competency has been demonstrated with manipulation of granulosa cells, trainees may then begin to assess the follicular aspirates for the presence of oocytes. Trainees should be instructed not to overfill the dishes and to gently swirl the fluid to help with identification of the oocytes. To begin, a realistic aim would be for trainees to work with around three to five aspirates before the experienced operator takes over. As speed and confidence build, trainees may gradually take over the entire process, with the dishes being checked a second time by the trainer. This checking procedure will require the use of a second heated workstation.

Observation of the oocytes by trainees can prove to be a time-intensive and demanding process at the beginning of the training period. Identification skills can only be improved by direct interaction within the procedure by trainees. Special attention should be given to oocytes with little or no cumulus cells and very immature oocytes that may appear with unexpanded cumulus and dark ooplasm with dense coronal layers.

We recommend that trainees should be able to carry out 10 consecutive procedures without misidentification or non-identification of an oocyte. If a mistake does occur, then the trainees must re-start the consecutive procedures. The oocyte retrieval process should be carried out in its entirety from identification of the patient through appropriate storage of the gametes.

4.6.2 Competency Assessment

A task-based competency assessment is used to show the minimum level of competence required (see Table 4.2). Competency must be shown in the practical task (including aseptic technique), performing within the operating procedure, record keeping, witnessing, quality control, communication, advice and information provision and performing within the regulatory framework.

4.7 Summary

Recommendations have been made to enable the technique of retrieval of oocytes from follicular aspirates within the embryology laboratory. Whilst local limitations and budgets may mean that it is not practical to follow all aspects covered, it is hoped that this guide will serve as a resource for those looking to initiate this practice. Additionally, we have aimed to provide a resource for those involved in training laboratory personnel from a relatively unskilled background and provided guidelines for assessment of competency.

References

1. Johansson, L. Handling gametes and embryos: oocyte collection and embryo culture. In *A Practical Guide to Selecting Gametes and Embryos*, ed. M. Montag (Boca Raton, FL: CRC Press, 2014).

2. Swain, J. E. Optimizing the culture environment in the IVF laboratory: impact of pH and buffer capacity on gamete and embryo quality. *Reprod Biomed Online* 2010; 18(6):799–810.

Chapter

5

Embryo Transfer for IVF
Training Protocol

Maria José de los Santos and Nicolás Prados

Introduction

From a practical point of view, the culmination of excellent work in the in vitro fertilization (IVF) laboratory ends with the perfect transfer of the right embryos into the right uterine cavity. Nowadays, despite other techniques having been described (tubal embryo transfers, trans-miometrial embryo transfers, etc.), the most accepted and extended technique, even for cleavage-stage embryos, is to leave the embryos inside of the uterine cavity through the cervical canal using a transcervical catheter.[1]

5.1 Background

As the final phase in a laborious assisted reproductive technology (ART) cycle, precise and careful technique in embryo transfer (ET) is crucial for ultimate success. This is actually quite a relevant procedure, and any difficulty at this precise time may spoil cycle outcome and significantly reduce the chances of pregnancy. Several factors may contribute to the efficacy of this procedure: physiological (i.e. uterine receptivity, embryo quality), anatomical (i.e. straightening of the utero-cervical angle, Müllerian duct malformations) or mechanical (i.e. dummy transfers, use of tenaculum).[2]

A published meta-analysis has shown that at the time of ET, there is no evidence for any clinical benefit offered by a full bladder, removal of cervical mucus or flushing the endocervical canal or endometrial cavity,[3] Nevertheless, based on our experience, these steps are performed in most cases because physicians feel more confident, and they facilitate the ET procedure using soft catheters in the vast majority of cases for transfer.

Even some embryological technical aspects, such as the presence of air bubbles inside the embryo catheter[4] and the use of a centre-well dish or microdrops to load embryos for ET,[5] do not seem to interfere with the final cycle outcome.

However, others aspects, such as traceability issues (i.e. witnessing procedures), must not be underestimated, because loss of traceability leads to one of the most common and undesirable adverse events in IVF.[6] This is actually one of the requirements for quality management systems (ISO 9001:2008) and the EU Directives followed by many IVF laboratories. ET requires participation and excellent communication among embryologists, physicians, nurses and patients.

This chapter focuses on laboratory practices, but it is also mandatory to remember that collaborative effort is involved and that each party has his or own complementary responsibilities that all contribute to make the technique a success.

This very simple procedure is actually under risk if several points are not considered or are undervalued. From a practical perspective, the main responsibility of physicians is to perform transfers in aseptic mode to avoid pelvic infection. This can be achieved by washing the cervix with either embryo culture medium or saline solution supplemented with 10% antibiotic. Performing atraumatic transfer is also mandatory as it has been shown that difficult embryo transfers are associated with lower live birth rates but not with higher ectopic or miscarriage rates. Performing atraumatic ETs requires plenty of skill and profound knowledge of the patient's cervix and uterine cavity before going ahead and will permit the most suitable catheter to be chosen for each patient[1,7] and awareness of any adverse events related to ETs. It has been shown that ET can be a physician-dependent technique; thus standardization of the technique and proficiency training are fundamental.[8]

Moreover, embryologists are responsible for ensuring proper embryo tracking in in vitro cultures, as well as for maintaining the embryos under the appropriate temperature, pH and osmolality conditions during embryo loading and the transfer itself in order to avoid using potentially toxic materials during handling.[9]

5.2 Technical Training and Testing

As with any other IVF laboratory procedure and in order to optimize clinical practice, the embryologists who perform ETs must pass a documented training process that confers a high proficiency level. This level of competency will allow embryologists not only to work without supervision but to also train other staff members in the laboratory.[10]

Only when individual pregnancy rates are compared with the laboratory average benchmark will an embryologist be ready to perform ETs without supervision. A basic understanding of the process involves

1. Comprehensive programme orientation
2. Reading and understanding the standard operating procedures
3. Observation of the ET procedures performed by qualified embryologists
4. Loading of discarded biological material without losing appropriate biological material

Working with supervision involves

1. Comprehensively understanding the procedure
2. The attainment of technical proficiency
3. The performance of 50 actual clinical cases of ET under supervision
4. Quality control (QC)/quality assurance (QA) testing (comparison of individual key performance indicators (i.e. pregnancy rates) with the laboratory average benchmark)

Autonomous work involves

1. Having similar individual key performance indicator (KPI) standards with the laboratory average benchmark (usually within 1 SD of the laboratory mean of a reference patient population i.e. women younger than 35 years of age, first cycle, no severe male factors). (QC data can be plotted as a Levey-Jennings chart to view data easily.)
b. Independence of procedure performance.
c. Independence in trouble shooting.

5.3 Reagents and Equipment

The following items will be required to perform ET:

- Heated laminar flow cabinet
- Cold lamina flow cabinet

- Stereomicroscope
- Incubator
- Pipette holder

Consumables include

- Embryo culture media (centre-well dishes)
- Transfer dish (centre well)
- Sterile disposable 10-ml pipettes
- Glass or plastic pipettes for embryo handling
- 1-ml syringe
- Mock transfer catheter
- Transfer catheter
- Sterile gauzes
- Latex gloves
- Clean wipes with low particle release (for cabinet cleaning)
- Benchtop cleaning disinfectant (3% H_2O_2, Oosafe, etc.)

5.4 Quality Control

All disposable items need to have a CE mark and undergo specific testing for both QC and QA purposes. More detailed information will be addressed in Chapter 12.

5.5 Procedure

5.5.1 Administrative Aspects

- Scheduling ET to avoid rushing between procedures
- Calling the patient to give the ET date/time and instructions according to each clinical policy (i.e. full bladder, preparation (day-to-day operation) or any other special considerations)

5.5.2 Practice Setup

On the day before the procedure

1. Check the number of ETs scheduled for that day.
2. Prepare transfer dishes (one per scheduled transfer) in a cold laminar flow cabinet.
3. Set up the cabinet with the items for preparing ET dishes in such a way as to avoid handing over dishes as this may facilitate microbial contamination.
4. Poor 1 ml of embryo culture into the central well and 4 ml into the outer ring of the dish.
5. Prepare a couple of extra ET dishes.
6. Label each ET dish with the patient's name.
7. Leave the dishes in the patient's incubator for gassing without labelling, should extra dishes be needed.

On the day of the procedure

1. Read and discuss the patient's clinical file and receive information from the embryologist who made the embryo evaluation and embryo selection for the transfer and cryopreservation to discuss any possible issue related to the ET.
2. Set up the cabinet for the ET by arranging items (i.e. pipettes, gauzes, etc.) in such a way as to avoid handing over the dishes as this may favour microbial contamination. The creation of an additional sterile zone in the flow cabinet using sterile surgical clothes may be considered but is not mandatory, provided that the handling of ET catheters is always sterile.
3. Warm the embryo catheter by placing it in the heated stage of the hood.
4. Inform and discuss with the practitioner general aspects of the patient cycle in terms of final number of embryos to be transferred (previously discussed with the patient during her cycle), cryopreservation and any further information, such as other tests performed (e.g. PGS, PGD, etc.).
5. Once the patient is in the operating room, double witness patient identity.
6. Bring the patient's embryos along with the embryo transfer dish to the heated cabinet.
7. Double-check the identification of the dishes for ET.
8. Wait for the practitioner to prepare access to the uterus.
9. Once the clinician is ready, special additional instructions are given to the embryologist (i.e. transfer according to a set procedure), and embryo loading is authorized. Connect the syringe to the catheter, and wash the warmed catheter twice with the culture medium of the external ring of the ET dish.
10. Load embryos into the catheter with a minimal volume (15–20 µl) (with or without air bubbles). Then bring embryos into the operating room.
    a. *Embryo loading with air bubbles.* After washing the catheter and ensuring that the catheter is full of culture medium, aspirate 10 µl of culture medium, 10 µl of air, 20 µl of the culture medium that contains embryos and 10 µl of air. Finish with 5 µl of culture medium in the catheter tip (Figure 5.1A).
    b. *Embryo loading without air bubbles.* After washing the catheter and ensuring that the catheter is full of culture medium, aspirate 10 µl more of culture medium and then ~20 µl more of embryo culture medium and embryos, and ensure that they remain in the catheter tip (Figure 5.1B).
11. Hand the catheter to the practitioner. Apply gentle mechanical pressure to the syringe plunger, if required, to flush the embryo into the uterine cavity.
12. After ET, double-check that no embryos are retained in the catheter.
13. Inform the practitioner about the double-check result.
14. If embryos are retained, inform the practitioner (see Table 5.1 for trouble shooting).
15. Discard the used material into appropriate containers.
16. Wash the flow cabinet to be ready for the next procedure.

5.6 Documentation

Documentation is another requirement of accredited laboratories. Therefore, only the latest version of standard operating procedures (SOPs) of ET and associated SOPs (e.g. the SOP for equipment verification) must be available. Other documents, such as declaration of follow-up and knowledge of the existence of SOPs, preventive and corrective actions or the KIP control document, are also necessary.

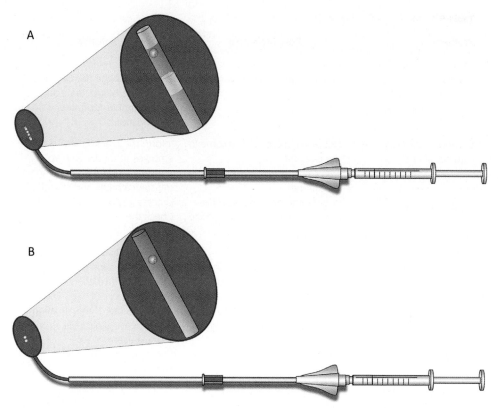

Figure 5.1 (A black and white version of this figure will appear in some formats. For the color version, please refer to the plate section.)

Records of the following items need to be kept:

1. Date and time of the ET
2. Operator's name
3. Name of the practitioner who performs the transfer
4. Number, developmental stage and quality of the embryos at the time of ET
5. Fate of the supernumerary embryos
6. Details about the procedure (e.g. difficulty, presence of blood, retained embryos, etc.)
7. Details of products and material in direct contact with embryos

5.7 Troubleshooting

Although strict compliance with established SOPs helps avoid problems, they may still appear, and it is important to be prepared to solve them without hesitation. Most problems associated with ET may be related to technical aspects while handling the embryos to be loaded. Other problems may not be related to the process itself (e.g. equipment or power failure). These can be solved in part by having an electricity backup, made available through a power generator or an interrupted power supply system. These solutions help critical equipment to continue working, as well as at least one laminar flow cabinet and a microscope, in order to finish the process undertaken in the laboratory at the time of power failure. Having certain equipment in reserve, such as a backup system, can also be very helpful.

Table 5.1 Troubleshooting during ET

Problem	Possible cause	Solution
Trouble while loading embryos into the catheter; embryos cannot be aspirated	Poor connection between the embryo catheter and syringe	Check the connection. If still not working, change the catheter. Record the brand name and batch number for further investigation.
Embryos retained in the catheter after ET	Not enough aspirated volume in the catheter Transfer done too quickly by the practitioner Poor connection between the embryo catheter and the syringe	Inform the practitioner. Transfer embryos to a new embryo transfer dish. Use a new embryo transfer catheter, and start the process again. Check the connection.
Blood in catheter after ET with retained and degenerated embryos	Traumatic ET Sensitive cervix In very few cases, especially in very traumatic ET, retained embryos may be degenerated. This is normally associated with the presence of plenty of blood. Uterine bleeding (very infrequent)	If embryos are degenerated, inform the practitioner and the patient. Use supernumerary embryos of the patient whenever feasible. Keep a record of this situation in the patient's clinical file as an adverse event. In case of uterine bleeding, cancel the ET.
Unexpectedly difficult transfer after embryo loading authorized by practitioner	False line may have been channelled. Straightening the utero-cervical angle not achieved No mock embryo transfer has been performed	Go back to the laboratory and leave embryos in the culture dish until access has been solved. Keep a record of this situation.

The technical problems that relate more to the procedure itself include

1. Trouble while loading embryos into the catheter
2. Embryos retained in the catheter after ET
3. Blood in the catheter after ET with retained and degenerated embryos
4. Unexpected difficult transfer after embryo loading authorized by the practitioner

Possible reasons and solutions are described in Table 5.1.

References

1. Pasqualini, R. S. and Quintans, C. J. Clinical practice of embryo transfer. *Reprod Biomed Online* 2002; 4(1):83–92.

2. Eytan, O., Elad, D. and Jaffa, A. J. Bioengineering studies of the embryo transfer procedure. *Ann NY Acad Sci* 2007; 1101:21–37.

3. Derks, R. S., Farquhar, C., Mol, B. W., Buckingham, K. and Heineman, M. J. Techniques for preparation prior to embryo transfer. *Cochrane Database Syst Rev* 2009; (4):CD007682.

4. Abou-Setta, A. M. Air-fluid versus fluid-only models of embryo catheter loading: a

systematic review and meta-analysis. *Reprod Biomed Online* 2007; 14(1):80–4.

5. Halvaei, I., Khalili, M. A., Razi, M. H., Agha-Rahimi, A. and Nottola, S. A. Impact of different embryo loading techniques on pregnancy rates in in vitro fertlization/ embryo transfer cycles. *J Hum Reprod Sci* 2013; 6(1):65–9.

6. de los Santos, M. J. and Ruiz, A. Protocols for tracking and witnessing samples and patients in assisted reproductive technology. *Fertil Steril* 2013; 100 (6):1499–502.

7. Schoolcraft, W. B., Surrey, E.S. and Gardner, D. K. Embryo transfer: techniques and variables affecting success. *Fertil Steril* 2001; 76(5):863–70 (Epub 2001/ 11/13).

8. Lopez, M. J., Garcia, D., Rodriguez, A., Colodron, M., Vassena, R. et al. Individualized embryo transfer training: timing and performance. *Hum Reprod* 2014; 29(7):1432–7.

9. Gianaroli, L., Plachot, M., van Kooij, R., Al-Hasani, S., Dawson, K. et al. ESHRE guidelines for good practice in IVF laboratories. Committee of the Special Interest Group on Embryology of the European Society of Human Reproduction and Embryology. *Hum Reprod* 2000; 15 (10):2241–6.

10. Keck, C., Fischer, R., Baukloh, V. and Alper, M. Staff management in the in vitro fertilization laboratory. *Fertil Steril* 2005; 84 (6):1786–8.

Chapter

6 ICSI for IVF
Training Protocol

Cristina Hickman

Introduction

Intracytoplasmic sperm injection (ICSI) is an insemination procedure that allows for a single sperm to be inserted directly into the ooplasm using a needle, therefore bypassing issues involving sperm that may be unable to reach an oocyte and/or bind to the zona pellucida. ICSI is traditionally indicated for male-factor infertility and/or following failed or low fertilization with conventional in vitro fertilization (IVF) in a preceding cycle. Because it is a technically demanding procedure, a structured and closely monitored training programme is required to achieve optimal success rates with ICSI. The objective of this chapter is to outline an ICSI training protocol by which the technical skills are acquired without compromising clinical outcome.

6.1 Background Knowledge Required

The first step in ICSI training is to establish the knowledge base required to perform ICSI. ICSI trainees are expected to have an understanding of the biology (i.e. anatomy of the oocyte and sperm and the fragility of the gametes with regards to environmental stressors, which gametes are suitable for treatment and which should be avoided), regulations (i.e. legal and ethical restrictions associated with ICSI) and the mechanics (i.e. equipment used to visualize the procedure and how to change the settings, equipment used for micromanipulation, consumables required) behind ICSI. The knowledge can be sourced from experienced ICSI practitioners, textbooks, publications, standard operating procedures (SOPs) and equipment manuals. The cognition competency can be established using multiple-choice questionnaires, case presentations, essays and/or oral *viva voce*. ICSI trainees should be able to grasp the knowledge and interpret the knowledge with regards to common scenarios they are likely to face as ICSI practitioners.

6.2 Consumables and Equipment

ICSI trainees should demonstrate their skill in preparation of ICSI dishes with media (generally, MOPS or HEPES based), polyvinylpyrrolidone (PVP) and oil. The media and PVP containing sperm should be shallow and positioned centrally in the dish to allow the micromanipulation tools to reach without obstruction from the dish sides. An understanding of the angle of the needle and holder is also required.

ICSI trainees should demonstrate their understanding of how to

- Optimize the settings of the inverted microscope to clearly visualize the oocyte and the sperm (including the sperm tail)
- Use the anti-vibration apparatus

- Set up the micromanipulation tools
- Manipulate the fine and coarse controllers of the micromanipulator
- Use the equipment safely whilst avoiding damage
- Optimize the settings of the various equipment involved with the ICSI procedure, load micro-tools, align the micromanipulator and create, pick up and control a small (around 2 μm) oil bubble inside the needle

6.3 Sperm Immobilization and Selection

Trainees should demonstrate their skill in selecting sperm, immobilizing it and picking up the sperm by the tail in a controlled manner and explain the reasons for selecting the sperm in a specific field of view based on motility and morphology. Immobilization may be confirmed by visual assessment of a kink in the tail and lack of motility and/or by moving the sperm into hypo-osmotic swelling solution (if the tail swells or coils, then immobilization was not achieved), thus demonstrating the ability to move immobilized sperm between drops.

Once competent in sperm immobilization, ICSI trainees should gain competence in more complex ICSI scenarios that require additional control of the needle. These include: severely oligospermic samples requiring searching for sperm in media and moving to PVP, samples with increased debris and cells, testicular biopsies, physiological ICSI (using sperm slow or pICSI dishes) and necrospermia. Trainees can practice using dishes already employed in treatment as these arise in the clinical setting during training. In cases where only immotile sperm are available for ICSI, ICSI trainees require competency in assessing sperm viability using theophylline, pentoxyfilline, the hypo-osmotic swelling test, laser-assisted immotile sperm selection and the sperm tail flexibility test (as described in Chapter 25).

6.4 Oocyte Injections

Surplus oocytes from treatment that are consented for use in training may be used for practicing injection, as well as oocytes that are not suitable for treatment (e.g. matured after ICSI or un-cleaved after ICSI). The unsuitability for treatment should be determined and documented by a member of staff other than the trainee. In some countries, injection of sperm into training oocytes is prohibited. Therefore, injection of oil droplets of a similar size to a sperm head and injection of training beads offer two useful alternatives.

To be deemed competent in oocyte injection, practitioners must demonstrate control of the movement of PVP in and out of the needle (without creating bubbles), control of movement of medium in and out of the holder, control of the positioning of the oocyte in the holder without using the needle by rolling the oocyte using medium propelled and sucked from and to the holder, controlled penetration of the needle into the oocyte, breakage of the oolemma via aspiration into the needle (with less than two oocyte lengths of aspiration), deposition of the oil droplet or bead into the oocyte and careful withdrawal of the needle. Injected oocytes should be cultured overnight, and at least 95% of oocytes should survive. Surviving oocytes may be re-injected, although survival rates are likely to reduce with number of days since collection and number of injections.

6.5 Monitoring ICSI Results

Once ICSI trainees have demonstrated competence in sperm selection and immobilization and oocyte injection (at least 50 normal injections with normal survival rates), the practitioner is then ready to start splitting clinical cases. In the first stage, a patient with large numbers of mature eggs (more than eight) would be selected, a trainee would inject one oocyte and the trainer would inject the remaining oocytes (minimum of 10 oocytes injected with normal performance, as determined by the trainer and the quality indicators). In the second stage, the trainer would inject five oocytes, whilst the remainder of the oocytes would be equally split between a trainee and the trainer. After the injection of 50 oocytes with normal performance, the trainee and trainer would split cases equally, with four or more oocytes (the third stage).

Normal performance should be determined based on supervision at the time of the ICSI, video assessment of the ICSI, comparison between the trainer and the trainee for the same patient (using the chi-square test). Minimum thresholds should be met, as described in Table 6.1, although it must be noted that these thresholds may vary between laboratories. Significant ($p < 0.05$) discrepancies between the performance of the trainer and that of the trainee may suggest issues that require further investigation to improve ICSI performance.

The indicators used to assess trainees should be objective and must be connected with a corrective measure. Different indicators are more sensitive to detecting issues with consumables, procedures and equipment (normal fertilization and degeneration rate), whilst others are more useful in rectifying suboptimal performance by individual technicians than assessing normal fertilization rates (e.g. degeneration rates, polyploidy rates, zero-pronucleate rates, cleavage arrest, low blastulation rates and high biochemical loss). Of these indicators, fertilization, polyploidy and degeneration rates have been identified as the most sensitive for monitoring individual technicians. Katz et al.[1] assessed several indicators every three months for one year after ICSI was first introduced in a laboratory and determined that fertilization rate (from 52% to 75%), degeneration rate (from 12% to 7%), polyploidy rate (from 17% to 10%) and implantation rate (6% to 12%) changed with experience, whilst pregnancy rate (~25%) and embryo arrest rate (~15%) did not, suggesting that the former set of indicators would be more useful for monitoring proficiency than the latter. In cases with a high number of oocytes processed through ICSI, the indicators assessed on day 1 represent a more sensitive indicator of ICSI proficiency than pregnancy rate; as in the case of poor fertilization rates, the number of embryos transferred can still be adjusted when sufficient eggs undergo ICSI. Individual technicians may be further assessed through observation by another skilled embryologist either live or by video using the criteria proposed by Ebner et al.[2] and Daniel et al.[3] This classification may be used to assess individual technicians and assist in training and improving individual performance over time.

6.6 Troubleshooting Poor Results

Once an indicator is identified as being outside the threshold limits, a corrective action must be implemented to achieve improvement in the quality of care. Understanding the common root causes of specific suboptimal quality control ICSI indicators may help to identify relevant technical corrective actions associated with ICSI technique to improve ICSI outcome. Evaluation of videos of the ICSI procedure may help to identify the appropriate corrective action.

6.6.1 High Degeneration Rate (>4%)

To avoid degeneration, the practitioner should ensure that

- The injection needle does not penetrate the opposing membrane, corrected by maintaining the needle between half and two-thirds of the diameter of the oocyte.

Table 6.1 Established Thresholds to Monitor ICSI Performance, Relevant Indicators to Assess Different Targets for Monitoring the ICSI Procedure and Relevant Action Plans to Lead to Improvement as Part of a Total Quality Improvement System

Indicator	Threshold	Target to access			
		Overall	Equipment	Consumables	Technician
Failure of fertilization in cycles with more than four injected oocytes	<1%	X			
Normal fertilization rate (two pronucleates only)	>60%		X	X	
Total fertilization rate (two pronucleates or more)	70–85%	X			
Zero-pronucleate rate	>25%				X
Degeneration rate	<4%		X	X	X
Polyploidy rate	<5%				X
Cleavage rate	>95%				X
Blastulation rate	60–75%				X
Clinical pregnancy rate (patient age dependent)	>30%	X			
Biochemical loss (patient age dependent)	<10%	X			X
Live birth rate	25–40% (depending on patient demographics)	X			

Table 6.1 (*cont.*)

Indicator	Threshold	Target to access			
		Overall	**Equipment**	**Consumables**	**Technician**
Type of comparison (relative to)		Threshold IVF Previous periods Other clinics	Other similar equipment (i.e. if more than one ICSI rig in the same laboratory)	Alternatives Previous batches	Threshold Previous periods Other technicians
Frequency of assessment		Monthly or quarterly	Quarterly and when new equipment is introduced	Between batches and when introducing alternatives	Monthly (sibling); quaterly (overall)
Action plan		Further investigation	Service, maintenance, replacement	Exclusion of defective batches/ alternative supplies	Staff training; sibling assessment; continual professional development

- Oil is not injected into the oocyte, which may be rectified by priming the needle with PVP rather than oil or cleaning the needle with the edge of the drop before injecting to remove oil bubbles.
- Minimum cytoplasm is withdrawn. Improved control of the syringes will allow for minimized cytoplasm withdrawal to less than 6 pl or a maximum of two widths of an oocyte, aiming for around one width.[4]
- Minimum PVP is injected into the oocyte by minimizing cytoplasm withdrawal and by bringing the sperm to the edge of the needle before penetrating the oocyte.[5] If the volume of PVP injected exceeds 6 pl, some surplus PVP may be re-aspirated as the injection needle is withdrawn, thus allowing the ooplasm organelles to tighten around the sperm and a reduction in the size of the breach during penetration.
- There is minimum vibration or movement of the injection needle whilst inside the oocyte,[3] which can be mediated by training in the use of anti-vibration equipment and training in maintaining the needle steady whilst inside the oocyte. When held by the suction pipette, the oocyte should be resting on the bottom of the dish to minimize movement during injection.
- Prior to injection, the needle is in the correct angle relative to the axis of the oocyte by observing an equilateral triangle-shaped indentation of the oolemma. The convexities at the site of invagination above and below the penetration point must be of equal length. The angle of the needle may be adjusted by raising or lowering it using the micromanipulator, twisting the needle or adjusting the angle of the needle, which should usually be set to the angle of the bend of the needle, usually 25 to 35 degrees.
- The oolemma is not excessively deformed due to difficulty of breakage whilst penetrating it. Difficult membrane breakage has been reported to occur in 6% of

injections, accounting for 28% of ICSI technical errors. In these cases, Ebner et al.[2] suggested using an adapted injection technique combining a pressing phase to the centre of the oocyte and a suction phase until the oolemma ruptured. Additionally, laser-assisted ICSI may be used.[6,7]

- Attachment of the ooplasm to the spike after withdrawal of the needle is avoided (reported to occur in less than 0.02% of injections[2]).
- The oocyte is tightly held by the holder, without visual deformation of the oolemma. Oocyte removal from the holding pipette during injection should be avoided (reported to occur in less than 0.02% of injections[2]).

6.6.2 High Polyploidy Rate (>5%)

To avoid inducing polyploidy, the practitioner should ensure that

- Only one sperm is injected into the oocyte. The needle should be cleaned with the edge of the drop before injecting to remove surplus sperm stuck on the outside of the needle. While injecting, only one sperm should be in the needle at any one time. The practitioner should also have a foolproof system to keep track of which oocytes have been injected to avoid double injections (e.g. numbering drops and using a counter, moving oocytes to specific drop positions before injection and a different position after injection).
- Morphologically abnormal sperm are avoided, particularly sperm with large or double heads.
- Damaging the spindle during injection is avoided. This can be identified when a second polar body is not extruded and instead forms a pronucleus, as described by Flaherty et al.[8] To avoid this, maintain the angle of the injection needle parallel to the axis of the oocyte, and position the polar body at 6 to 7 or 11 to 12 o'clock (ideally at 7 o'clock[9,10]), and the needle injects at the 3 o'clock position to minimize the chances of damage to the meiotic spindle during injection. This maximizes the distance between the likely spindle location and the needle.

6.6.3 High Zero-Pronucleate Rate (>25%)

To avoid a failed fertilization, the practitioner should ensure that

- The tail of the immobilized sperm has a permanent crimp, making the tail kinked, looped or convoluted. Surgically retrieved sperm have different membrane characteristics than ejaculated sperm, so a more aggressive technique is necessary to immobilize them – the sperm tail is rolled backwards and forwards with a needle. Insufficient sperm immobilization has been reported in 3% of ICSIs (accounting for 13% of ICSI technical errors).[2]
- The oolemma is broken. Breakage of the oolemma is evidenced by a sudden quivering of the convexities at the site of invagination above and below the penetration point, sometimes accompanied by a sudden proximal flow of the cytoplasm and sperm up the injection needle.
- The sperm is not deposited into a vacuole. Repositioning the oocyte on the holder may be required to find an optimal sperm deposition site.
- The sperm is not expelled from the oocyte during cytoplasmic leakage. The sperm should be injected past the tip of the injecting needle. After the needle is withdrawn, the

technician should observe the penetration point of the oolemma to ensure that the sperm does not leak out. If for any reason the sperm does not remain inside the ooplasm, then the injection should be repeated. In some cases, the sperm remains attached to the spike of the injection needle during release of the gamete into the ooplasm. If this occurs, the injection needle should be rotated to release the sperm, as described by Ebner et al.[2] If sperm release does not occur, then the sperm may be carried out into the perivitelline space, in which case it should be removed and a different sperm re-injected. Cytoplasmic leakage has been demonstrated to be practitioner influenced.[3] Evaluation of a higher incidence of cytoplasmic leakage should be rectified with training. The technique of breaking the membrance and positioning the sperm past halfway in the oocyte may reduce the incidence.[3] Rejection of sperm in the perivitelline space has been reported to occur in 3% of oocytes injected (accounting for 13% of ICSI technical errors).

- A minimum amount of PVP is deposited into the oocyte (around 1 to 2 pl, maximum 6 pl).
- The angle of the injection needle is parallel to the axis of the oocyte.
- The positioning of the polar body is either at 10 to 12 or 6 to 8 o'clock.
- The time the needle is within the ooplasm is kept to a minimum (less than 50 seconds[3]).
- The time oocytes are kept out of the incubator for the ICSI procedure is minimized. The injection procedure should take around two minutes per oocyte. The number of oocytes in the dish at any one time will vary depending on the quality of the sperm and oocytes and the skill of the technician. The technician should aim to keep the oocytes out of the incubator for a maximum of 15 minutes. To achieve this, the technician may choose to split the case with other technicians, select and immobilize the sperm before adding the oocytes into the dish and/or minimize the number of oocytes in the dish at any one time. There is also the option to change the medium used to hold the oocytes when outside the incubator to a medium that can sustain physiological conditions for longer.
- Sperm damage during immobilization and/or loading into the injection needle is avoided. The sperm tail should be compressed or slashed close to but avoiding the midpiece. After the sperm is immobilized, it may remain firmly attached to the bottom of the dish. In these cases, discard the sperm. When picking up the sperm with the injection needle, take care not to damage the head as it enters the needle.
- Viable sperm are selected. Indications of viability used by the ICSI technician are motility, progression and morphology, respectively. Intracytoplasmic morphologically selected sperm injection (IMSI) may be used to increase the chances of selecting a viable sperm.
- Sperm is deposited inside the oocyte. Attachment of the sperm to the pipette has been reported in 5% of injections (accounting for 24% of ICSI technical errors[2]).

6.6.4 Low Cleavage Rate (<90%), Low Blastulation Rate (<60%), High Biochemical Loss (>20%)

To promote cleavage, the ICSI technician should

- Maintain the angle of the injection needle parallel to the axis of the oocyte;
- Minimize the time oocytes are kept out of the incubator for ICSI procedure and
- Select sperm most likely to be viable.

6.7 Conclusion

ICSI is a technically demanding procedure that has a high impact on the success rates of an IVF clinic. For this reason, it must be taught properly in the beginning to ensure technical skills with immobilization and injection. Once in practice, it should be monitored closely to detect and eliminate technical factors that may negatively affect its performance. Over time, trainees gain experience and confidence in a closely monitored programme, reassured that their training will not negatively affect the overall results of the clinic.

References

1. Katz, E., Watts, L. D., Wright, K. E., Bennett, F. C., Litz, J. L. et al. Effect of incremental time experience on the results of in vitro fertilisation with intracytoplasmic sperm injection (ICSI). *J Assist Reprod Genet* 1996; 13 (6):501–4.

2. Ebner, T., Yaman, C., Moser, M., Sommergruber, M., Jesacher, K. et al. A prospective study on oocyte survival rate after ICSI: influence of injection technique and morphological features. *J Assist Reprod Genet* 2001; 18(12):623–8.

3. Daniel, C. E., Hickman, C., Wilkinson, T., Oliana, O. Gwinnett, D. et al. Maximising success rates by improving ICSI technique: which factors affect outcome? *Fertility and Sterility* 2015; 104(3):e95–6.

4. Dumoulin, J. M., Coonen, E., Bras, M., Bergers-Janssen, J. M., Ignoul-Vanvuchelen, R. C. et al. Embryo development and chromosomal anomalies after ICSI: effect of the injection procedure. *Hum Reprod* 2001; 16(2):306–12.

5. Tsai, M. Y., Huang, F. J., Kung, F. T., Lin, Y. C., Chang, S. Y. et al. Influence of polyvinylpyrrolidone on the outcome of intracytoplasmic sperm injection. *J Reprod Med* 2000; 45(2):115–20.

6. Nagy, Z. P., Liu, J., Joris, H., Bocken, G., Desmet, B. et al. The influence of the site of sperm deposition and mode of oolemma breakage at intracytoplasmic sperm injection on fertilization and embryo development rates. *Hum Reprod* 1995; 10 (12):3171–7.

7. Rubino, P., Viganò, P., Luddi, A. and Piomboni, P. The ICSI procedure from past to future: a systematic review of the more controversial aspects. *Hum Reprod Update* 2016; 22(2):194–227.

8. Flaherty, S. P., Payne, D., Swann, N. J. and Mattews. C. D. Aetiology of failed and abnormal fertilization after intracytoplasmic sperm injection. *Hum Reprod* 1995; 10(10):2623–9.

9. Blake, M., Garrisi, J., Tomkin, G. and Cohen, J. Sperm deposition site during ICSI affects fertilization and development. *Fertil Steril* 2000; 73(1):31–7.

10. Nagy, Z. P., Oliveira, S. A., Abdelmassih, V. and Abdelmassih, R. Novel use of laser to assist ICSI for patients with fragile oocytes: a case report. *Reprod Biomed Online* 2002; 4(1):27–31.

Chapter

7

Embryo Assisted Hatching for IVF

Training Protocol and Method

Mina Alikani

Introduction

The zona pellucida surrounding in vitro–grown human embryos may be breached to facilitate the process of hatching following in vitro culture, either to promote implantation or in preparation for removal of cells for pre-implantation genetic testing. This technique is referred to as 'assisted hatching' (AH). To breach the zona pellucida, a chemical method (acidified Tyrode's solution (AT)) or, more commonly now, a laser-assisted method may be used. Since publication of the first studies on AH, multiple variations of the technique for selected and unselected patient populations have been attempted by practitioners around the world. However, results have not been consistent, and application in unselected patients has been repeatedly shown to fail to improve implantation. Proper training, patient selection and methodology therefore are important to the clinical success of AH when applied to improve implantation or to facilitate embryo biopsy. Complete removal of the zona pellucida to avoid trapping has been proposed as an alternative to partial breach.

7.1 Background

A critical early step in the process of implantation in the human is contact between the trophectoderm of the blastocyst and the endometrium. The shedding of the zona pellucida is a prerequisite to this contact, and therefore to embryo implantation; the uterus plays a prominent role in this process.[1] Experimental evidence in several species suggests that in vitro culture alters the dynamics of 'hatching', putting more energy demands on the embryo.[2,3] Human embryos grown in vitro have variable hatching ability, but nearly all embryos with an artificial opening of an appropriate size in the zona pellucida can be persuaded to hatch through that opening if they reach the blastocyst stage[4], earlier than their non-manipulated counterparts and even in the presence of zona pellucida abnormalities (Figure 7.1A–D).

Since the first randomized, controlled trials (RCTs) of assisted hatching,[5] it has been clear that not all embryos or patients would benefit from AH. The method was shown to be effective in poor-prognosis patients but not in young patients with a good prognosis for pregnancy,[5,6] perhaps reflecting the already high incidence of implantation in the latter group. It is also now clear that not all techniques are effective in facilitating hatching. Following attempts at partial zona dissection, zona 'drilling' using AT was selected as a method of choice due to the consistency in the size and shape of the holes.[5] Although with the introduction of lasers into assisted reproductive technology (ART) laboratories this method has been slowly replaced with a laser-assisted method, not all laser methods have been properly investigated or validated. Laser-assisted 'zona thinning' is one such example.

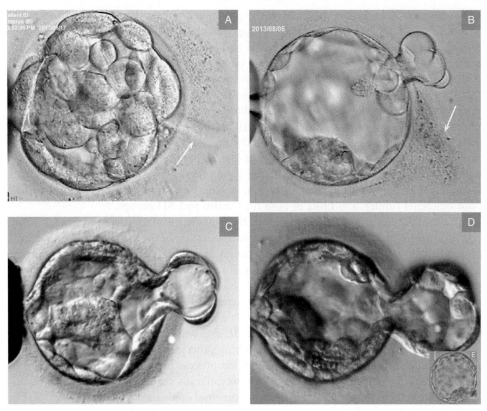

Figure 7.1 Embryos with laser-assisted hatching. (A) Day 5 embryo with abnormally thick zona pellucida, breached with the laser (arrow). (B) Day 5 embryo with trophectoderm cells protruding through the laser breach in a multi-layered abnormal zona pellucida. (C and D) Day 5 embryos hatching through a breach introduced in the zona pellucida using a laser on day 3 of development. Note the thickness of the zona pellucida compared with the day 5 embryo shown in the inset (E) with an un-manipulated zona pellucida. (A black and white version of this figure will appear in some formats. For the color version, please refer to the plate section.)

A detailed study in the mouse has shown that laser-assisted zona thinning without breaching the inner zona pellucida does not facilitate hatching of mouse embryos.[7] Moreover, time-lapse monitoring of the manipulated embryos has demonstrated that even in its least invasive form, that is, ablation of half the thickness of the zona pellucida over one-quarter of the zona circumference, the method may disrupt the hatching process in multiple significant ways.[7] Evidence also shows that embryos with thinned zonae not only hatch as frequently as un-manipulated embryos, but they also often do so from an area outside the thinned zone.

Despite the obvious influence of the method of AH on the viability and hatching ability of the embryo,[7,8] this confounder has been minimally considered in systematic reviews of AH published to date; nonetheless, the reviews have concluded that clinical pregnancy increases following application of AH in certain patients, including frozen embryo transfer and poor-prognosis groups.[9,10]

In the United Kingdom, guidelines issued by the National Institute for Health and Clinical Excellence (NICE) stipulate that 'Assisted Hatching is not recommended because it has not been shown to improve pregnancy rates' (www.nice.org.uk/guidance?action=byID& r=true&o=10936). This is certainly one interpretation of the published data, albeit an erroneous one.[9,10] In the United States, the Practice Committee of the American Society for Reproductive Medicine (ASRM) published new guidelines for AH in 2014.[11] The committee's recommendations were primarily based on the meta-analysis of Carney et al.,[9] which concluded that AH was associated with an increase in clinical pregnancy rate (CPR) in patients with poor prognosis, as well as an increased risk of multiple pregnancy. However, there was insufficient evidence to show that AH improved live birth rates (LBR). The discrepancy between these two findings – that is, an increase in clinical pregnancy and multiple pregnancy, no increase in miscarriage rates, but unchanged LBR – was not addressed in the Cochrane Review nor by the Practice Committee, but this is clearly of interest. Close examination suggests that it is due to the heterogeneous nature of the trials that reported live birth data: trials including good prognosis or unselected patients, using laser zona thinning or partial zona dissection, including as few as 20 patients and reporting poor outcomes (under 10% LBR) in both the control and AH groups.[11]

The Practice Committee also referred to the study of Ge et al.[14] as the largest RCT on AH and pointed out that the study showed that application of the procedure had no impact on implantation rate, CPR or LBR. It is important to emphasize, however, that the average age of the patients in that trial was 31.08 ± 4.68 years, and more than 80% of the patients had either tubal or male-factor infertility – in other words, the study included good-prognosis patients and would not have been expected to show improved outcomes in the study group.[5] Furthermore, the method used for AH was laser zona thinning of a quarter of the embryo without breaching the zona pellucida; as discussed earlier, this method has been shown to be ineffective in facilitating the hatching process.[7,15,16]

Interestingly, examination of the implantation process in an in vitro model has shown that significantly more 'assisted hatched' mouse embryos than naturally hatching blastocysts attained stable attachment to human endometrial epithelial cell monolayers.[12] AH in these experiments entailed complete removal of the zona pellucida using AT solution.[12] Indeed, complete zona removal as a means of improving implantation has been vigorously advocated recently,[13] although it remains to be clinically validated.

What is perhaps a fortunate by-product of a 20-year experience with AH for improved implantation is that it is a reliable, reproducible and safe technique to be used in conjunction with embryo biopsy at any stage. Current trophectoderm biopsy methodologies involve AH on day 3 of development to allow herniation of the trophectoderm through the hole, which, in turn, facilitates removal of cells from the herniated segment. Although it is possible to open the zona pellucida immediately before trophoectoderm biopsy on day 5 or 6 of development, the procedure is more complicated and risks damage to the embryo proper. Moreover, the absence of an opening in the zona obliges the embryo to spend more energy on expansion and accumulation of fluid in the blastocoelic cavity, which may be a significant deviation from the in vivo hatching process.[2,3]

7.2 Training

The only validated approach to AH is the full breach of the zona pellucida. Either a laser or acidified Tyrode's solution may be used for this purpose. Both methods should be mastered first by practicing on animal embryos or discard human embryos. Of course, there is more flexibility with animal embryos in that further embryonic development can be assessed properly. Manipulated mouse embryos, for instance, may be maintained in culture until the hatching blastocyst stage and be reasonably expected to form blastocysts at rates that are equivalent to non-manipulated or sham-manipulated embryos. Any reduction in development potential of the manipulated embryos would be attributable to problems with the procedure, and would have to be investigated. With human embryos, continued observation is limited because discard embryos are not expected to have further development potential.

The main issue with use of the laser by non-experts is excessive use of energy and, in some cases, introduction of an inappropriately sized hole in the zona. Increased pulse duration (which determines the peak temperature at the focal point as well as the surrounding medium) could jeopardize cellular integrity and should be avoided.[17] With respect to the use of AT, the most frequently encountered difficulty is failure of zona dissolution due to failure to effectively expel the solution. This problem arises as a result of dilution of the AT solution and increased pH (above 2.5), which renders it ineffective. The problem should be addressed during the training period. If it is nonetheless encountered while performing a clinical case, the operator should immediately address it either by reloading the needle with AT solution or, if the problem cannot be diagnosed quickly, stop the procedure, return the embryo(s) to the incubator and troubleshoot the entire setup before attempting the procedure again. Possible blockage of the needle as well as failed suction as a result of a dirty tool holder should be investigated.

Having to switch between objectives (e.g. 10× and 20×) after the AH needle is lowered in the manipulation drop can lead to dilution as well. It is therefore quite important that the operator can position and locate the needle at 20× without having to return to lower magnification. This is achieved by practice but requires awareness of the problem and deliberate aim to avoid it.

7.2.1 Patient and Embryo Selection

It is important to keep in mind that at the time AH was proposed as a method to improve implantation,[3] and for several years after, routine culture of embryos to the blastocyst stage was not possible, embryo transfer was performed primarily on day 2 or 3 of development and comprehensive chromosome screening was still many years away from clinical application. The introduction and widespread use of extended culture, as well as the possibility of euploid embryo selection at the blastocyst stage, have changed the treatment calculus and provided new options to patients. These and other relevant factors should be considered before recommending AH.

As a general guideline, the suggested criteria for application of AH include

- All frozen/thawed or vitrified/warmed embryos
- All day 3 embryos from patients ≥ 38 years of age, except oocyte recipients (blastocyst biopsy for pre-implantation genetic screening (PGS) is an option)
- All day 3 embryos from patients with a follicle-stimulating hormone (FSH) level ≥ 10 mIU/ml or an anti-Müllerian hormone (AMH) level <0.8 ng/ml (blastocyst biopsy for PGS is an option)
- All day 3 embryos from patients with previous unexplained implantation failure (blastocyst biopsy for PGS is an option)
- All day 3 embryos with slow development (six or fewer cells)
- All day 3 embryos with significant fragmentation ($\geq 15\%$ by volume)
- All embryos with abnormal or thick zonae
- All day 3 embryos to be biopsied on day 5 or 6 of development

7.3 Reagents, Supplies and Equipment

7.3.1 Laser-Assisted Hatching

- HEPES-buffered medium, protein supplemented
- Washed mineral oil
- Incubator
- Laminar flow hood
- Dissecting microscope
- Infrared laser optical system (usually delivered through a 25× objective)
- Computer loaded with laser software
- Inverted microscope equipped with micromanipulators
- Anti-vibration table
- Marker
- Diamond pen
- Manipulation dishes
- Holding micropipette (120–150 μm OD; 25–30 μm ID)
- Plastic tip, 200 to 300 μm
- Pipetter
- Pipette tips, sterile

7.3.2 Additional Material for Chemical-Assisted Hatching

- Acidified Tyrode's solution
- Plastic tubing assembled for mouth suction (with air filter and mouthpiece)
- AH micropipette (10–12 μm OD)

7.4 Quality Control

- Use sterile technique throughout the procedure.
- Check laser alignment before each procedure.
- Always keep the laser power level at 100%.
- Irradiation times should be as low as the procedure allows.

Note: An incorrectly aligned laser puts material at risk of irreversible damage due to misdirected radiation. The alignment should be checked using the same dish as that used for the actual manipulation because dish thickness and height affect alignment. Confirm that the microscope and computer display are 'parfocal', meaning that the image is simultaneously in focus on both. If not, adjust as required. Keep in mind that analog cameras are preferred over digital cameras to avoid lags. If the microscope is equipped with a 1.5× magnification changer, confirm that the changer is either completely engaged or completely disengaged. Magnification changers can be used with the laser, but the laser must be realigned if the magnification changer setting is changed, as laser alignment will be altered with engagement of the magnification changer. If a magnification changer is used for alignment, it must also be used for the actual procedure.

7.5 Laser-Assisted Hatching

7.5.1 Preparations

1. Use one flat culture/manipulation dish (per two embryos to be manipulated) for each patient to have AH.
2. Using a 100-µl pipetter, make two 20-µl drops of micromanipulation medium (preferably HEPES-buffered medium supplemented with protein). Cover with washed mineral oil, and keep warm until use, either in a no-CO_2 incubator or, with the lid tightly closed, in a CO_2 incubator. This preparation may be done several hours ahead of the procedure.
3. It is recommended that a holding pipette be placed on the left-side tool holder to secure the embryo during the procedure and allow deliberate positioning and selection of an area for ablation. This will reduce the speed of the procedure but will increase its safety and accuracy.
4. Check laser alignment.

7.5.2 Laser Alignment Check

1. To check how well the laser is aligned with the scope, mark an ink-line target on the inside surface of the dish bottom using a dry-erase ink marker.
2. Select a pre-determined (pre-tested) irradiation time. Irradiation times vary substantially for different laser models and even between different units of the same model. Thus, each laboratory should test and determine the appropriate pulse length, keeping in mind that total irradiation energy (hence heat) as well as opening size is determined by pulse duration and laser power.[17]
3. Ablate an area of the dry-erase ink line, and check that the target is at the centre of that area. Otherwise, adjust as necessary.
4. Repeat to confirm and accept the setting to lock the alignment.
5. If the laser is perpendicular to the stage/target surface, the laser will be more focused and effective. The more off-centre the laser, the less focused and less effective it becomes, in turn, requiring more energy to be used.
6. Increasing irradiation times should generate visually different sized ink ablation areas.

7.5.3 Procedure

1. Identify the patient whose embryos are to be subjected to AH.
2. Locate the patient's dishes, and remove them from the incubator to a laminar flow hood.
3. Transfer a maximum of two embryos from the culture dish wells into the manipulation dish, one embryo per drop. *Do not put more than one embryo in a drop or attempt to manipulate embryos while in group culture! This is poor practice that can prolong manipulation time, expose multiple embryos to changing environmental conditions and lead to stress and embryo damage.*
1. Position the first embryo in the centre of the field, and lower the holding pipette into the drop (if using).
2. Increase suction, and secure the embryo on the holding pipette (if using).

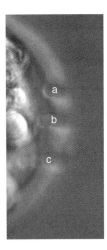
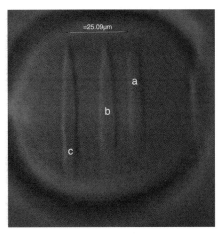

Figure 7.2 Laser-assisted hatching in a mouse embryo to demonstrate the shape and dimensions of the opening (a–c). (A) Side view of three openings, each cutting further into the pervitelline space. (B) Top view of the same openings after removal of the cells/fragments. The deeper the cut (a–c), the longer the corresponding opening in the zona pellucida (a–c). (A black and white version of this figure will appear in some formats. For the color version, please refer to the plate section.)

4. Position the embryo so that the zona is in the path of the laser beam and touching the bottom of the dish.
5. Focus on the zona pellucida.
6. Fire the laser two to three times (allowing a short time in between pulses so that you can visualize and verify the area of ablation) while moving the stage slowly and in a straight line to ablate the full width of the zona from the outside-in and through the inner zona. This will generate an ellipsoid opening with the minor axis of approximately 15μm and a major axis of about 25μm.
7. Move the stage gently in order to relocate the embryo away from the area where the laser was used.
8. Release the embryo, and raise the holding pipette.
9. Place the manipulation dish under the microscope, and wash the embryos one at a time with at least three fresh culture drops before placing back in the original dish (or a new dish).
10. Return the culture dish with the embryos to the incubator.
11. Complete the appropriate paperwork.

Note: Representative micrographs of laser-manipulated zonae are shown in Figure 7.2 to demonstrate the dimensions of the breach created by the laser.

7.6 Chemical-Assisted Hatching

7.6.1 Preparation

1. Use one manipulation dish (per two embryos to be manipulated) for each patient to have AH.
2. Using a 100-μl pipetter, place two 20-μl drops of manipulation medium at the centre of the dish. Place one 20-μl drop of acidified Tyrodes solution towards the top of the dish. Cover with mineral oil immediately. Circle the AT solution clearly with a marker on the bottom of the dish. Keep warm until use, either in a no-CO_2 incubator or, with the lid tightly closed, in a CO_2 incubator. This preparation may be done several hours ahead of the procedure.

3. Place a holding pipette on the left tool holder and an AH needle on the right tool holder and align.
4. Attach the suction unit to the tool holder holding the AH needle.

7.6.2 Procedure

1. Identify the patient whose embryos are to be subjected to AH.
2. Locate the patient's dishes, and remove them from the incubator to a laminar flow hood.
3. Transfer a maximum of two embryos from the culture dish wells into the manipulation dish, one embryo per drop. *Never put more than one embryo in a drop or attempt to manipulate embryos while in group culture! This is very poor practice and will lead to embryo damage.*
4. Place the manipulation dish on the warm stage of the inverted microscope; position it so that the border of the AT drop (on the right) is in the centre of the field.
5. Lower the needle, and load it with AT solution by strong suction.
6. Raise the needle completely out of the drop once the level of solution is easily visualized in the needle and approaches the bend in the tool.
7. Position the first embryo in the centre of the field, and lower the holding pipette into the drop.
8. Increase suction, and secure the embryo on the holding pipette.
9. Position the embryo so that the area at the 3 o'clock position is either free perivitelline space or occupied by cytoplasmic fragments.
10. Focus on the zona pellucida, making certain that both the outer and inner boundaries are in sharp focus.
11. Lower the AH needle into the drop while keeping a gentle positive pressure on the solution column, and quickly move the needle adjacent to the outer zona at the 3 o'clock position.
12. Immediately increase the positive pressure and expel AT solution against the zona while moving the needle up and down along the outer zona covering a distance of about 20 to 30 μm.
13. The outer zona should begin dissolving quickly (1–2 seconds); the thin inner zona may be more resistant to the acid, but it should 'break' easily. Watch closely as this layer moves inward and then eventually breaks.
14. As soon as the inner zona is broken, start gentle aspiration to remove excess AT solution and reduce the acid concentration around the blastomeres.
15. Move the stage gently in order to relocate the embryo away from the area where AT was expelled.
16. Raise the AH needle.
17. Release the embryo, and raise the holding pipette.
18. Repeat the procedure for the second embryo (if applicable).
19. Remove the manipulation dish from the microscope, and place it on the warm surface of the hood.
20. Wash the embryos one at a time with at least three fresh culture medium drops before placing them back in the original dish (or a new dish).
21. Return the culture dish with the embryos to the incubator.
22. Complete the appropriate paperwork.

7.7 Acknowledgement

Mr. Tim Schimmel is gratefully acknowledged for performing assisted hatching on discarded human and mouse embryos in order to provide the micrographs in Figure 7.2 of this chapter.

References

1. McLaren, A. Can mouse blastocysts stimulate a uterine response before losing the zona pellucida? *J Reprod Fertil* 1969; 19:199–201.

2. Gonzales, D. S. and Bavister, B. D. Zona pellucida escape by hamster blastocysts in vitro is delayed and morphologically different compared with zona escape in vivo. *Biol Reprod* 1995; 52(2):470–80.

3. Montag, M., Koll, B., Holmes, P. and van der Ven, H. Significance of the number of embryonic cells and the state of the zona pellucida for hatching of mouse blastocysts in vitro versus in vivo. *Biol Reprod* 2000; 62 (6):1738–44.

4. Malter, H. E. and Cohen, J. Blastocyst formation and hatching in vitro following zona drilling of mouse and human embryos. *Gamete Res* 1989; 24:67–80.

5. Cohen, J., Alikani, M., Trowbridge, J. and Rosenwaks, Z. Implantation enhancement by selective assisted hatching using zona drilling of human embryos with poor prognosis. *Hum Reprod* 1992; 7:685–91.

6. Cohen, J. Assisted hatching: indications and techniques. *Acta Eur Fertil* 1993; 24:215–19.

7. Schimmel, T., Cohen, J., Saunders, H. and Alikani, M. Laser-assisted zona pellucida thinning does not facilitate hatching and may disrupt the in vitro hatching process: a morphokinetic study in the mouse. *Hum Reprod* 2014; 29:2670–9.

8. Cohen, J. and Feldberg, D. Effects of the size and number of zona pellucida openings on hatching and trophoblast outgrowth in the mouse embryo. *Mol Reprod Dev* 1991; 30:70–8.

9. Carney, S. K., Das, S., Blake, D., Farquhar, C., Seif, M. M. et al. Assisted hatching on assisted conception (in vitro fertilization (IVF) and intracytoplasmic sperm injection (ICSI)). *Cochrane Database Syst Rev* 2012; 12:CD001894.

10. Martins, W. P., Rocha, I. A., Ferriani, R. A. and Nastri, C. O. Assisted hatching of human embryos: a systematic review and meta-analysis of randomized controlled trials. *Hum Reprod Update* 2011; 17:438–53.

11. Practice Committee of the American Society for Reproductive Medicine and Practice Committee of the Society for Assisted Reproductive Technology. Role of assisted hatching in in vitro fertilization: a guideline. *Fertil Steril* 2014; 102:348–51.

12. Singh, H., Nardo, L., Kimber, S. J. and Aplin, J. D. Early stages of implantation as revealed by an in vitro model. *Reproduction* 2010; 139:905–14.

13. Vajta, G., Rienzi, L. and Bavister, B. D. Zona-free embryo culture: is it a viable option to improve pregnancy rates? *Reprod Biomed Online* 2010; 21(1):17–25.

14. Ge, H. S., Zhou, W., Zhang, W. and Lin, J. J. Impact of assisted hatching on fresh and frozen-thawed embryo transfer cycles: a prospective, randomized study. *Reprod Biomed Online* 2008; 16:589–96.

15. Cohen, J. and Alikani, M. Evidence-based medicine and its application in clinical preimplantation embryology. *Reprod Biomed Online* 2013; 27:547–61.

16. Chailert, C., Sanmee, U., Piromlertamorn, W., Samchimchom, S. and Vutyavanich, T. Effects of partial or complete laser-assisted hatching on the hatching of mouse blastocysts and their cell numbers. *Reprod Biol Endocrinol* 2013; 11:21.

17. Douglas-Hamilton, D. H. and Conia, J. Thermal effects in laser-assisted pre-embryo zona drilling. *J Biomed Opt* 2001; 6 (2):205–13.

Chapter

8

Embryo Biopsy for IVF
Training Protocol

Oriol Oliana, Cristina F. L. Hickman, Jonathan Lo and Dawn A. Kelk

Introduction

Pre-implantation genetic screening (PGS) of embryos involves confirming the chromosomal status of the embryo through assessment of biopsied cells. Most miscarriages and failed implantations are believed to be due to abnormal chromosomal status. Possessing the correct chromosome complement increases the ability of an embryo to implant and result in a live birth. Historically, biopsies occurred at the cleavage stage. With more cells being able to be biopsied at the blastocyst stage, representing a smaller proportion of the embryo, blastocyst biopsy is currently regarded as a safer procedure with increased sensitivity for detecting mosaics. Therefore, as the benefits of blastocyst biopsy became more evident, blastocyst biopsy has gradually become the method of choice in most in vitro fertilization (IVF) laboratories. As a technical procedure, lack of blastocyst biopsy skills has been an obstacle for some clinics to adopt this practice. This chapter outlines a structured methodology to train a biopsy practitioner to acquire the competency to confidently perform this procedure in a consistent manner that is safe for the embryos whilst maximizing the chance of pregnancy.

8.1 Background Knowledge

To acquire the knowledge base for blastocyst biopsy, trainees must demonstrate awareness of the concepts concerning the biology of the embryo, the equipment and consumables used and the technical and procedural choices to ensure the safety of the embryo throughout the procedure (Table 8.1). This information can be presented to trainees via graphical presentations summarizing the literature, videos of example biopsies and observation of real-time cases. The knowledge acquisition can be assessed by means of essays, verbal discussions or written examinations. Biopsy trainees should be able to understand and interpret the knowledge with regards to common scenarios they are likely to face as biopsy practitioners.

Examples of knowledge competencies that must be acquired include

- Understanding of the benefits of trophectoderm biopsy compared with polar body and cleavage biopsy
- Understanding of the possible genetic results: euploid, aneuploid, no result, partials, mosaics, affected, unaffected
- Understanding of the clinical implications of the possible genetic results, including the chance of pregnancy when transferring an euploid embryo and the chance of multiple pregnancy when transferring multiple euploid embryos
- Awareness of the chances of an euploid embryo in a cycle decreasing with age and increasing with the number of embryos biopsied and embryo quality

Table 8.1 Template Training Record with Necessary Competencies for Sign-Off

Knowledge competence		Biopsy technical competence		
Competency description	Performance	Competency description	No. of times to be performed	Performance
Understanding of the benefits of trophectoderm biopsy versus polar body or blastomere biopsy	☐	Familiar with required consumables	Once	☐
Understanding of genetic results: euploid, aneuploid, no result, partials, mosaics	☐	Biopsy dish preparation	Once (if ICSI trained)	☐
Chance of pregnancy and chance of no embryo transfer versus age	☐	Microscope setup	Once	☐
Understanding of chances of chromosomally normal embryo versus number of blastocysts and maternal age	☐	Micro-injector aspiration stability	Five	☐
Trophectoderm versus ICM	☐	Laser calibration	Once	☐
Implications of too many cells removed	☐	Identification of embryos suitable for biopsy	Twenty	☐
Trophectoderm cells versus fragments	☐	Paperwork for biopsy (biopsy form)	Once	☐
Implications of too many laser pulses	☐	Traceability/ witnessing	Fifteen	☐
Understanding of the legal and ethical restrictions	☐	Positioning the ICM	Ten	☐
Holder size	☐	AH-expanded blastocysts	Fifteen	☐
Bevelled versus flat biopsy needle	☐	Able to count trophectoderm cells (three to six cells)	Twenty	☐
Importance of testing and calibrating the laser	☐	Able to recognize lysed cells	Five	☐

Table 8.1 (cont.)

Knowledge competence		Biopsy technical competence		
Competency description	**Performance**	**Competency description**	**No. of times to be performed**	**Performance**
Understanding of which embryos can be biopsied and which not	☐	Able to recognize cell junctions and apply the laser to them	Twenty	☐
Understanding of the implications of no result	☐	Cell biopsy at 3 o'clock	Ten	☐
Investigations to perform if no result rate or implantation of normal embryo is suboptimal	☐	Cell biopsy at 12 o'clock	Ten	☐
Biopsy key performance indicators (KPIs)	☐	'Flicking' biopsy	Ten	☐
Tubing technical competence		Early blastocysts biopsied	Ten	☐
Competency description	**Performance**	Expanded blastocysts biopsied	Fifteen	☐
Determining cell viability	☐	Non-hatched embryos biopsied	Fifteen	☐
Sterility preservation	☐	Hatched embryos biopsied	Fifteen	☐
Primer drop volume and visualizing cells inside PCR tube	☐	Able to biopsy all blastocyst stages	Once	☐
Cooling and DNA stability	☐	Blastocysts re-expansion rate	≥95%	☐
Traceability	☐	Total number of embryos biopsied	Fifty	☐
Fifteen samples tubed	☐	Troubleshoot common biopsy problems (i.e. strings, laser not responding)	Once each	☐
≥95% of biopsied samples amplified	☐	Pack biopsies for transportation	Once	☐
Supervisor signature				
Patient numbers for traceability purposes				

- Understanding of the importance of not disturbing the inner cell mass and positioning the inner cell mass as far as possible from the laser
- Understanding of the preference for collecting several cells in order to increase the detection of mosaic embryos and that removing too many cells may be detrimental to embryo viability (optimally three to six cells)
- Ability to differentiate between a cell and a fragment and awareness that fragments may have a different ploidy to the embryo and should therefore be avoided
- Understanding that lasers generate heat and pose a risk to cell viability and therefore that lasers should be used conservatively and away from the inner cell mass
- Understanding of the legal and ethical restrictions regarding trophectoderm biopsy in the country where the biopsy is taking place

8.2 Consumables

Trainees must have an understanding of the importance of sterility for the embryo and a DNase-free environment for the biopsy and that gloves must be worn throughout the procedure to avoid contaminating the biopsy. Trainees should understand the choice of consumables used for biopsy:

- Embryos should be biopsied in HEPES- and/or MOPS-based medium (rather than bicarbonate) in order to maintain the pH during the procedure.
- Polyvinylpyrrolidone (PVP) may be useful for coating the outside of the holder and priming the inside of the biopsy pipette to reduce the chance of biopsies sticking to the micro-tools.
- Use of the same oil and dish used for intracytoplasmic sperm injection (ICSI).
- Holder with a bend angle that fits the settings of the micromanipulation equipment (the holder should be larger (OD 120–150 μm, ID 25–30 μm) than usually used for ICSI, particularly if blastocysts are expanded).
- Flat blastomere biopsy needle (ID 30–40 μm), either flat or bevelled (although certain procedures are not possible with bevelled needles).
- 200- to 290-μm pipetters that are DNase free.

Trainees also should understand the choice of consumables used for tubing:

- DNAse-free phosphate-buffered saline (PBS) solution
- DNAse-free 100- to 145-μm pipetter

8.3 Dish Preparation

When demonstrating competency in dish preparation for biopsy, trainees must prepare at least 10 dishes under supervision, meeting the following criteria:

- Media drops should be located centrally on the dish to ensure easy access by the angled micro-tools.
- Drops that will contain embryos must be numbered with the embryo number to ensure that embryos and biopsies are traceable.
- If multiple embryos are biopsied within the same dish, buffer drops must be present between drops containing embryos to minimize the chance of drops containing embryos merging.

- Buffer drops may be used for washing embryos from a bicarbonate medium into a HEPES and/or MOPS medium, reducing medium contamination and maintaining optimal pH.
- Drops must be at least 20 μl to avoid the holder aspirating so much medium that the drop containing the embryo dries up.
- Drops must be less than 50 μl and sufficiently spaced to reduce the chance of drops merging.
- When moving the dish between stations, the drops must not merge.

8.4 Equipment Setup

Trainees must demonstrate competency in using the equipment necessary for biopsy:

- The temperature of the heated stage must be constant and maintained between 36 and 38°C, as measured directly in the drop.
- The inverted microscope should be configured such that the cell junctions are clearly visible.
- The holder and biopsy needle should be aligned, allowing for embryos to be held anchored to the bottom of the dish, without dragging the tools on the dish and with the embryo, holder and biopsy needle being in the same focal plane.
- Trainees must be confident in using the micro-manipulator, demonstrating control of the suction and aspiration of both the holder and the biopsy needle.
- Trainees must demonstrate competence in checking the calibration of the laser and calibrating the laser if and when necessary.
- Trainees must demonstrate the ability to modify the laser settings with regards to size, number of shootings and pathway.

8.5 Blastocyst Material for Training

Blastocysts not suitable for treatment may be used for biopsy training only when permission is given by the gamete providers. To avoid a conflict of interest, the unsuitability for treatment should be determined and documented by a member of staff other than a trainee. Typical examples are three-pro-nuclear (3PN) blastocysts and surplus embryos that the patient requested in writing to donate for training, whether fresh or cryopreserved.

Good-quality mouse blastocysts are a good model for biopsy training as the behaviour of the cells during biopsy is similar to that of human blastocysts, yet mouse embryos are more readily available, allowing for larger numbers to be used for intensive training sessions. In order to acquire the confidence and competence required for blastocyst biopsy, it is beneficial to biopsy multiple embryos in the same day (preferably 25 to 50 blastocysts at different expansion stages over two consecutive days).

Different embryos respond to biopsy in different ways, so the strategies for blastocyst biopsy may slightly differ depending on the characteristics of the target embryo. Large numbers of biopsies are therefore required in training so that trainees may gain awareness of the expected variation in practice. This will allow trainees to experience good and poor practice and to apply the technical skills learnt from one biopsy to another, thus increasing the speed at which trainees progress in the biopsy learning curve.

8.6 Choosing Embryos for Biopsy

Trainees must be able to competently grade blastocyst expansion, inner cell mass and trophectoderm[1] and identify which embryos are suitable for biopsy, as well as the optimal timing for biopsy. Poor-quality blastocysts with an expanded blastocoel cavity[2] and even morulas[3] may be considered for biopsy, although blastocyst biopsy criteria must be validated on-site and may vary between clinics. Time-lapse videos of blastocyst expansion are useful tools for teaching and assessing the understanding of the local criteria in order to reach consistency between different practitioners in the same laboratory. Trainees should demonstrate awareness that embryos may be cultured for longer (even overnight) for the opportunity to increase expansion and/or trophectoderm cell number.

8.7 Traceability

Trainees must demonstrate competence in requesting a witness to verify that the embryo being biopsied and the biopsy are traceable (including embryo number and date and time of transfer) whenever an embryo or biopsy moves from one vessel to another.

8.8 Priming Micro-Tools

Trainees should demonstrate competence in priming needles and holders:

- Priming the needle with PVP whilst the meniscus is still visible
- Coating the outside of the holder with PVP and priming the holder with medium
- Demonstrating fine control of the meniscus of the biopsy and holder pipettes
- In between embryos being biopsied, emptying the biopsy needle into a spare drop and reloading with fresh PVP (to avoid contamination between samples)

8.9 Positioning of the Blastocyst

Trainees should be able to demonstrate sufficient control with the holder suction and aspiration to rotate the blastocyst without using the biopsy needle to position the blastocyst in the optimal position for biopsy:

- The inner cell mass (ICM) should be located as far as possible from the biopsy location (usually at the 3 o'clock position).
- The 9 o'clock position would ideally have a perivitelline space between the trophectoderm cells and the zona pellucida.

8.10 Breaching the Zona Pellucida

Trainees should be competent at assisted hatching on day 3 or day 4, which is technically easier than breaching the zona pellucida at the time of biopsy. However, since hatching may occur insufficiently or at the incorrect location, it is important that trainees also be competent at breaching the zona pellucida at the time of biopsy. In order to reduce cell damage with the laser, trainees should demonstrate competency in

- Using the laser at the correct pulse size (7–12 μm), avoiding use of the laser directly on cells
- Positioning the embryo so that there is a natural perivitelline gap at 9 o'clock;
- Shooting the cell junction to induce collapse

- Nudging the trophectoderm with the biopsy needle to either induce collapse or create a perivitelline gap
- Putting the biopsy pipette in contact with the embryo and gently expelling medium inside the perivitelline space to induce detachment of the trophectoderm from the internal wall of the zona pellucid, making the embryo collapse and facilitating the final zona breaching
- Staggering the zona pellucida following a small slit in the zona to create an artificial perivitelline gap

Trainees also should have an awareness that in the event that the laser is malfunctioning or not available, embryo biopsy should not take place, and embryos should be cryopreserved for a later biopsy, if required.

8.11 Picking Up Cells

Trainees should demonstrate competence in picking up cells using the biopsy needle via a controlled gentle suction:

- ICM cells should not be touched by the biopsy needle.
- Cells should be counted as they enter the biopsy needle (three to six cells).
- Suction should be controlled to avoid cell lysis.
- Whilst aspirating cells into the biopsy needle, the needle should be gently pressed against the embryo to avoid lysing the cells during suctioning.
- After holding the biopsy slightly, the cells should be released from the biopsy needle to allow for lasering of the cell junctions.

8.12 Applying the Laser on the Cell Junction

Trainees should demonstrate

- An ability to apply laser pulses on cell junctions whilst applying pressure on the cells by slightly increasing suction and pulling back the needle
- A minimum number of pulses used (aiming for around five pulses, not exceeding 10)
- An awareness that the heat generated by the laser might compromise cell viability in the embryo and/or DNA integrity in the biopsy
- Lasering in the correct focal plane to ensure accuracy of the laser pulse
- Lasering away from the ICM
- Critical assessment of the number of embryos to be biopsied given the quality of the blastocyst

8.13 Disconnecting the Biopsy from the Embryo

Different techniques are available to approach the trophectoderm biopsy (see Figure 8.1). The traditional approach locates the cells to biopsy at 3 o'clock, and with the aid of the laser and aspiration control, the cells are released. However, there are other alternatives that should be taught. 'Mechanical biopsy' consists of a rapid flick between the holding and the biopsy pipettes as the biopsy pipette holds the cells. For embryos with a large number of cells that would require an increased number of laser pulses, placing the herniated area at 12 o'clock reduces the cell surface tension. Trainees should be able to control and decide what the best approach is for any given case.

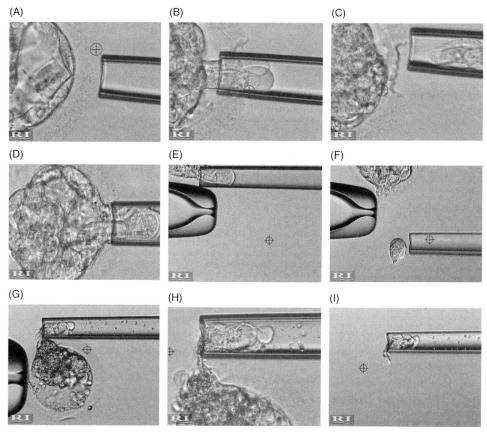

Figure 8.1 Different methods of trophectoderm biopsy. (A black and white version of this figure will appear in some formats. For the color version, please refer to the plate section.)

8.14 After the Biopsy

Once the biopsy is detached from the embryo, trainees should demonstrate competence in

- Positioning the embryo in the bottom of the drop and the biopsy in the top of the drop (at 40× magnification)
- Determining whether the biopsy cells are intact (membrane visible) or lysed and recording the result on the biopsy form
- Washing the embryo in bicarbonate medium and returning it to a post-biopsy dish prior to cryopreservation
- Washing the biopsy with four drops of PBS and then loading it into a labelled tube already containing a drop of PBS
- Visualizing the biopsy inside the tube (the tubing procedure is best supervised using a screen connected to the microscope so that the supervisor can also see the biopsy inside the tube)
- Placing the tube in a frozen polymerase chain reaction (PCR) block right after each sample has been tubed to preserve DNA integrity
- Storing the samples in a −20°C freezer (with −80°C ideal for a long storage period)

Biopsied embryos should be cultured further to assess re-expansion, and at least 95% of blastocysts should survive. Time lapse is a useful tool to assess survival and re-expansion rates. Re-biopsy of surviving blastocysts may be attempted, although survival rates are likely to be reduced compared with fresh embryos.

8.15 Progression in Clinical Cases

After biopsying 50 blastocysts at various stages of expansion, tubed biopsies should be assessed for PCR amplification (with less than 5% failing to amplify), and the embryos should be cultured overnight (with a greater than 95% survival rate). Once these target thresholds are met, trainees may progress to splitting clinical cases where there are at least four embryos suitable for biopsy or an uneven split in the ratio 1:3, with the better quality embryos being biopsied by the supervisor. After 10 consecutive clinical embryos are biopsied (where the supervisor observes good technique and KPIs are maintained), trainees can then be promoted to splitting in a ratio of 1:1. Once ongoing pregnancies are confirmed, trainees may progress to performing whole clinical cases. The KPIs are monitored continuously and regularly.

8.16 Troubleshooting Suboptimal KPIs

Normal performance should be determined based on supervision at the time of biopsy and retrospective video assessment. To be signed off, trainees should meet the following KPI thresholds:

- From at least 20 supervised biopsies, re-expansion rates should be equal to or higher than 86% (two hours after biopsy).
- The time length of the biopsy should be fewer than three minutes per sample.
- Ninety-five per cent of biopsies should amplify.
- Biopsies should consist of between three and six cells.
- There should be a less than 15% miscarriage rate.
- There should be a 60% live birth rate per transfer (this proportion may vary between clinics; an increased success rate compared to non-PGS cycles is expected).

Once an indicator is identified as being suboptimal, a corrective action must be implemented to achieve improvement in the quality of care. All biopsies should be filmed. Evaluation of videos of biopsy procedures may help identify the appropriate corrective action.

In the event of low survival/re-expansion rate ($<$86%) and/or increased miscarriage rate ($>$15%) or decreased clinical pregnancy rate (fewer than cycles without biopsy), a review of the biopsy videos is necessary to assess

- Aspiration control
- That a maximum of six cells are collected from a single blastocyst
- The timing of blastocyst biopsy in terms of expansion
- Vibration during biopsy
- Whether the size of the zona pellucida breach was not too large or too small (in fact, the aperture created to get access to the trophectoderm cells should be smaller than the pipette used for biopsy)
- Whether use of the laser was excessive
- Whether the ICM was inappropriately disrupted (mechanically or by laser pulses)

- Whether blastocyst was firmly held during biopsy, without spinning
- Whether environmental conditions are embryo safe (i.e. toxicity, temperature, air quality, light)
- Whether the micro-tools are angled correctly

In the event of a high rate of no PCR amplification ($>5\%$), the following corrective actions are applicable:

- Review the tubing technique to ensure that biopsied cells are correctly washed and visualized within the tube.
- Review the biopsy videos to assess
  - Suction power at the time of pulling the cells from the embryo, as this could lyse the cells with the consequent DNA lost
  - Length and number of laser pulses (excessive use of the laser may compromise DNA integrity in the biopsy)
  - Biopsy integrity
  - Lasering only of cell junctions (lasering of cells should be avoided)

8.17 Conclusion

Trophectoderm biopsy is a technically demanding procedure that requires well-trained embryologists. By following this structured training protocol, trainees would gain experience and confidence in a closely monitored programme, reassured that their training will not negatively affect the overall results of the clinic.

References

1. Gardner, D. K. and Schoolcraft, W. B. In vitro culture of human blastocysts. In *Toward Reproductive Certainty: Fertility and Genetics Beyond*, ed. R. Jansen and D. Mortimer (pp. 378–88) (Carnforth, UK: Parthenon, 1999).

2. Capalbo, A., Ubaldi, F. M., Cimadomo, D., Maggiulli, R., Patassini, C. et al. Consistent and reproducible outcomes of blastocyst biopsy and aneuploidy screening across different biopsy practitioners: a multicentre study involving 2,586 embryo biopsies. *Hum Reprod* 2016; 31(1):199–208.

3. Kort, J. D., Lathi, R. B., Brookfield, K., Baker, V. L., Zhao, Q. et al. Aneuploidy rates and blastocyst formation after biopsy of morulae and early blastocysts on day 5. *J Assist Reprod Genet* 2015; 32(6):925–30.

9

Vitrification for IVF
Training Protocol

Andrew Dorfmann

Introduction

During the past decade, vitrification has become a routine method of cryopreservation in the human embryology laboratory and is the preferred method in many in vitro fertilization (IVF) laboratories around the world. Many laboratories have adopted this method. This change has been based on both voluminous reports in the literature[1,2] and the superior outcomes achieved within these laboratories. Vitrification involves a rapid cooling and later rapid warming of specimens after equilibration in various combinations of cryoprotectant solutions. Most laboratories have found these methods to be quite robust, repeatable and successful. However, one difficulty of adopting vitrification of oocytes and embryos is that the techniques, while not extremely difficult to master, can be highly technician dependent and require both training and extensive practice before they can be applied appropriately in a clinical setting. There are many variations of the protocols used for vitrification (which are treated elsewhere in this book), any one of which can be successful in the right hands. This chapter focuses only on training. If training is done carefully and methodically and is followed up with an appropriate amount of practice, technicians can learn the methods and carry them out in a successful and repeatable way.

One of the most important aspects of training, particularly in this modern era of embryology, is giving the new embryologist the appropriate foundation and understanding of the underlying principles that make these methods work. There is a tendency to approach these methods as 'cook book' recipes, which may work in the short term and can expedite training to a certain degree. However, it is crucial for the modern embryologist to understand the biological and physical principles that make vitrification work. In this way, technicians will understand what changes in protocol might affect and which ones should not be altered without thorough experimentation. It is highly recommended that this aspect of education should be built into any training process.

9.1 Background

Vitrification is not a new concept in cryobiology. It first surfaced in the context of reproductive medicine in the 1980s when Fahy, Rall and others[3,4] published a number of papers describing the use of vitrification for cryopreserving mouse embryos. However, prior to this, it was a serious line of research in cryobiology for many years. However, the fear of using high concentrations of cryoprotectants and the multiple early successes with controlled-rate freezing quickly eclipsed vitrification as a clinical method, and it was put on the backburner until 1999, when Kuleshova et al.[5] published their landmark paper describing the first successful birth use of vitrification applied to human oocytes. This spurred a rapid succession of work and publications beginning around the year 2000 (for examples, see Kuwayama,[6] Chian et al.[7] and Cobo et al.[8]).

Vitrification is the solidification of a liquid solution into a non-crystalline (amorphous) solid known as a 'glass'. Vitrification works by rapidly cooling a solution past its glass transition temperature T_g and increasing viscosity while eliminating ice crystallization. The trick is to use a combination of extremely rapid cooling and high enough solute concentration to 'run past' the glass transition temperature without ice crystal formation.[9] The significance for biological systems is that vitrifying cells can minimize or eliminate membrane damage that may occur from chilling injury or osmotic stress. Interestingly, the molecular and structural contents of cells are left largely unaffected by the change in temperature. As in most cryopreservation strategies, solutions are made using so-called cryoprotectant molecules.

There are two main groups of cryoprotectant molecules: small membrane-permeable molecules (e.g. dimethyl sulfoxde (DMSO), ethylene glycol and propanediol) and large polymeric molecules (e.g. sucrose and trehalose). The most common methods of vitrification typically involve gradually increasing concentrations of ethylene glycol and DMSO together to induce vitrification as the cell(s) rapidly cools. Conversely, most warming protocols reverse the process by using solutions of large sugar molecules to protect the cells from osmotic stress as the solutions dilute out the permeable molecules and gradually re-introduce water molecules into the cells as they warm past the glass transition temperature.

For vitrification to be effective, both cooling and warming rates must be kept high to avoid ice crystallization. The process can be further enhanced if the solutions surrounding the cells are highly viscous. This viscosity reduces osmotic damage from water molecules moving back and forth across the membrane in response to the introduction or elimination of the cryoprotectant molecules. This last point is one that technologists must keep in mind as they begin to work physically with the delicate cell types involved in mammalian reproduction, especially human oocytes. Accuracy is required, as is speed, but equally important is to handle the specimens gently to help avoid osmotic stress.

9.2 Equipment and Supplies

Vitrification as a procedure will be treated elsewhere in Chapter 20. However, in order to perform and later train embryologists to perform vitrification, there is a certain basic set of tools and reagents that must be available in the laboratory:

1. Stereo microscope(s)
2. Higher-powered phase contrast or Hoffman inverted microscope(s)
3. Ample supply of liquid nitrogen
4. Styrofoam containers or other insulated containers for handling liquid nitrogen on the bench
5. Hemostats
6. Various sterile plastic ware (specifics will depend on the particular protocol used)
7. Vitrification device (either 'open' or 'closed')
8. Vitrification media (below are examples only – these solutions are available from many suppliers with different formulations):

a. Equilibration solution (ES). The base medium can be any acceptable HEPES- or MOPS-based modified IVF medium. Medium M199 is often used:

    i. 7.5% ethylene glycol

    ii. 7.5% DMSO

b. Vitrification solution (VS):

    i. 15% ethylene glycol

    ii. 15% DMSO

9. Warming medium:

a. Thaw solution (TS): 1M sucrose or trehalose

b. Dilution solution (DS): 0.5 M sucrose or trehalose

c. Washing solution (WS): no cryoprotectant, only base medium with protein support

10. Timers, preferably multichannel

11. Mouse embryos, one- or two-cell embryos

12. Human oocytes and embryos:

a. Initial training phase – discarded/unused oocytes

    i. Immature germinal vesicle (GV) or metaphase-I (MI) stage oocytes

    ii. Unfertilized oocytes

b. Final clinical training phase:

    i. Blastocycsts

    ii. Oocytes

9.3 Training Protocol

The process of training will vary from laboratory to laboratory, but certain principles should always be applied. We generally recommend the following sequence when training new staff in any aspect of embryology, but for vitrification training, these steps are essential. Training should be deliberate and methodical. Data should be kept at each step, and moving from one step to the next should not be allowed until the results are equivalent to the most experienced embryologist in the laboratory.

1. New technologists should be given time to study materials in advance of their bench training:

a. The biological and physical basis of cryopreservation. This material should be agnostic as to the specific protocol used in the laboratory, and instead, it should focus on the common principles shared by all methodologies. Consider these excellent recent reviews:

    i. Principles of cryopreservation,[10]

    ii. The principal variables of cryopreservation: solutions, temperatures and rate changes,[11]

    iii. Principles of cryopreservation by vitrification, Fahy and Wowk.[9]

b. The specific written protocol used in your laboratory.

2. Physically learning the protocol:

   a. Begin with mouse one- or two- cell embryos. Unless you have access to a mouse colony at your facility, these can be purchased from various suppliers either cryopreserved or fresh in embryo culture medium. If cryopreserved, you must first thaw the embryos and let them re-equilibrate prior to use. Working with mouse embryos has several distinct advantages

      i. They are plentiful and can be used without any special permissions.
      ii. Generally speaking, they may be heartier than human material, so as a starting point they will survive well, giving new embryologists confidence as they move forward in their training.
      iii. These embryos should also be able to survive multiple rounds of vitrification and warming, so they can be re-used several times.

   b. Trainees should work through the entire protocol several times using mouse embryos under the watchful eye of a fully experienced embryologist who is familiar with the technique and has demonstrated the ability to successful vitrify and warm human material. Once the trainer is satisfied, the practice phase should begin.

      i. Trainees should, over the course of days or weeks, depending on how much time can be allotted for training, practice the protocol over and over until they are reaching a nearly 100% recovery and survival of mouse embryos. The results from each round should be recorded and analyzed by a laboratory supervisor or the laboratory director.
      ii. If one- or two-cell embryos are used for this part of the training, they should be cultured for five days, and blastocyst formation rates should be noted and compared with control samples (embryos not vitrified and warmed). The rate of blastocyst formation should be comparable between mouse control embryos and mouse embryos that have been vitrified and warmed. Survival alone should not be the only test endpoint. Each laboratory must develop its own standards for blast formation. There is no absolute percent blastocyst formation that can be given in a text, but we have found that a good embryology laboratory should be able to grow mouse embryos from the two-cell to blast stage at a rate of at least 90%. But the true test in this context is that the trainees doing vitrification and warming should be nearly equal in blast formation to whatever the laboratory's established baseline for control is.
      iii. Once the desired proficiency has been achieved, it is time to move on to human material.

3. Human oocyte and embryo training:

   a. Phase 1: Discarded human material

      i. In every embryology laboratory, there is material, typically oocytes, that either are not mature enough to inseminate, that have failed to fertilize or that arrest during their development too early to be frozen or vitrified for future use, which will inevitably be thrown away. This material can be used to help trainee embryologists to understand the physical appearance of human oocytes and embryos as they go through the vitrification and warming cycle. Since human material is slightly larger than mouse material, this typically is perceived as being easier by most trainees.

ii. Assessing this phase can be tricky. This material is by nature of poor quality. Therefore, survival rates may be lower than expected, and of course, there is no way to judge development. The main goal at this point is to get trainees comfortable with handling human material. The more the protocols are burned into muscle memory, the better trainees will do when they begin their last and final phase of training.

b. Phase 2: Working with actual clinical specimens:

i. Partial cases

(1) The first step in trainees becoming fully adept at vitrification is to have them work alongside fully trained and experienced embryologists. We have found that the best way to move this forward is to assign a particular trainee to a specific trainer in the laboratory and have them work together as a team (a sort of mentor relationship) on large cases with expected good prognosis. These are typically donor oocyte patients or young good-prognosis patients with whom there will likely be both high numbers of good-quality embryos and a high likelihood of success. Our approach to this is to start with trainees handling a small percentage of the blastocysts to be vitrified (generally about 20%).

(2) We then gradually move to 50% of the blastocysts. It is important to follow the outcomes of the thaws as they come up, but the downside here is that the expected implantation and pregnancy rates on these initial fresh cases is high, so it may take a significant amount of time before the outcomes of these vitrification attempts are known. Therefore, it is critical for the assigned trainer to assess the trainee's proficiency. In the end, we must rely on this judgement quite heavily. It may be many months or years before we can get an accurate data-driven answer to the progress of training at this phase.

ii. Full clinical cases:

(1) Once trainer and any supervisors in charge of this process feel that the trainees are fully prepared to move forward, the decision can be made to have the trainee embryologists work with all the embryos on a given case. Again, it is best to start with good-prognosis patients such as donor oocyte patients and patients younger than 35 years of age with expected good outcomes. The data will be available more quickly and can be analyzed on a more reasonable time horizon.

(2) Over time, the trainees' data should be carefully tracked – as all the embryologists in a given laboratory should be – both for survival and for implantation and pregnancy rates.

9.4 Conclusion

Vitrification is now a routine and important procedure in most embryology laboratories. Though the method is not unreasonably difficult to learn and master, the results from it are quite dependent on the skill and experience of the technical staff carrying it out. Therefore, it is critical for the training of new embryologists learning these methods to be careful and methodical. Each laboratory should set out a rigorous training programme and ensure that when new staff are hired and need to be trained, the pathway is adhered to, and records are kept. If this is done correctly, trainees can master the techniques in a reasonable amount of time, and results for the patients in each programme will remain high.

References

1. Vajta, G. Vitrification in human and domestic animal embryology: work in progress. *Reprod Fertil Dev* 2013; 25 (5):719–27.

2. Cobo, A. and Diaz, C. Clinical application of oocyte vitrification: a systematic review and meta-analysis of randomized controlled trials. *Fertil Steril* 2011; 96(2):277–85.

3. Fahy, G. M., Levy, D. L. and Ali, S. E. Some emerging principles underlying the physical properties, biological actions and utility of vitrification solutions. *Cryobiology* 1987; 24:196–213.

4. Rall, W. F. Factors affecting the survival of mouse embryos cryopreserved by vitrification. *Cryobiology* 1987; 24:387–402.

5. Kuleshova, L., Gianaroli, L., Magli, C. Ferraretti, T. and Trounson, A. Birth following vitrification of a small number of human oocytes: case report. *Hum Reprod* 1999; 14:3077–9.

6. Kuwayama, M. Highly efficient vitrification for cryopreservation of human oocytes and embryos: the Cryotop method. *Theriogenology* 2007; 67:73–80.

7. Chian, R. C., Huang, J. Y., Gilbert, L., Son, W. Y, Holzer, H. et al. Obstetric outcomes following vitrification of in vitro and in vivo matured oocytes. *Fertil Steril* 2009; 91:2391–8.

8. Cobo, A., Remohi, J., Chang, C. C. and Nagy, Z. P. Oocyte cryopreservation for donor egg banking. *Reprod Biomed Online* 2011; 23:341–6.

9. Fahy, G. M. and Wowk, B. Principles of cryopreservation by vitrification. In *Cryopreservation and Freeze-Drying Protocols, Methods in Molecular Biology*, ed. W. F. Wolkers and H. Oldenhof (pp. 21–62). 2015.

10. Pegg, David E. Principles of Cryopreservation. In *Cryopreservation and Freeze-Drying Protocols,* ed. J. G. Day and G. N. Stacey (pp. 39–57) (Totowa, NJ: Humana Press, 2007), doi: 10.1007/978-1-59745-362-2_3.

11. Leibo, S. P. and Pool, T. B. The principal variables of cryopreservation: solutions, temperatures, and rate changes, Fertility and Sterility, 2011; 96(2):269–276.

Chapter

10

Mouse Embryo Assay for Quality Control in the IVF Laboratory

Dean E. Morbeck

Introduction

Ensuring proper quality control (QC) in the laboratory is critical to the success of any in vitro fertilization (IVF) programme, as the environment of the laboratory can alter the quality of the embryos produced. The ultimate role of the embryology laboratory is to maintain the inherent viability of the gametes and embryos in an environment outside the female reproductive tract.[1,2] There is a need for objective, sensitive and reproducible methods and assays for testing materials for embryo toxicity as well as growth promoting and inhibiting factors. The manufacturers test commercially available IVF media and plastic ware and provide the results of their testing with the shipment of supplies. It may be advisable to test media and supplies upon arrival to confirm that nothing occurred during shipping. The suitability of various reagents and materials for use in human IVF can be tested using a range of bioassays. While the most used bioassays for QC in IVF laboratories are the human sperm survival assay and the mouse embryo bioassay (MEA), the one-cell MEA has been consistently shown to be the most sensitive.

10.1 Background

The selection of a proper bioassay should be based on which culture medium, contact material or electrical equipment is tested, as well as the availability of bio-specimens.

10.1.1 Mouse Embryo Assay

The MEA is the most widely used bioassay to test for toxicity and functionality testing of media, plastic ware and laboratory equipment that may come in contact with gametes and embryos. MEA is the 'gold standard' of bioassays for detecting toxic and suboptimal raw materials, media and contact materials. Key elements of this assay include the mouse strain used and various endpoints.[3] An inherent limitation of the MEA is the relative lack of sensitivity of the primary endpoint of expanded blastocysts. Expanded blastocysts can form from a few blastomeres and are not always associated with viability, a fact confirmed with a more objective endpoint such as cell number.[9] The acceptable threshold for optimal embryo growth can be based on individual set criteria, for example, culture conditions, the developmental marker, the transgene/reporter gene and test items. Differentiation of cells within the blastocyst can be evaluated via confocal microscopy or immunohistochemistry.

Generally, in the MEA, embryos are divided between a control group, which is exposed to a neutral/control medium, and a test group, which is exposed to the potentially toxic medium or device for human assisted reproduction. Inferences on toxicity are based on differences in successful development between the two groups.

More specifically, the MEA follows a stratified (mouse), randomized (embryo), balanced (equal numbers per group, per mouse) design.

The sensitivity of the MEA is the most common reason for choosing it as a QC assay, and the one-cell MEA is more sensitive than the two-cell MEA[10-13] or human sperm motility assay (HSMA).[12] Nonetheless, it is unclear whether the sensitivity of this assay is sufficient to detect toxins relevant to the human IVF laboratory. The strain of mouse used for production of embryos is another variable that could improve assay sensitivity. Classes of mouse strains used include genetically identical inbred mice, genetically diverse outbred mice and hybrid mice created by a cross between different inbred strains. Hybrid strains, the industry standard for QC testing, are foremost because they are not prone to the two-cell block observed with outbred and many inbred strains, as well as because they respond well to super-ovulation and produce embryos that have a consistent and high potential to develop to blastocysts.[14] Inbred or hybrid mice are less sensitive to known embryo toxins than outbred mice.[15] Outbred mice are more sensitive to adverse conditions and thus may be more suitable for human embryos.[1,16] Embryos from outbred mice develop to the blastocyst stage at a rate (40–60%) comparable to that of human embryos (30–50%), presenting a sensitive QC model that is both sensitive and difficult to maintain. The low and variable blastocyst rates of embryos from outbred mice make their routine use impractical.

Exact timings of mouse embryo development in the one-cell assay using time-lapse imaging provides a new and highly sensitive assay that is capable of detecting toxins that are not detected using blastocyst rates alone.[17] We know that mouse embryos develop more slowly in vitro than in vivo, and this rate of development is affected by the quality of culture conditions. Perhaps the most sensitive measure of mouse embryo development is the time of blastulation, a marker that is not available without time-lapse imaging. Other useful parameters include duration of the second and third cell cycles and synchrony of the second and third cell divisions. Through time-lapse microscopy it is possible to apply different culture condition (i.e. media, oxygen, temperature, air quality, oil) and use the morphokinetic analysis of cell divisions tested against a control for each assay.

10.2 Equipment and Supplies

- Water bath (37°C)
- Test tube rack, timer, stylet, scissors
- Cryopreserved one-cell murine embryos
- Stereomicroscope with heated plate
- Heating block for tubes
- CO_2 incubator at 37°C; CO_2 set to 5% to 7% to obtain pH of 7.2–7.3
- 35-mm embryo culture dish
- Stripper pipetter
- Stripper pipette tips (120–150 μm in diameter)
- Gloves (non-powder)
- A simple salt solution for embryo culture such as human tubal fluid (HTF)
- HTF-HEPES
- Polyvinyl alcohol (PVA), Sigma P8136–250G
- Light mineral oil
- MEA worksheet

10.3 Setup (Day −1)

- Prepare and filter warming (HTF-HEPES) and testing media (HTF) containing 0.1 mg/ml PVA.
- Prepare 20-μl drops of HTF-PVA under mineral oil in a 35-mm culture dish (control). Prepare a minimum of four drops: three for rinsing and one for performing the test.
- Prepare 20-μl drops of HTF-PVA exposed to test items (or a different oil) in a separate dish. Prepare a minimum of four drops: three for rinsing and one for performing the test.
- Place prepared dishes in an incubator for overnight equilibration.

10.4 Setup (Day 0)

- Pre-warm all equipment to the appropriate temperature.
- Pipette 7 ml modified human tubal fluid (mHTF)–PVA into one 35-mm dish, and allow it to reach room temperature.
- Prepare workstation near water bath with timer, test tube rack, stylet, scissors and empty 35-mm dish.

10.5 Bioassay Procedure

1. A minimum of 10 embryos is required for each test item, and the optimal number is 30 per test. Embryos are supplied in groups of 10 or 20 per straw.
2. Expose the straw to room-temperature air for two minutes. Rest the straw horizontally on a test tube rack so that it is surrounded by room-temperature air. The straw can be placed anywhere or supported in any way as long as it rests horizontally and nothing touches the area containing the embryos.
3. Place the straw in a 37°C water bath for one minute.
4. Remove the straw from the water bath, and gently wipe it dry.
5. Expel the contents of the straw as a single drop into a sterile 35-mm Petri dish in the following manner: With scissors, remove the lower heat seal. Remove the upper heat seal by cutting to bisect the cotton plug at the PVA section. Using the stylet, push down on the remaining cotton plug, expelling the contents of the straw into a sterile Petri dish. To make sure that no liquid remains, push the plug to the very end of the straw.
6. Using an embryo-handling pipette and working quickly, pick up all the embryos and transfer them to room-temperature mHTF-PVA. Place embryos at the top of medium, allowing them to sink to rest on the bottom of the dish. Leave embryos undisturbed at room temperature for 10 minutes.
7. Rinse the handling tip thoroughly in mHTF-PVA (control medium), and proceed to transfer embryos in groups of 10 or more to the test dishes while working on a heated stage.
8. Expel embryos in the first rinse drop, and then expel the remainder of the mHTF-PVA in the thaw dish.
9. Pick up fresh HTF-PVA from the next rinse drop, and then move the embryos from the first to the second drop. Repeat steps 8 and 9 until the final drop. Thorough rinsing is critical to minimize the carryover of protein from the freeze medium.
10. Using zoom or an inverted microscope, view the embryos to determine the number of viable zygotes. Record total and time on the MEA worksheet.
11. Assess embryo development at 24, 48, 72, 96, 120 and 144 hours after thawing. During the first 48 hours, record exact cell numbers. After 48 hours, indicate stage of blastocyst

(or morula) and hatching. For the final two assessments at 120 and 144 hours, blastocysts either remain expanded with some contraction or are completely regressed.

12. The QC standard is greater than 75% development to the blastocyst and/or hatching blastocyst stage at 96 hours for the one-cell assay. An enhanced assay is used for mineral oil, where more than 50% of embryos should remain as expanded blastocysts at 144 hours.

13. If the standard is not met, re-test. After two failed tests, reject the product. Items failing two tests will be discarded and not used for patient purposes.

References

1. Bavister, B. D. Culture of preimplantation embryos: facts and artifacts. *Hum Reprod Update* 1995; 1(2):91–148.

2. Leese, H. J. Metabolic control during preimplantation mammalian development. *Human Reproduction Update* 1995; 1:63–72.

3. Punt–van der Zalm, J. P. E. M., Hendriks, J. C. M., Westphal, J. R., Kremer, J. A. M., Teerenstra, S. et al. Toxicity testing of human assisted reproduction devices using the mouse embryo assay. *Reproductive BioMedicine Online* 2009; 18(4):529–35.

4. Bavister, B. and Andrews, J. C. A rapid sperm motility bioassay procedure for quality control testing of water and culture media. *J In Vitro Fert Embryo Transf* 1988; 5:67–75.

5. Critchlow, J. D., Matson, P. L., Newman, M. C. et al. Quality control in an in-vitro fertilization laboratory: use of human sperm survival studies. *Hum Reprod* 1989; 4:545–9.

6. Stovall, D. W., Guzick, D. S., Berga, S. L. et al. Sperm recovery and survival: two tests that predict *in vitro* fertilization outcome. *Fertil Steril* 1994; 62:1244–9.

7. Alvarez, J. G. and Storey, B. T. Spontaneous lipid peroxidation in rabbit and mouse epididymal spermatozoa: dependence of rate on temperature and oxygen concentration. *Biol Reprod* 1985; 32:342–51.

8. Claassens, O. E., Wehr, J. B. and Harrison, K. L. Optimizing sensitivity of the human sperm motility assay for embryo toxicity testing. *Hum Reprod* 2000; 15:1586–91.

9. Lane, M. and Gardner DK. Differential regulation of mouse embryo development and viability by amino acids. *J Reprod Fertil* 1997; 109:153–64.

10. Davidson, A., Vermesh, M., Lobo, R. and Paulson. R. Mouse embryo culture as quality control for human in vitro fertilization: the one-cell versus the two-cell model. *Fertil Steril* 1988; 49:516–21.

11. Scott, L. F., Sundaram, S. G. and Smith, S. The relevance and use of mouse embryo bioassays for quality control in an assisted reproductive technology program. *Fertil Steril* 1993; 60:559–68.

12. Hughes, P. M., Morbeck, D. E., Hudson, S., Fredrickson, J., Walker, D. L. et al. Peroxides in mineral oil used for in vitro fertilization: defining limits of standard quality control assays. *J Assist Reprod Genet* 2010; 27:87–92.

13. Morbeck. D.E., Khan, Z., Barnidge, D. R. and Walker, D. L. Washing mineral oil reduces contaminants and embryotoxicity. *Fertil Steril* 2010; 94:2747–52.

14. Suzuki, O., Asano, T., Yamamoto, Y., Takano, K. and Koura, M. Development in vitro of preimplantation embryos from 55 mouse strains. *Reprod Fertil Dev* 1996; 8:975–80.

15. Khan, Z., Morbeck, D. E., Walker, D. L. et al. Mouse embryos and in vitro stress: does mouse strain matter? *Fertil Steril* 2010; 94:S58.

16. Gardner, D. K., Reed, L., Linck, D., Sheehan, C. and Lane, M. Quality control in human in vitro fertilization. *Semin Reprod Med* 2005; 23(4):319–24.

17. Wolff, H. S., Fredrickson, J. R., Walker, D. L. and Morbeck, D. E. Advances in quality control: mouse embryo morphokinetics are sensitive markers of in vitro stress. *Hum Reprod* 2013; 28(7):1776–82.

Sperm Survival Assay for Quality Control in the IVF Laboratory

Marius Meintjes

Introduction

The purpose of the human sperm survival assay (HSSA) is to test disposables, media and reagents for potential sources of cytotoxicity in a human assisted reproductive technology (ART) laboratories before their use in in vitro fertilization (IVF)/andrology procedures. The contact bioassay is a cornerstone of a successful and safe ART laboratory, and in many countries, the use of a contact bioassay is required by law. When using a bioassay in the laboratory, it must be useful rather than just fulfilling a legal requirement. This means that the assay should be able to detect very subtle levels of toxicity consistently without any false-negative or false-positive results. Several alternative contact bioassays have been described that may fulfil these requirements, but they are not all equally affordable, accessible and practical to execute. The use of human sperm in a contact bioassay is inexpensive and convenient, as well as invaluable for consistent quality assurance in ART laboratories. If used appropriately, the HSSA is sensitive, repeatable, readily available and each sample acts as its own control.

11.1 Background

It is considered a standard of practice and required by law in most developed countries to test all materials with a bioassay that may come into direct or indirect contact with human gametes in the ART laboratory.[1] The ultimate responsibility for testing belongs to the local ART laboratory, but commercial providers of ART products are now also required to provide bioassay information with all certified ART products. At the discretion of the laboratory director, these results may be accepted in lieu of re-performing the testing in-house. However, best practice still suggests that ART laboratories should perform at least some of their own bioassay testing for several reasons.

Companies have different standards of quality and use a wide array of bioassays to verify their standard of quality. Their assays may not be as sensitive as assumed, and their standards may be lower than those assumed for optimal screening and performance of products in the ART laboratory. Secondly, bioassays performed at the point of manufacture do not take into account interferences that may affect the quality of the product between production and the point of use, such as shipping, packing and handling conditions. Furthermore, it is not always possible to use all human ART-certified products in the laboratory, even though we should aspire to do so. Some products may be certified for clinical use but at a standard inferior to that required for an ART laboratory. Therefore, all products may not have been adequately tested by the industry and subsequently mandate careful testing in our own laboratories.

When using a bioassay in the laboratory, we want to ensure that the test is actually useful, meaning that it should be able to detect very subtle levels of toxicity. Some products intended for use in the ART laboratory should actually fail from time to time. A good bioassay should not only be sensitive but also robust, repeatable and consistent in its ability to detect compromised contact materials. Furthermore, the test should be relatively easy to use and as cost and time efficient as possible. Even though the bioassay can be validated by participating in an external proficiency-testing programme, real-life requirements of a trusted in-house bioassay often exceed the conditions simulated by proficiency-test samples.

In general, three main types of bioassays are encountered in ART laboratories: the mouse embryo assay (MEA),[2] the HSSA[3] and the hamster sperm survival assay.[4,5] The MEA is plagued by inconsistency, variable sensitivity, a lack of consensus on measured endpoints, high cost, availability of biological material and many variables such as mouse strain, embryo stage and culture conditions.[6] The hamster sperm survival assay, in turn, is hampered by the availability of epidydimal hamster sperm, cost to consistently have material available and overall cumbersomeness. If used appropriately, the HSSA is sensitive, repeatable, readily available and each sample act as its own control.

11.2 Equipment, Reagents and Supplies

- Preference should be given to a standard upright phase contrast microscope with a 20× objective and a 10× eye-piece for an overall magnification of 200×.
- Human tubal fluid (HTF) with HEPES (mHTF) + 0.3% human serum albumin (HSA; control medium) (Note A) stored at 4°C per manufacturer's expiration date; stored at 37°C for 2 days once designated for use (Note B).
- Isolate or other commercial ART-certified colloidal gradient stored at 4°C per manufacturer's expiration date; stored at room temperature for 1 day once designated for use (Note C).
- Sterile culture tubes, 5 and 15 ml (Note D).
- Freshly prepared human sperm (liquefied at room temperature and optimized for motility using a gradient).
- General andrology laboratory supplies such as pipettes, pipette tips and sperm counting chambers.
- Selected disposables, media and reagents to be tested.

11.3 Quality Control

1. All materials and supplies used to perform the HSSA should have passed a previous HSSA and should be known to be non-toxic.
2. Keep a current inventory log, which should list all contact materials received in the laboratory. The log should also indicate when each item was tested, whether it failed or passed the HSSA and specifics on the expiration date. At the commencement of the HSSA, record the lot number, expiration date and date received. At the completion of the HSSA, document the date the product was placed in use and the passing HSSA results.
3. Always run the assay with a positive control (e.g. previously tested control medium plus a piece of known toxic latex glove) and a negative control (e.g. previously tested control medium alone). The negative control (sperm and control medium only) should have a

Sperm Survival Assay

Consult Laboratory Director if an item does not pass. Record any passing items into the Inventory of Supplies and Reagents notebook.

Item being tested	Lot #	Tube #	Day 0 Date 1/09/06	Day 1 Date 1/10/06	Day 3 Date 1/12/06	Day 4 Date 1/13/06	Day 4 Average	S.I.	Pass	Fail
Negative Control	------	1,2	93.93	77.81	82.84	74.76	75	100	X	
Positive Control	------	3,4	93.93	0.0	0.0	0.0	0	0		X
P-1	1279	5,6	93.93	86,78	87,87	81,80	80.5	107	X	
G-1	500395	7,8	93.93	84,84	80,72	74,76	75	100	X	
G-2	500391	9,10	93.93	81,81	78,90	75,77	76	101	X	

Action taken with failed item(s):_____

Prepared by:_____   Date: _1-13,06_

Reviewed by _____ 7   Date: _2/3/06_

Figure 11.1 Sample HSSA.

greater than 75% survival index, and the positive control (sperm, control medium and toxic material) must have 0% motility after five days of incubation for a valid assay.

4. No results are reported unless quality control measures are within normal limits. Items repeated due to a failing result must have two of three passing scores to be considered passing and useable.
5. Retain records for a minimum of two years (see Figure 11.1).

11.4 Procedure

1. Select a sperm sample that may yield the highest possible number of sperm to be used for testing (at least a normal sample). Also, more than one sample can be pooled to increase the number of sperm in the final prepared sample (Note E).
2. Separate sperm from semen, and optimize the percent motility by using a one- or two-layer colloidal gradient so that a minimum of 70% motility is obtained.
3. Adjust the final sperm concentration to 2×10^6/ml motile sperm using the control medium.
4. Place 0.5-ml aliquots of the final sperm sample (at 2×10^6/ml motile sperm or 1×10^6 total motile sperm per test tube) in Falcon 5-ml culture tubes. Cap loosely (Note F).
5. *Disposables:* Place a piece of the disposable to be tested in the designated pair of culture tubes (every item is tested in duplicate)(Note G) pre-loaded with 0.5 ml of control medium and 1×10^6 total motile sperm. Multiple test items can be loaded in a single test tube to maximize the number of items that can be tested in a single HSSA (Note H).
6. *Media:* Centrifuge the culture tube with the sperm suspension for eight minutes at 300xg to remove the control medium. Now add 1 to 2×10^6 motile sperm in 0.1 to 0.2 ml of control medium to 0.5 ml of the medium to be tested.
7. *Reagents:* Examples of reagents are culture oil, polyvinylpyrrolidone (PVP), protein and hyaluronidase. Prepare the test tubes as for disposables in step 5. For protein, supplement unsupplemented mHTF with the test concentration of protein; for example, supplement mHTF with 0.5% HSA or 10% serum substitute supplement (SSS). For oil,

perform the test with an oil overlay. For PVP and hyaluronidase, the control medium–sperm suspension as in step 5 can be spiked with 0.1 ml of the test product (Note I).

8. Incubate loosely capped tubes at room temperature for 5 days (Note J).
9. Sample and assess each culture tube on days 2, 4 and 5 for the percent motility (progressive and non-progressive) (Note K).

11.5 Evaluating Results

1. The progressive motility on the fifth day is used to calculate a survival index:

$$\text{Survival index} = \frac{\%\ \text{progressive motility of test}}{\%\ \text{progressive motility of negative control}}$$

2. A survival index of 0.75 or greater is considered a passing score for items tested.

11.6 Notes

A. Some minimal protein supplementation is required to ensure lubrication for the sperm to demonstrate motility. Higher concentrations of protein are discouraged as they may mask subtle toxic effects of the test medium or supplies. The use of complex proteins such as SSS is discouraged because it can directly inhibit sperm motility.

B. In general, any atmosphere-buffered medium can work to include medium buffered with HEPES, phosphate, zwitter ions, MOPS or a combination of these. Interestingly, even bicarbonate-buffered medium used at regular atmospheric conditions, as specified for this test, may give good results. The pH of bicarbonate-buffered medium at atmospheric conditions typically settles at about 7.8, which is not much different from that of seminal fluid. P-1 medium from Irvine Scientific is an excellent control medium.

C. The goal is to optimize the percent motile sperm. Any commercial gradient and gradient protocol can be used at the discretion of the testing facility to ensure the maximum number and percentage of motile sperm available for the HSSA. Swim-up procedures are not recommended as they typically yield lower total numbers of sperm and reduce the functional life span of the sperm (five days needed).

D. Several options exist for supplies. The brand is less important than the principle of using tested, non-toxic control supplies. The actual testing should be performed in a small tube (5 ml) to optimize use of the available sperm, ensuring that a maximum number of tests can be performed with a finite number of sperm. Snap-cap tubes allow for loose capping. The HSSA is performed without an oil overlay for five days. Airtight capping may result in the loss of sperm motility over time due to the lack of atmospheric gas circulation. Without capping, evaporation may result in significant osmolarity changes and the premature loss of sperm motility.

E. Establish donors from whom you can dependably obtain 90% motility after preparation and whose sperm can survive for five days at room temperature. Use sperm from the same donor or the same combination of donors for the entire assay.

F. Cap loosely to prevent evaporation and subsequent osmolarity changes. Make sure to keep and store the test for these five days away from excessive drafts as found inside a running laminar flow hood or beneath an air-conditioning supply duct.

G. Run all tests in duplicate and average the results. If the results differ by more than 15% motility, consider the test invalid.

H. Samples of multiple disposables can be pooled in a test tube (or individual test) to maximize the number of contact materials that can be tested with a single prepared sperm sample. Should this test tube pass the test, multiple items can be signed off as passed. Be aware that should such a combination tube fail the sperm survival assay, the result will be confounded by the number of disposables in that tube. However, a second, follow-up sperm survival assay can then identify the specific disposable responsible for this test failure.

I. Not all test scenarios or test products can be accounted for in this protocol. In some scenarios, the laboratory must use its own initiative to design and modify the test conditions to mimic conditions as close as possible to the actual use of products in the ART laboratory. However, make every effort to attain a five-day assay, as subtle toxicities frequently only manifest on day 4 or 5 of the HSSA. Certain media optimized for blastocyst culture cannot be tested successfully for five days without dilution. For example, sequential blastocyst-stage culture medium should be diluted 1:4 with mHTF to reap the benefit of a five-day HSSA.

J. Room temperature is defined as 22 to 26°C. Be aware that some building air-conditioning units may disengage after hours and result in overheating during the summer months or cold shock during the winter. Make sure to keep the test tubes away and isolated from cold metal surfaces such as a stainless steel laboratory bench. Styrofoam tube racks or tube racks placed on non-metal isolated surfaces (e.g. a Styrofoam or thick plastic sheet) can be helpful to keep the test within the targeted temperature range for the five days. The HSSA should never be performed at 37°C as sperm will be depleted of energy and not survive for five days.

K. Some non-progressive motility will be noted towards the end of the five-day test period. Non-progressive motility should be counted and given the same value as progressive motility.

L. Maintain sterile technique throughout the procedure as even slight contamination will result in failure of a test. Such a failure may incorrectly be interpreted as a quality failure of a specific contact material. Testing each product in duplicate will safeguard against and assist in identifying the unintentional contamination of a single tube – one tube will pass the assay, and the other will fail.

M. Adhere to all general laboratory safety precautions during the procedure as any sperm sample, even after cleaning it up with a gradient, should be considered a biohazard.

N. Classify all waste as biohazard, dispose of it in a biohazard bag at the point of generation and remove daily.

O. All control specimens should be tested in the same manner as the tested items.

11.7 Limitations of Procedure and Troubleshooting

1. The test is only as good as the donor sample after gradient preparation.
2. Execution of a usable HSSA depends on the availability of sperm donors.
3. Due to the variability of test samples, initiative should sometimes be used to customize the five-day HSSA for problematic materials. Some culture media (e.g. blastocyst culture medium) and materials (e.g. vitrification solution) are inherently difficult to test over five days, and innovative limited exposure or dilution techniques must be applied to the satisfaction of the laboratory director, still guaranteeing a valid test. However, the testing of standard embryo, oocyte and sperm handling media as well as for routine contact materials can easily be standardized.

4. If the entire assay fails:
   a. Repeat the entire assay as quickly as possible.
   b. Identify anything that could possibly cause the assay to fail, such as

   i. Control medium or common supply item that might not have been tested with a prior HSSA
   ii. Poor sperm quantity or motility yield after the gradient preparation and/or poor sperm quality
   iii. Specific sperm donor whose sperm lacks the ability to survive at room temperature for five days
   iv. Technical error such as uncapped tubes, dilution error of sperm or reagents
   v. Inappropriate dilution or exposure of a problematic contact material or medium such as vitrification solutions
   vi. Environmental cause such as high or low room temperatures after hours, cold or warm bench surfaces or air drafting over tubes
   vii. Fungal or bacterial contamination
   viii. Call the medium manufacturer to check on any complaints from other people using the same medium

5. When repeating the assay, try to use a different control medium (known to have passed a previous HSSA) and run parallel to the control medium of the recently failed HSSA, even if the current control medium also has passed previously.
6. Do not use any disposable, medium or reagent that failed this HSSA until the assay is repeated.

References

1. Carrell, D. T. and Cartmill, D. A brief review of current and proposed federal government regulation of assisted reproduction laboratories in the United States. *J Androl* 2002; 23:611–17.

2. Gorrill, M. J., Rinehart, J. S., Tamhane, A. C. and Gerrity, M. Comparison of the hamster sperm motility assay to the mouse one-cell and two-cell embryo bioassays as quality control tests for in vitro fertilization. *Fertil Steril* 1991; 55 (2):345–54.

3. de Jonge, C. J., Centola, G. M. Reed, M. L., Shabanowitz, R. B., Simon, S. D. et al. Andrology lab corner: human sperm survival assay as a bioassay for the assisted reproductive technologies laboratory. *J Androl* 2003; 24:16–18.

4. Bavister, B. and Andrews, J. C. A rapid sperm motility bioassay procedure for quality control testing of water and culture media. *J In Vitro Fertil Embryo Trans* 1988; 5(2):67–75.

5. Rinehart, J. S., Bavister, B. D. and Gerrity, M. Quality control in the in vitro fertilization laboratory: comparison of bioassay systems for water quality. *J In Vitro Fertil Embryo Trans* 1988; 5 (6):335–42.

6. Davidson, A., Vermesh, M., Lobo, R. A. and Paulson, R. J. Mouse embryo culture as a quality control for human in vitro fertilization: the one-cell versus the two-cell model. *Fertil Steril* 1988; 49:516–21.

7. Claasens, O. E., Wehr, J. B. and Harrison, K. L. Optimizing sensitivity of the human sperm motility assay for embryo toxicity testing. *Hum Reprod* 2000; 15 (7):1586–91.

8. Critchlow, J. D., Matson, P. L., Newman, M. C., Horne, G., Troup, S. A. et al. Quality control in an in vitro fertilization laboratory: use of human sperm survival studies. *Hum Reprod* 1989; 4(5):545–9.

Chapter

12

Quality Control in the IVF Laboratory
Continuous Improvement

Georgios Liperis and Cecilia Sjöblom

Introduction

The performance of the embryology laboratory is of imperative importance for the successful outcome of an in vitro fertilization (IVF) cycle. The development and viability of gametes and embryos can be compromised by small fluctuations in their environment, so it is crucial to establish optimal culture conditions at which gametes and embryos are attained and maintained. In order to ensure and maintain these very specific conditions, quality control (QC) routines need to be established with quality specifications for each quality parameter. These parameters are assessed on a daily, weekly, monthly or annual basis to determine whether they meet certain specifications, followed by any necessary fine-tuning to bring the levels back within the acceptable limits of uncertainty of measurement.

12.1 Background

In the recent years, most laboratories are required to employ QC programmes, with the usefulness of such programmes being demonstrated by optimal laboratory performance along with effective troubleshooting when problems such as low fertilization rates or low pregnancy rates arise.[1] In addition, QC schemes can be vital in assessing and validating new methods and techniques to ensure that quality of service to the patients is not compromised. A QC programme includes monitoring of all parameters that can affect the outcome of the process. These include, but are not limited to, staff, equipment, culture media, consumables, protocols and environmental parameters such as temperature, pH, medium, osmolality, air quality and contamination.

Temperature is a key parameter for embryo culture, and the importance of maintaining 37°C during all aspects of human in vitro procedures was established in 1969.[2] Fluctuations in temperature have been shown to disrupt spindle and chromosomal organization in human oocytes, leading to chromosomal abnormalities in the developing embryos.[3] Determining the optimal temperature range for embryo culture has been challenging owing to the inaccuracy of most temperature measuring devices.[4] Optimal temperature is assumed to be between 36.7°C and 37.0°C, with an increase or decrease from this range considered critical.

The human embryo is also highly susceptible to oscillations in the pH of the culture medium, known as the 'external pH' (pHe).[5] The pHe depends on the association/disassociation of compounds in the medium, and due to the logarithmic scale of pHe, small variations in factors that affect the balance of compounds in solution, such as temperature, can lead to rapid change.[6] It is therefore crucial that a constant temperature be maintained to avoid changes in pH.

Maintenance of pH is particularly difficult outside the incubator, where preliminary data in mice have shown that an increase of pHe during manipulations outside the incubator had a significant impact on mouse blastocyst development and altered gene expression profiles.[7] In addition, even though embryos can regulate their pH to a certain extent, oocytes lack this capacity.[8] pH is known to affect the embryo actin cytoskeleton filaments and mitochondrial localization,[9] and it is possible that oocytes are affected in a similar manner. There is likely no single optimal value for pHe, but rather a range of pHe values from 7.2 to 7.4 is known to support the development of embryos.[10,11] However, a 0.2 change in pHe can result in a 60% change in proton (H^+) concentration; therefore, it is vital to maintain the pHe range as narrow as possible. A range of 7.27 to 7.32 at 37°C can be more acceptable, but ultimately, recommendations from the media manufacturers must be taken into account (Note A).

The pHe is a result of the balance of concentrations of CO_2 in the incubator and the amount of bicarbonate in the medium. Since the medium manufacturer sets the bicarbonate concentration, the CO_2 concentration is used to regulate the set point of medium pHe, with the two having an inverse relationship.[5] Defining the most suitable CO_2 concentration is difficult because apart from CO_2 and bicarbonate, there are other contributors to the set point of pHe, for example, protein source and concentration as well as the elevation of the laboratory. This is why stipulating a specific CO_2 value for the culture environment might be problematic. In addition to CO_2, some laboratories maintain low oxygen during embryo culture (5–7%) in order to improve embryo quality.[13] A low oxygen environment is created either by supplying the incubator with pre-mixed gas or by suppressing the atmospheric oxygen using nitrogen.

The presence of particles, volatile organic compounds (VOCs), microbes and perfumes can be harmful to gametes and embryos.[14] Even small levels of VOCs in an IVF laboratory have been shown to have detrimental effects on pregnancy rates.[15] It is therefore important to have an air filtration system that can eliminate airborne pathogens by efficiently filtering hydrocarbon pollutants, VOCs and chemically active compounds and that the efficacy of the system is monitored. Moreover, close attention has to be given to infection control of the clean room laboratory.

In addition to the physical and environmental conditions, the performance of equipment and staff will affect the outcome of the embryology processes and should be considered a part of the routine QC. A successful QC programme requires validations and ongoing monitoring of all these parameters, but appropriate consideration has to be given to the uncertainty of measurements, for which there is a place in risk management.

12.2 Reagents, Supplies and Equipment

All equipment needs to be calibrated to international standards minima annually.

12.2.1 Temperature

- Thermocouple device
- PT100 probes (one for each incubator)
- Surface probe
- Micro-probe (type K)
- Digital thermometer
- Temperature data loggers
- Liquid-in-glass thermometer

12.2.2 pH

- Blood gas analyzer
- Functioning pH meter with temperature compensation/automatic temperature compensation with pH electrodes and electrode calibration standards (4, 7, 10).

12.2.3 CO_2 and Gas Mixtures

- Blood gas analyzer
- Gas sensors

12.2.4 Air Quality

- Particle counter
- Photo-ionization monitor

12.3 Quality Control Procedure

12.3.1 Temperature

The temperature of the culture environment needs to be consistent during manipulations and handling outside the incubator and culture within the incubators (Note B). Manipulation and handling outside the incubator involve the use of microscope heated stages, laminar flow hood heated surfaces and warming blocks. The set temperature of these devices needs to be determined firstly by a series of measurements of the temperature inside a specific dish or tube alongside the corresponding surface temperature (Note C). The aim is to determine the set surface temperature (as shown on the equipment display) required to maintain 37.0°C inside the medium dish/tube. The final settings will vary depending on the type of culture dish used, conductivity, oil overlay and so on. If more than one type of dish is used on the heated surface, this validation of set point needs to be repeated for each type of dish, and consideration should be taken for the risk of overheating in one dish compared to the other. Usually the resulting set point for the heated stage or block is higher than 37.0°C. After the set point is determined, the corresponding surface temperature (measured using a surface probe) can be used for the temperature mapping.

Having determined the set point for the heating device, there can be significant variations between different heated areas. For each of the heated stages and surfaces, temperature mapping is required to indicate temperature variations. Temperature mapping is conducted every three months, with the temperature being measured at different locations to reveal which locations support the desired temperature, with these locations marked as 'safe to use' and the rest marked as 'not suitable for use' (Note D). Following validation, daily routine QC measurements can be done on the 'safe to use' areas with the use of a standard surface probe.

Maintaining a constant temperature inside the incubator is crucial for successful embryo culture. Incubator types include the standard large box incubator that can have a single inner door or multiple inner doors and the smaller bench-top incubators that can recover faster after opening and closing the door. Risk assessment is required to identify the number of dishes the incubator can support without temperature loss.

Regardless of model, all incubators require temperature mapping over a period of 24 hours to determine possible temperature inconsistencies under different conditions over time (Note E). Similarly to the heated surfaces, temperature mapping is performed when a new incubator is installed and every three months thereafter, positioning dishes or tubes in different locations around the chamber (Note C).

For daily temperature monitoring of incubators, constant accurate readings are essential. The type K micro-probe used for temperature mapping can be affected by electromagnetic fields and is therefore susceptible to errors and lack precision to detect differences of $\pm 0.1°C$ at $37°C$. For this purpose, more accurate platinum sensor PT100 probes are used in all incubators. These probes can be connected daily either to a thermocouple for manual daily readings (noted in a log book) or to a continuous monitoring system, where the temperature data are obtained and transferred via a wireless connection to a base station. The data are checked daily in comparison to the instrument display and weekly to verify that there are no fluctuations over time. In addition, external control is achieved by activating alarm options that include remote alarms such as Short Message Service (SMS) and alarm relay if temperatures fall outside the acceptable range.

Daily temperature measurements (or continuous) should also include laboratory ambient room temperature (RT; normally $23 \pm 2°C$; Note F) and refrigerator and freezer temperatures (set according to media manufacturers' recommendations). The log book recordings should include current, minimum and maximum temperatures and staff signature.

12.3.2 pH

A narrow acceptable pHe range is crucial for a thorough QC programme that aims to optimize the culture system. It is essential to verify the pH weekly for the culture medium in use and for all incubators. Moreover, pH should be checked every time a pre-mixed gas cylinder is replaced or before a new lot of culture medium is taken into use. Media are equilibrated in dishes or loosely capped tubes overnight before testing, with the exception of handling media. Handling media are warmed to $37°C$ in a capped tube placed in a warming block.

Monitoring pH using a blood gas analyzer provides highly accurate measurements. After start-up calibration (according to the manufacturer's instructions), the pre-equilibrated culture medium is loaded into the blood gas analyzer, and a pH reading is usually obtained together with other blood gas parameters (Note G). The traditional method of using a bench-top pH meter to measure the pH might not be completely accurate if it is not used quickly and efficiently, and consideration also must be taken of the negative effect of high protein levels in the medium on the pH probe. Alternatively, specialized pH meters can measure continuous pH inside the incubator under the same volume and conditions to which the embryos are exposed, but these pH meters are less accurate.

12.3.2.1 Calibration and pH Measurements Using a pH Meter

1. Calibrate the pH meter according to the manufacturer's instructions. Set the pH meter to $37°C$, or place the automatic temperature compensation probe inside a tube containing water in a warming block.
2. Place freshly aliquoted calibration standards into capped tubes.
3. Allow the standards to reach $37°C$.

4. Place the pH electrode into standard pH 4. When the pH is stabilized and calibrated, rinse the electrode with de-ionized H_2O and gently blot it dry. Repeat the process by first placing the electrode into standard pH 7 followed by standard pH 10.

5. After calibration, place the electrode back into standard pH 7 and verify the reading (~6.98 ± 0.02). If the reading is not within the range, repeat the calibration.

6. Remove the test tube containing medium from the incubator, and cap the tube quickly. Place the tube on a warming block at 37°C, and place the electrodes into the medium. When the reading stabilizes, record it (Note H).

7. Repeat the process for the other tube of the same medium, and average the two readings

8. Repeat the process for all different media used and for all incubators.

9. When all measurements are completed, cover the electrodes with a 3 M KCL solution.

Records for the calibration are kept together with maintenance records for the probe and probe performance. If the measured values differ significantly from the target values, electrodes must be replaced. Cleaning of electrodes with detergents can cause damage, and the electrodes are not always efficient; therefore, electrodes have to be replaced after 12 months of use.

12.3.3 CO_2 and Gas Mixtures

Daily monitoring of the incubator CO_2 concentration (and O_2 when applicable) is required. The CO_2 set point can vary between incubators and is determined (adjusted, if needed) according to the weekly pH verification. If all the measurements of pH are within the acceptable range, no further action is required. However, if the pH for a particular incubator is out of range, the CO_2 level is adjusted to raise or lower the pH (Note I). The pH can also be affected by gas quality and possible leaks. Certificates from the gas company must be provided, including gas purity and specifications in compliance with international standards. Checks for leaks must be conducted on a yearly basis (Note J).

A blood gas analyzer that has been through two levels of external liquid QC (provided by the manufacturer) can be used for accurate readings of CO_2 and O_2 levels in the culture medium, along with pH readings. Before testing, a set of two tubes with culture medium is equilibrated for 24 hours in each incubator.

A number of CO_2 measuring devices are available. If the daily QC is done using such a device, it needs to be calibrated against a standard certified gas before and after each series of readings (Note K). Thermal conductivity sensors are calibrated in an H_2O saturated atmosphere, and the incubator doors must not be opened for at least 15 minutes before taking a reading. Infrared sensors can also determine the CO_2 and O_2 levels with the benefit of not requiring high humidity levels to function. Portable devices exist that can take simultaneous CO_2, O_2, relative humidity and temperature readings (Note L). Some of the newer technology incubators come with built-in gas and temperature sensors and readings that can be reviewed and downloaded. Alternatively, external CO_2 and humidity sensors for each incubator can be used in conjunction with multi-input data loggers (automated monitoring and alarm system, as for temperature).

Whichever instrument is used, CO_2 and O_2 measurements are taken daily, and records are kept for all incubators. The values obtained have to correspond to both the set point and the incubator display. For bench-top incubators that use pre-mixed gas, accurate control of the gas mixture sometimes is not possible due to the potential blocking of the tubing by condensation, resulting in lower pressure and reduced reserve volume. In this case, the measurement of pH is crucial to verify the pre-mixed gas. In addition, for this type of incubator, the purge rate of the incoming gas needs to be monitored (set at approximately 15–25 ml/ml).

12.3.4 Air Quality

Clean, ultrapure air is required in the IVF laboratory. This is achieved by the heating, ventilation and air-conditioning (HVAC) system, along with an air-handling unit that exchanges air automatically. Positive air pressure, where the laboratory has 10 to15 Pa more than the adjacent rooms, is required to avoid air from adjacent rooms entering the laboratory. The temperature must not fluctuate significantly between seasons (±1°C), and the HVAC system should be adjusted when necessary. The HVAC system aids in cooling the air and removes humidity. The relative humidity levels in the laboratory should be between 40% and 60% to minimize fungal growth.

The number and size of particles per cubic meter of air can define how clean the air is. In order to remove airborne contaminants, high-efficiency particulate air (HEPA) filters are placed in the ceiling of the laboratory. Laminar flow hoods also contain HEPA filtration, and all filters are checked and replaced regularly. The norm for particulate and micro-organism contamination is set by the European Union Cells and Tissue Directive,[16] which suggests that particle counts and microbial colony counts have to be equivalent to Grade A with a Grade B background (Note M).

Pre-filters along with activated carbon filters and potassium permanganate filters are also required to maintain the quality of the air inside the laboratory by absorbing VOCs (Note N). Stand-alone filtration units can also be used for this purpose.

12.3.5 Contamination and Infection Control

Although antibiotics are used in the culture medium, and embryologists apply stringent aseptic techniques, there is still a risk for contamination if the environment is not controlled. The laboratory is cleaned and decontaminated daily, with all surfaces rinsed with sterile water to remove any toxic residue from laboratory disinfectants (preferably commercially available embryo-tested spray or 70% ethanol). All incubators are cleaned and autoclaved every three to six months.

12.3.6 Other Parameters

The subject of routine QC can be limitless, and while this chapter aims to capture the core items, there are still others that apply to certain laboratories and certain circumstances. For example, if a laboratory is weighing a sperm sample to determine the volume, then the QC needs to incorporate the routine weighing of standard weights. It should also be acknowledged that monitoring of staff performance is a crucial part of QC, but its processes are very much specific to each individual laboratory. It is therefore important to assess each process and ask, what parameters can affect the outcome of this process? All these parameters will need to be included in the routine QC process.

12.3.6.1 Monitoring Standard Operating Procedure

All parameters need to be monitored (frequency in parentheses). The monitoring log book needs to include measurement value, acceptable range and action taken when a measurement falls outside the given range. Each entry requires a staff signature.

1. Temperature measurements of the 'safe to use' heated areas of all heated devices (daily)
2. Temperature measurements of all incubators (continuously or daily)
3. Check of temperature data loggers (daily and weekly for continuous systems)
4. Ambient room temperature (daily)
5. Refrigerator and freezer temperatures (daily)
6. Temperature mapping for heated devices and incubators (every three months and for all new equipment before put into use)
7. pH measurements (weekly or for new medium LOT and new pre-mixed gas bottle)
8. CO_2 concentration for all incubators (daily or continuously)
9. O_2 concentration for all incubators (daily or continuously when low-oxygen culture is applied)
10. Positive pressure (daily)
11. Laboratory humidity (daily)
12. Particle count (twice daily, at rest and in operation)
13. VOCs (daily)
14. Contact plates or swabs of all work surfaces (three times a month) (Note O).
15. Active air samplers and settlement plates (three time a month) (Note P)

12.4 Notes

A. All commercial embryo culture media have a recommended pH, ranging from 7.1 to 7.45. Some manufacturers recommend the same range for all their media, while others have different ranges for different media.
B. An alternative option is the use of an IVF chamber – an isolated system with integrated temperature and gas control along with air filtration that has no interaction with its external environment.
C. Thermocouple device with micro-probe or surface probe validated to an accuracy of ±0.1°C along with a dish that is set up under the same conditions as the gametes/embryos are held (type of dish, volume of medium and oil overlay, position of droplets).
D. If the temperature mapping reveals that the locations that are more commonly used by embryologists fall outside the desired temperature range, an alternative option is to change the set temperature of the heated surface accordingly and re-map temperatures until the desired areas correspond to the correct temperatures.
E. Temperature mapping is also required for tube holders that are used during the oocyte pickup. If transport incubators are also used, temperature mapping is required for all the tube insertion points under the exact conditions under which gametes/embryos are transferred.
F. The laboratory RT could be debated, with some saying higher temperatures decrease the risk of cooling when samples are held outside the incubators. However, it must be considered that higher RT also increases the risk for bacterial/fungal contamination.
G. Blood gas analyzers can be expensive, but most IVF laboratories, which are embedded in larger hospitals, can make use of the hospital analysers located in the central laboratory or emergency/maternity department. Using medium rather than blood will not alter the accuracy of the measurement or damage the equipment.
H. A tight seal between the electrode and the walls of the test tube is required for accurate measurements. A rubber gasket can be placed around the electrode to create a seal and stabilize pH readings.

I. Because of their inverse relationship, raising CO_2 levels is used to lower pH and lowering CO_2 levels is used to raise pH until it reaches the predetermined acceptable range.

J. Certified gas purity values can have a range between ±1% for alpha standard and ±2% for beta standard of the actual concentration value. In certain countries where gas cylinders are not certified, there are situations where the O_2 levels are between 5% and 20% according to the gas provider, which essentially means that the embryos are cultured in ambient O_2 conditions.

K. Certified standard gas, 5% CO_2/5% O_2, is provided in a small bottle that can be held in the laboratory and comes with a certificate of accuracy. Alternatively, certified pre-mixed gas for incubators can be used, but this requires pressure reduction (as per device instructions) in order to avoid damaging the measuring device.

L. If a thermal conductivity sensor is used to monitor, the incubator humidity might need to be increased to make sure that the sensor is functioning (>90% humidity is required). On the contrary, if the humidity of the air inside the laboratory is high, it might need to be reduced.

M. Grade A criteria: maximum permitted number of particles per cubic metre is 3,520 for particles that are 0.5 μm or greater in size and a maximum of 20 for particles that are 5.0 μm or greater in size. These criteria apply at rest and in operation, and an area that is at least 1 m^3 is required for accurate readings.

N. The levels of VOCs should not exceed the 0.5 ppm. If there are any levels above the 0.5 pprm margin, then passive absorption on a gas chromatography column is used by opening one side of the column and leaving it open for one week before sending the column for analysis. The results can indicate the amount and type of molecule(s) so that appropriate actions can be taken.

O. Contact plates, such as replicate organism detection and counting (RODAC) containing sabouraud dextrose agar (SDA, for detection of fungus) and trypticase soy agar (TSA, for detection of bacteria), should be used for surfaces, and swabs should only be used for surfaces that are not flat or are in hard-to-reach areas. Zero colonies for Grade A areas.

P. Active air sampling is done by drawing a pre-determined volume of air using a large syringe or similar and expelling it over SDA and TSA plates. Settlement plates are located at crucial operative sites, such as flow hoods, ET table, ICSI rig and so on and are exposed for four hours during full laboratory operation. Zero colonies for Grade A areas.

References

1. Wikland, M. and Sjoblom, C. The application of quality systems in ART programs. *Mol Cell Endocrinol* 2000; 166:3–7.

2. Brinster, R. L. In vitro cultivation of mammalian ova. *Adv Biosci* 1969; 4:199–233.

3. Almeida, P. A. and Bolton, V. N. The effect of temperature fluctuations on the cytoskeletal organization and chromosomal constitution of the human oocyte. *Zygote* 1995; 3(4):357–65.

4. Higdon, H. L., 3rd, Blackhurst, D. W. and Boone, W. R. Incubator managements in an assisted reproductive technology laboratory. *Fertil Steril* 2008; 89(3):703–10.

5. Swain, J. E. Optimizing the culture environment in the IVF laboratory: impact of pH and buffer capacity on gamete and embryo quality. *Reprod Biomed Online* 2010; 21:6–16.

6. Swain, J. E. and Pool, T. B. New pH-buffering system for media utilized during gamete and embryo manipulations for assisted reproduction. *Reprod. Biomed Online* 2009; 18:799–810.

7. Koustas, G. and Sjoblom, C. Epigenetic consequences of pH stress in mouse embryos. *Hum Reprod* 2011; 26:i78.

8. Fitzharris, G. and Baltz, J. Regulation of intracellular pH during oocyte growth and maturation in mammals. *Reproduction* 2009; 138:619–27.

9. Squirrell, J. M., Lane, M. and Bavister, B. D. Altering intracellular pH disrupts development and cellular organization in preimplantation hamster embryos. *Biol Reprod* 2001; 64:1845–54.

10. Swain, J. E. Is there an optimal pH for culture media used in clinical IVF? *Hum Reprod Update* 2012; 18(3):333–9.

11. Quinn, P. and Cooke, S. Equivalency of culture media for human in vitro fertilization formulated to have the same pH under an atmosphere containing 5% or 6% carbon dioxide. *Fertil Steril* 2004; 81:1502–6.

12. Graves, C. N. and Biggers, J. D. Carbon dioxide fixation by mouse embryos prior to implantation. *Science* 1970; 167:1506–8.

13. Peng, H., Shi, W., Zhang, W., Xue, X., Li, N. et al. Better quality and more usable embryos obtained on day 3 cultured in 5% than 20% oxygen: a controlled and randomized study using the sibling oocytes. *Reprod Sci* 2015; pii:1933719115602761.

14. Morbeck, D. E. Air quality in the assisted reproduction laboratory: a mini-review. *J Assist Reprod Genet* 2015; 32(7):1019–24.

15. Boone, W. R., Johnson, J. E., Locke, A. J., Crane, M. M., 4th and Price, T. M. Control of air quality in an assisted reproductive technology laboratory. *Fertil Steril* 1999; 71(1):150–4.

16. Directive 2003/23/EC of the European Parliament and of the Council of 31 March 2004 on setting standards of quality and safety for the donation, procurement, testing, processing, preservation, storage and distribution of human tissues and cells. *Official Journal of the European Union*, L 102, 7.4.2004, pp. 48–58, available at http://europa.eu.int/eur-lex/en/oj/.

Chapter

13

Setup Procedures for Optimizing Performance in the IVF Laboratory

Klaus E. Wiemer

Introduction

Optimization of procedures routinely performed in a clinical human in vitro fertilization (IVF) laboratory have become increasingly important due to the increase in complexity of procedures now performed in the laboratory. The addition of new technologies requiring more oversight has increased dramatically within the last decade. As a result of incorporating these new technologies, safe and efficient operation of the IVF laboratory has become increasingly complex and requires a substantial understanding of processes within the laboratory. In today's modern IVF laboratory, the amount of staff time to perform every increasingly complicated case has more than doubled.[1] Similarly, the amount of time required to prepare for these cases has increased dramatically as well. In many instances, the increase in complexity of laboratory procedures has not translated into hiring of new staff but the creation of challenges to improve efficiency within the laboratory. The current guidelines for allocation of staff are based upon cycle numbers performed on an annual basis, not complexity of cases performed.[2]

This chapter describes how we have organized our daily laboratory activities to improve efficiency, maintained high quality and reduce the likelihood of errors.

13.1 Duties Related to Starting Up the Laboratory

The initial morning hours within the IVF laboratory prior to starting patient care provide for a very unique opportunity to establish critical standards. This is due to the fact most laboratories have not had any activities occur during the overnight period to confound values. This is the ideal time period to establish critical surface temperatures on heated surfaces, surface temperatures of bench-top incubators, pH values in incubators, O_2/CO_2 values in box-type incubators, nitrogen levels in cryostorage units and temperatures in refrigerators/freezers. We have found that the 'true values' of heated equipment as well as critical equipment such as incubators are best recorded in the morning prior to use. We have found that incubator values, after the incubators had been closed all night, best represent the conditions to which embryos are most likely being exposed. Previous experience has shown that measurement of values after breaching the incubator environment provides little value in terms of assessing what conditions embryos are actually being exposed to. We have also found that measuring liquid nitrogen values in the morning provides an accurate measurement of the liquid nitrogen within each tank and provides a more accurate value to gauge individual nitrogen use and integrity of the tank in question. These measurements are useful to gauge whether the vacuum within certain tanks is breaking down and thus is more susceptible to a catastrophic event. For more details on

Table 13.1 Opening and Closing Checklist

Month:_____   Year: _____

	Opening checklist:	Bring in trash cans	Perform opening QC	Check clinical tasks in eIVF	Check gasses (if low-order)	Triple gas switched over?	Closing checklist:	Complete daily/data-entry checklist	Change water in humidifying jar	Turn off all scopes/wipe oculars	Wipe hood (1% 7x, dH 2O, methanol)	Wipe stripper handles	Clean rubber bulbs- air dry	Empty biohazard	Take out trash/ shred bin	Put up schedule for next day	Check that PR O2 is off	Do time out!!	Restock plastics/14-ml tubes	Turn on coda towers and hood	Turn off monitors
1																					
2																					
...																					
31																					

the measurements taken in our laboratory, as well as frequency, please refer to Tables 13.1, 13.2 and 13.3.

To maximize staff efficiency and reduce delay in staff time to start embryo evaluations in the morning, we have one staff member come in 30 to 45 minutes prior to everyone else so that tasks associated with starting the laboratory up are completed prior to arrival of the rest of staff. We have a policy to have one person perform the start-up tasks consecutively for one week in order to reduce any potential technician effect when measuring such values as temperature and pH values. Having one person perform these duties allows that person to better understand trends and patterns for each piece of equipment. In short, it allows each staff member the opportunity to understand intimately the characteristics of each piece of equipment in the laboratory. This policy has been useful in helping staff study aberrant patterns with equipment and make judgement calls if equipment values are starting to drift or if equipment used for measuring values merely needs calibration.

13.2 Maintaining Efficiencies during the Day

The complexity of IVF cases continues to grow every day at ever-increasing rates. We no longer can assume that patients will follow more traditional lines of therapy. For example, we can no longer assume that a patient will even have a transfer in a fresh cycle but rather is going to bank zygotes for use in conjunction with pre-implantation genetic diagnosis (PGD)/pre-implantation genetic screening (PGS) at a later time. As a result, we have developed a patient embryology process checklist system that allows us to effectively use our time and materials wisely (see Table 13.4). It also allows us to develop a checklist that is specific to the particular patient. The process of developing a meaningful checklist within

Table 13.2 Embryology Laboratory Daily Monitor

Date	Time	Tech	Dish oven	Tube warmer			Warming oven	Hoods			Stage warmer		Air table		Temperature	Humidity
				Micro.	Retrieval	PR		6 inch, left	6 inch, right	3 inch	1	2	1	2		
1																
2																
...																
31																
Ranges			36–38°C	36–38°C			36–38°C	36.0–40.0°C			36.8–42.5°C	36.8–42.5°C	>100 psi	>100 psi	19–27°C	>15%

Greyed-out days = weekends and holidays. They may not be monitored. Reviewed by: _____ Date: _____

Table 13.3 Media Prep Daily Monitor

Date	Time	Tech.	Temperatures						Liquid nitrogen			Magnehelic		Tanks
			Room, ambient	Refrigerator			Freezer, actual	Media oven	Tank 1	Tank 2	Tank 3	HVAC gauge		filled
				Min.	Max.	Actual						F1	F2–5	
1														
2														
…														
31														
Ranges			19–27°C	2°C	8°C	2–8°C	0 to −27°C	35.5–38.5°C	>27 cm	>27 cm	>27 cm	0.05–0.3 inch H_2O	0.5–1.0 inch H_2O	

Greyed-out days are weekends and holidays and may not be monitored. Reviewed by:_____ Date:_____

91

Table 13.4 Daily Patient Checklist

Series # _____ Page # __ of ___	Doe, Jane	Doe, Jane	Doe, Jane	Doe, Jane
Day −1	Date: Incubate egg rinse/hold dishes Retrieval/oil tubes Flush/rinse in warming oven			
Day 0	Date: Sperm prep Retrieval Oocyte freeze/thaw Culture dishes ICSI/INSEM			
Day 1	Date: Clean eggs, check fertilization Microdrop Change Over Discard excess sperm Zygote freeze/thaw PM check			
Day 2	Date: Cleavage check Prep blast dishes TRF medium			
Day 3	Date: Embryo evaluation Assisted hatching Blast changeover Embryo transfer			
Day 4	Date: Day 4 check Day 5 FET dish TRF MEDIA			
Day 5	Date: Day 5 check Blastocyst transfer Blastocyst freeze			
Day 6	Date: Day 6 check Blastocyst freeze Send final report Billing sheet			

our centre begins with the person compiling all the material in order to prepare the embryology laboratory sheets. During the process of procuring all the patient's information and treatments, the embryologist can place the specific embryology procedures on the checklist. In this manner, the checklist becomes the organizational 'heart and soul' of that patient's treatment. We have found that by making one person responsible for the entire embryology chart, we have reduced the incidence of preparing unnecessary culture dishes, for example. In this manner, a patient checklist greatly reduces unnecessary tasks and improves staff efficiency. Our checklist has also helped us to gauge the amount of daily setup required for a specific day. The daily checklist allows us a quick over view of duties that need to be performed that day.

To ensure that we are efficient in preparation for upcoming cases, we have a very set schedule in which we review all upcoming patients. For example, all patients are reviewed at between 12:00 and 12:30 every day as a group, and a senior member from the laboratory is present for this review. During this review, the number of patients who are being triggered is determined, and the upcoming transfer schedule is determined. Nursing has an internal checklist to ensure that all documents are signed and in the chart so that the embryology staff do not have to perform these tasks. The embryology laboratory determines the retrieval schedule and transfer schedule. Retrieval times are based somewhat on the treatment plan of the patient. For example, we schedule oocyte and zygote vitrification at the end of the retrieval schedule to ensure that we freeze the oocytes at the correct time. For zygote cryopreservation cases, we also schedule these towards the end of retrieval schedule so that we are sure that we can cryopreserve the resulting zygotes less than 24 hours after retrieval. intracytoplasmic sperm injection (ICSI) patients are scheduled so that ICSI can be performed three to six hours after retrieval; typically these are the first cases of the day. With proper scheduling, this corresponds to time slots that are available right after transfers. Once the upcoming schedule has been determined, one person is then tasked to put the charts together and develop the patient-specific checklists prior to any culture dish preparation. Once the upcoming schedule is finalized, tasks are assigned whenever possible to ensure that all work is completed in a timely manner. Tasks are assignment based upon a person's experience and skill sets.

Although the modern laboratory has become increasingly complex, we have found it to be imperative to set up culture dishes at approximately the same time on a daily basis. In the past, the busyness of the day would not allow a consistent time to prepare dishes. We found that this was affecting the pH values of our various culture systems and also was affecting our ability to use embryo morphology as a biomarker to gauge how our culture systems were performing.[3] In order to have consistent culture conditions within our laboratory, we have found that dishes need to be prepared no later than 12 noon to 1 in the afternoon. This fits well with our centre because it allows culture dish preparation to occur during the time retrievals are being performed, and the person assigned can serve as a witness for moving gametes to new dishes or for witnessing biopsy cases. We have found with our current case load and number of incubator openings, having culture dishes in the incubators by 12 noon to 1 PM, ensures consistent pH values regardless of incubator openings for the following day.

Another very important aspect to preparation of culture dishes is to ensure that our plastic ware has had sufficient time to off-gas and/or is rinsed prior to use. Unpublished studies in our laboratory have found that allowing embryo culture dishes at least 48 hours to off-gas prior to use allows materials such as aldehydes and styrenes to dissipate from the dishes prior to use. These compounds are commonly used in the production of plastic ware used for embryo culture. We know from previous studies in our laboratory that these materials are very soluble in oil and can accumulate in the oils used for embryo culture. The process of off-gassing culture dishes is very easy. We remove the dishes from their sleeves at the end of the day after all tasks have been completed, and these dishes are stacked inside a laminar flow hood with the air on high to expedite the off-gassing process. We had found in the past that the presence of the compounds would affect embryo development in a very inconsistent manner. In other words, it was not apparent all the time and was very difficult to isolate. We found in mouse studies that overall embryo development was impaired, characterized by slower rates of development and lower rates of blastocyst development with lower numbers of cells within these blastocysts. In a similar fashion, prior to making off-gassing a policy, we often noted erratic development of human embryos cultured in dishes that were not off-gassed prior to use.

The subject of aliquoting media is a controversial topic because its impact on embryo development can be sporadic. In the past, we used to aliquot all of our media into previously QC tested plastic ware when we received media from the manufacturers. We found that embryo development was often erratic, and it was very difficult to reduce this variation. We found one lot of 4-ml snap-cap tubes to be a real issue despite off-gassing. However, once we rinsed the tubes with protein-free human tubal fluid (HTF), the erratic effects decreased dramatically. In a small study we did in our laboratory, we found that mouse embryos tended to develop better and have higher cell counts if we rinsed our 4-ml tubes with medium prior to storage of embryo culture medium (for up to five days). However, we noted that human embryo development was slightly less than optimal when we stored medium in rinsed 4-ml tubes when compared to medium straight from the bottle despite our results with mouse embryos. As a result, we no longer store any medium used directly for embryo culture or sperm preparation in plastic ware. We take all media for embryo culture straight from the culture medium bottle. The exception for this is medium used for sperm preparation. In these cases, we thoroughly rinse our QC-tested tubes with HTF prior to overnight incubation of this medium for sperm preparations the following days. Media used for egg collections and transfers are placed in rinsed QC-tested tubes the day prior to retrievals as well. Medium that comes in direct contact with embryos is never aliquoted prior to use.

Another controversial area is oil washing and handling. Oils used for embryo cultures are not well defined and are often the source contaminants that can affect embryo development.[4,5] We also have established that oils can contain peroxides as well as aldehydes that may affect human embryo development. As a result of the findings of Morbeck et al.,[5] as well as our own laboratory findings, we now wash all oils used for embryo culture with protein-free culture medium. In addition, we store all oils in the dark to reduce peroxidase activity. Oil that is washed with culture medium is stored in the refrigerator. We wash all our oils used for embryo culture at least 73 hours prior to use. We do not remove the medium from the oil-containing bottles because it settles to the bottom and does not interfere with dish preparation.

For preparation of dishes, we do not have the hood on as we have found that the water components in the medium will evaporate quickly and will increase the solute concentrations and thus potentially affect embryo development. We clean the hood thoroughly with 6% ultrapure hydrogen peroxide prior to making dishes; we wear masks and use gloves when preparing culture dishes. We try not to use syringe filters, if possible, because the adhesives used to bond the elements will often leach into the product being filtered. If something requires filtering, we wash the filter by passing 4 to 5 ml of protein-free medium through the filter prior to use.

13.3 Ending the Day on a 'Good Note'

In our experience, the afternoon of the day can present many unique challenges in terms of ensuring optimal efficiencies in the laboratory. Mental exhaustion becomes more apparent in the afternoons and can lead to loss of focus as well as loss of productivity. Unlike other laboratory disciplines, the time required to complete one's tasks may be more open ended and can depend of the complexity as well as number of cases to complete. During the afternoon periods, many laboratories are performing complex tasks such as ICSI, embryo cryopreservation and blastocyst biopsy. All these tasks require sharp mental focus. For this reason, whenever possible, we try to rotate staff who have been performing complex tasks with staff performing less complex tasks. In many laboratories (including ours) this is often a luxury, so we use monitors to witness all procedures. We use verbal confirmations in conjunction with visual witnessing of samples and/or procedures to ensure accuracy.

Staff members not involved in complex procedures will begin to confirm that all paper work is completed for the day. Other staff will begin to perform our 'shut down' procedures (see Table 13.1.) These tasks are designed to ensure that all duties intended to be completed on that day have indeed been completed. Perhaps the most important task we perform at the end of the day is called 'time out'. During this phase of the laboratory shutdown, we physically check each incubator to ensure that oocytes have been inseminated or injected, dishes have been made, embryos have been moved accordingly and transfer media prepared. Not only is this a verbal process but also a visual one. We want to use both verbal and visual confirmations that tasks specific for each patient have been completed. By using a combination of our daily patient checklist (Table 13.4) and our end of the day checklist (Table 13.1), we have improved staff efficiency by assigning tasks to appropriately trained staff and have increased staff utilization remarkably.

13.4 Summary

As mentioned previously, the complexity of IVF cases has increased dramatically in the last several years. This increase in complexity has not necessarily increased the hiring practices of IVF clinics. To date, the staffing recommendations for a human IVF laboratory are based upon cycle volume not cycle complexity. As a result, we have had to become increasingly organized within the laboratory and improve staffing efficiencies. We have found that using checklists such as those discussed within this text has greatly improved personnel efficiencies, all the while ensuring that our QC/quality assurance (QA) programmes are not compromised. Developing patient-centric/specific checklists has helped us to assign tasks to appropriately trained staff and helped to organize our days within the laboratory. Incorporating set times to review and schedule patients has also helped us to set up corresponding culture dishes with appropriate time to ensure that dish equilibration is consistent. In addition, the use of off-gassed plastic ware, rinsed plastic ware and washed oils is essential to provide optimal conditions for embryo development. The use of our 'time out' at the end of the day has proven to be priceless. This list has afforded us one more additional step to ensure that we reduce the potential for errors that could go unchecked.

In conclusion, we feel that the use of checklists and the organization of daily activities into various tables have improved staffing efficiencies and have helped to make our staff more accountable, thus reducing errors. As our field becomes more complex, improving efficiencies will become more paramount.

References

1. Alikani, A., Go, K. J., McCaffrey, C. and McCulloh, D. H. Comprehensive evaluation of contemporary assisted reproduction technology laboratory operations to determine staffing levels that promote patient safety and quality care. *Fertil Steril* 2014; 102:1350–6.

2. Practice Committee of the American Society for Reproductive Medicine. Revised guidelines for human embryology and andrology laboratories. *Fertil Steril* 2008; 90 (Suppl. 3): S45–59.

3. Lundin, K. and Ahlström, A. Quality control and standardization of embryo morphology scoring and viability marker. *Reprod Biomed Online* 2015; 459–71.

4. Hughes, M. P., Morbeck, D. E., Hudson, S. B. A., Fredrickson, J.R., Walker, D.L et al. Peroxides in mineral oil used for in vitro fertilization: defining limits of standards quality control assays. *J Assist Reprod. Genet* 27:87–92.

5. Morbeck, D. E., Khan, Z., Barnidge, D. R. and Walker, D. Washing mineral reduces contaminants and embryotoxicity. *Fertil Steril* 2010; 94:2747–52.

Chapter

14

Sperm Preparation for Therapeutic IVF

Verena Nordhoff and Sabine Kliesch

Introduction

Spermatozoa have to be separated from seminal fluid to omit negative influences and to ensure best assisted reproductive technology (ART) results. Several preparation techniques exist that can be used to enrich the best motile and morphologically normal spermatozoa: (1) simple washing, (2) swim-up (with or without washing step) and (3) density gradient centrifugation. Every technique has its advantages and disadvantages, and also, the final attribution of the sample (e.g. usage for intrauterine insemination, in vitro fertilization or intracytoplasmic sperm injection) has to be taken into account. Simple washing is optimal for high sperm numbers in normozoospermic patients. Swim-up gives excellent results in normozoospermic and moderate oligoasthenoteratzoospermic (OAT) samples, and density gradient centrifugation is preferred if a sample is moderate to severe OAT. Epididymal aspirated samples can be prepared either by swim-up or by density gradient. Testicular sperm extraction samples have to be processed differently, as steps dissociating the tissue have to be executed first. Depending on the presence of an obstructive or a non-obstructive azoospermia, rather a mechanical or enzymatic preparation should be chosen. Good-quality sperm preparation is a prerequisite for the highest success rates in ART.

14.1 Background

Semen, naturally a perfect mixture of fluids and cells for executing fertilization of an oocyte, cannot be used for ART as it is. There are three major points that have to be considered before using ejaculated spermatzooa for ART. First, semen consists of different fractions: one fraction of spermatozoa from the testes and another fraction of seminal fluid from accessory glands such as the epididymides, seminal vesicles and prostate.[1] Although seminal fluid is important in aiding spermatozoa to penetrate the cervical mucus,[2] some substances such as prostaglandins and zinc may hinder sperm from achieving a pregnancy, for example, in intrauterine insemination (IUI) cycles, where sperm do not pass physiological selecting barriers.[3] Therefore, preparation of semen samples is necessary and of great importance.

Additionally, possible negative effects may be caused by non-sperm cells from the seminal fluid. These cells naturally would never enter the female tract and have to be omitted by quick (normally within one hour) separation of spermatozoa from the seminal fluid. The separation will yield a fraction of highly motile and morphologically normal spermatozoa of good quality. Processing of semen is necessary and should always be done in a controlled manner exhibiting the highest-quality standards. The preparation will lead to the best-quality sperm selection and will help to provide high success rates in ART.

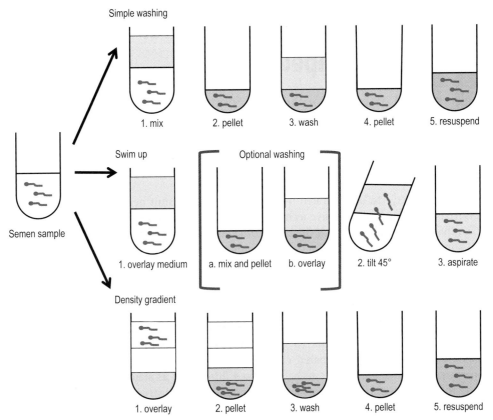

Figure 14.1 Schematic presentation of sperm preparation techniques (for exact procedure, see respective sections). (A black and white version of this figure will appear in some formats. For the color version, please refer to the plate section.)

For correct semen preparation, the World Health Organisation (WHO) has recently published the fifth edition of the *Laboratory Manual for the Examination and Processing of Human Semen*.[4] This chapter will describe the main techniques for sperm preparation and processing. However, it is not meant to be a replacement for the WHO handbook. The explanations given here should rather be seen as a technical note, and wherever specific questions are raised, the WHO handbook should always be considered, as it is of overriding importance.

The most used semen preparation techniques are simple washing, swim-up and density gradient centrifugation (Figure 14.1). Which technique is chosen for what purpose is determined mostly by the nature of a semen sample (Table 14.1).

1. Simple washing is used mostly for normozoospermic semen samples as it is a quick and not very cumbersome technique. Basically, the motility of sperm is used as they will swim into the overlayed medium. Although it does not gives the highest numbers of sperm, at least they are selected for the highest forward progression.

2. A swim-up procedure is carried out when sperm parameters are within the normal range. This preparation method will not give the highest recovery rates in comparison with density gradient centrifugation, but the technique is quick and easy to perform and will lead to a highly enriched fraction of motile spermatozoa.[5,6] An additional washing

Table 14.1 Comparison of Different Sperm Preparation Techniques and Their Advantages and Disadvantages

Technique	Spermatozoa quality	Advantage	Disadvantage
Simple washing	Normozoospermia Epididymal spermatozoa (low numbers)	Quick and easy Yields high number of spematozoa	Only for sperm counts with high sperm numbers Not useful for samples with contamination (other cells, debris or blood cells)
Swim-up (direct or including a washing step)	Normozoospermia Moderate OAT Epididymal spermatozoa (moderate to high numbers)	Quick and easy Good rates of highly progressive motile spermatozoa	Lower recovery rates compared to DG
DG centrifugation	Moderate to severe OAT Epididymal spermatozoa (moderate to high)	High numbers of motile spermatozoa Best removal of debris or other cell types from the semen sample	Difficult to standardize High-molecular-weight compounds of unknown influence Costs more (DG solutions have to be purchased)
Mechanical mazeration	Obstructive TESE	High numbers of possibly motile spermatozoa Easy and quick	Not useful in severe non-obstructive cases
Enzymatic digestion	Obstructive and non-obstructive TESE	Best release of low numbers of tissue-bound spermatozoa	High contamination with other cells, debris or blood cells (secondary a DG might be of help, but loss has to be taken into account)

Note: OAT= oligoasthenoteratozoospermia; TESE = testicular sperm extraction.

step before swim-up is an elegant way to minimize or remove substances from the seminal plasma (e.g. zinc) as these factors might have a negative influence on sperm quality. However, there are some reports that say a washing step before swim-up might cause peroxidative damage to sperm membranes.[7]

3. Density gradient (DG) centrifugation is often used for lower sperm concentrations, lower sperm motility or lower sperm morphology (e.g. OAT) to facilitate an enrichment of high numbers of motile spermatozoa mainly for in vitro fertilization (IVF) or intracytoplasmic sperm injection (ICSI). DG reaches not only an optimal selection of good spermatozoa but also reduces debris, leucocytes and other cells from the ejaculate. Two different density solutions are used that consist of colloidal silica coated with silane of high molecular mass and low osmolality, a lower gradient with high density (80% v/v) and an upper gradient with low density (40% v/v). The semen is placed on top, and spermatozoa are enriched by centrifugation through the gradient into a sometimes loose pellet at the bottom of the tube. However, standardization, especially for the centrifugation step, is the crucial point using DG centrifugation.

Another important issue is the preparation of epididymal or testicular spermatozoa. Both sperm types can be retrieved during standard surgical techniques, but the success rate depends on the function of the testes.

14.1.1 Epididymal Spermatozoa

In azoospermic patients (only obstructive cases), it might be possible to retrieve epidymal fluid with spermatozoa from the enlarged epididymis. The fluid should be collected with as few as possible contaminating erythrocytes or other cells. If sperm numbers are high, either a DG or a swim-up might be the best choice for preparation. If sperm numbers are low, a simple washing step is more appropriate.

14.1.2 Testicular Spermatozoa

Spermatozoa can be retrieved by open biopsy using a conventional testicular sperm extraction (TESE) or a microsurgical TESE using a microscope.[8] In an obstructive azoospermic patient a biopsy will most likely give high rates of spermatozoa, whereas in non-obstructive cases, where testis function is compromised, the microsurgical retrieval of foci with spermatogenic activity can be quite elaborate. In these patients, the expected sperm numbers might be very low and the discovery quite laborious and time-consuming. Therefore, these specimens should always be handled with care. TESE material is often contaminated with erythrocytes, and a washing step before preparation and a DG step after preparation might be of help. Tissue-bound spermatozoa are released either by mechanical mazeration or, in addition, by enzymatic digestion. The latter is more important in cases of non-obstructive azoospermia where sperm numbers are low.

14.2 Reagents, Supplies and Equipment

14.2.1 Simple Washing

- Balanced salt solution or a commercially available sperm preparation medium supplemented with protein (e.g. human serum albumin (HSA)), ready to use medium, pre-incubated at 37°C, without CO_2 if with HEPES; if without HEPES use 5–6% CO_2 (see Note A)
- Incubator
- Sterile test tubes of 6- or 13-ml volume (Note B)
- Centrifuge (up to 500×g)
- Pipettes with variable volumes (2–200 μl and 100–1,000 μl) and corresponding sterile tips
- Neubauer chamber for sperm concentration
- Microscopic slides and coverslips for evaluation of motility
- Microscope for evaluation of concentration, motility and morphology

14.2.2 Direct Swim-Up (Optional with Additional Washing Step)

- Balanced salt solution or a commercially available sperm preparation medium supplemented with protein (e.g. HSA), ready to use medium, pre-incubated at 37°C, without CO_2 if with HEPES; if without HEPES use 5–6% CO_2 (see Note A)
- Incubator
- Sterile test tubes of 6- or 13-ml volume (Note B)

- Centrifuge (up to 500×g)
- Pipettes with variable volumes (2–200 μl and 100–1,000 μl) and corresponding sterile tips
- Neubauer chamber for sperm concentration
- Microscopic slides and coverslips for evaluation of motility
- Microscope for evaluation of concentration, motility and morphology

14.2.3 Discontinuous Density Gradient Centrifugation

- Balanced salt solution or a commercially available sperm preparation medium supplemented with protein (e.g. HSA), ready to use medium pre-incubated at 37°C, without CO_2 if with HEPES; if without HEPES use 5–6% CO_2 (see Note A)
- Gradient media (commercially available, use according to manufacturer's protocol), either ready to use or must be diluted with an iso-osmotic medium according to manufacturer's recommendations
- Incubator
- Sterile test tubes of 6- or 13-ml volume (Note B)
- Centrifuge (up to 500×g)
- Pipettes with variable volumes (2–200 μl and 100–1,000 μl) and corresponding sterile tips
- Neubauer chamber for sperm concentration
- Microscopic slides and coverslips for evaluation of motility
- Microscope for evaluation of concentration, motility and morphology

14.2.4 TESE Preparation

14.2.4.1 Mechanical Technique

- Balanced salt solution or a commercially available sperm preparation medium supplemented with protein (e.g. HSA), ready to use medium, pre-incubated at 37°C, without CO_2 if with HEPES; if without HEPES use 5–6% CO_2 (see Note A)
- Incubator
- Two tuberculin syringes with fine needles; alternatively, glass slides
- Sterile test tubes of 6- or 13-ml volume (Note B)
- Sterile Petri dish of 6 to 10 cm (Note B)
- Centrifuge (up to 500×g)
- Pipettes with variable volumes (2–200 μl and 100–1,000 μl) and corresponding sterile tips
- Microscopic slides and coverslips for evaluation of motility
- Microscope for evaluation of spermatozoa

14.2.4.2 Enzymatic Technique

- Collagenase type 1A from *Clostridium histolyticum* (commercially available) or ready-to-use collagenase solution
- Balanced salt solution or a commercially available sperm preparation medium supplemented with protein (e.g. HSA), ready to use medium, pre-incubated at 37°C without CO_2 if with HEPES; if without HEPES use 5%-6% CO_2 (see Note A)
- Incubator

- Sterile test tubes of 6- or 13-ml volume (Note B)
- Centrifuge (up to 500×g)
- Pipettes with variable volumes (2–200 µl and 100–1,000 µl) and corresponding sterile tips
- Microscopic slides and coverslips for evaluation of motility
- Microscope for evaluation of spermatozoa

14.3 Quality Control

The andrology laboratory should implement a quality assurance programme to prove that its results are accurate and correct. Both internal and external quality control must be implemented in the laboratory, as suggested by the WHO.[4]

Reagents should only be used until their expiry date to omit possible influences on sperm that might have an effect on ART outcome. The centrifugation step for the DG should be validated before clinical application. Time and speed of the centrifuge may have to be adjusted to local equipment and supplements.

14.4 Procedures

14.4.1 Simple Washing

1. Mix semen well (e.g. stirring with a glass rod).
2. Transfer sample to a test tube (divide into several test tubes if sample is of high volume).
3. Add an equal amount of pre-incubated medium.
4. Mix gently by tilting the closed test tube.
5. Centrifuge at 300 to 500×g for 5 to 10 minutes.
6. Gently aspirate or decant the supernatant.
7. Add 1 ml of pre-incubated equilibrated medium to pellet.
8. Gently re-suspend the pellet by flicking the tube or by gentle pipetting up and down.
9. Centrifuge again at 300 to 500×g for 3 to 5 minutes.
10. Gently aspirate or decant the resulting supernatant.
11. Re-suspend the pellet with fresh equilibrated medium to a final volume of 0.5 to 0.7ml (for IUI, the amount should not be higher than 0.5 ml; for other purposes, volume can be higher).
12. Determine sperm concentration and, if necessary, motility and morphology (according to WHO[4]).

14.4.2 Direct Swim-Up (Optional with Washing Step)

1. Mix semen well (e.g. stirring with a glass rod).
2. Transfer 1 ml of sample to a test tube (divide into several test tubes if sample is of high volume).
3. Pipette 1.0 to 1.2 ml medium onto the semen sample (overlaying is easier than underlaying).
4. Place the test tube angled at 45 degrees in the incubator (to reach a higher surface area).
5. Incubate for one hour at 37°C (depending on desired concentration, duration can be reduced: high concentration, low incubation time; low concentration, high

incubation time; try not to exceed one hour as zinc and other seminal plasma components may diffuse into the medium, which might create problems for the spermatozoa[5]).

6. After incubation, gently aspirate the top 0.5 to 0.7 ml of the medium.
7. If the sample is very high in concentration, dilute with equilibrated medium (if sample is used for IUI, better to decrease incubation time than to use additional dilution; amount of inseminated fluid placed into uterus is limited).

   a. (Optional) A variation on the procedure is to centrifuge the sample at 300 to 500×g for 5 minutes and to re-suspend the pellet in 0.5 ml medium.

8. Determine sperm concentration and, if necessary, motility and morphology (according to WHO[4]).

With washing step:

1. Mix semen well (e.g. stirring with a glass rod).
2. Transfer sample to test tube.
3. Add an equal amount of the medium:

   a. Mix gently by tilting the closed test tube.
   b. Centrifuge at 300 to 500×g for 5 to 10 minutes.
   c. Carefully aspirate or decant the supernatant.
   d. Add 1 ml of equilibrated medium to pellet.
   e. From here follow preceding steps, starting at step 4.

14.4.3 Discontinuous DG Centrifugation

1. Prepare DG layers: place 1 ml of 80% gradient medium into a test tube; then add 1 ml of 40% medium on top of first layer.
2. Mix semen well (e.g. stirring with a glass rod).
3. Transfer 1 ml of semen gently to the pre-layered gradient media (divide into several test tubes if sample is of high volume).
4. Place test tube carefully into centrifuge, and centrifuge at 300 to 400×g for 15 to 30 minutes.
5. Aspirate the supernatant, leaving the sperm pellet.
6. The sperm pellet is washed by adding 5 ml of equilibrated medium and re-suspend by gentle pipetting (Note C).
7. Centrifuge again at 200×g for 4 to 10 minutes.
8. Re-suspend the pellet in 0.5 to 0.7 ml of medium (depending on ART procedure to be performed).
9. Determine concentration and, if necessary, also motility and morphology (according to WHO[4]).

14.4.4 Epididymal Sperm from MESA

Microsurgical epididymal sperm aspiration (MESA) samples are prepared by swim-up (for technique, see Section 14.4.2) or DG (for technique, see Section 14.4.3) if sperm numbers are high. If number and motility are impaired in a MESA sample, a simple washing step (for technique, see Section 14.4.1) is to be preferred.

14.4.5 TESE

14.4.5.1 Mechanical Method

1. Incubate freshly retrieved or frozen tissue (frozen in a cryoprotective agent often containing glycerol) in equilibrated medium for up to 30 minutes to remove contaminating red blood and other cells.
2. Remove tissue from the test tube, place into a Petri dish and, if necessary, add some culture medium.
3. Macerate tissue either with fine needles or glass slides until a suspension of small pieces of tissue is reached.
4. Transfer suspension to tube, and centrifuge at between 100 and 300×g for 10 minutes.
5. Gently discard supernatant.
6. Gently re-suspend the pellet by flicking the tube or by pipetting.
7. Centrifuge again at between 100 and 300×g for 10 minutes.
8. Re-suspend the pellet either in remaining culture medium or add 0.2 to 0.5 ml of fresh medium.

14.4.5.2 Enzymatic Method

1. Incubate freshly retrieved or frozen tissue (frozen in a cryoprotective agent often containing glycerol) in equilibrated medium at 37°C for 30 minutes.
2. Prepare collagenase solution by dissolving 0.8 mg of collagenase type 1A in 1 ml of culture medium or use ready-to-use collagenase.
3. Add tissue to collagenase and incubate at 37°C for 1.5 to 2 hours, vortex every 30 minutes (some tissue might not be resolved; these are remnants of tubular structure in cases of testicular dysfunction).
4. Centrifuge at 100 to 300×g for 10 minutes.
5. Gently discard the supernatant.
   a. (Optional) 1a subsequent DG centrifugation is possible (see Section 14.4.3; however, it is only advisable if TESE sample contains high sperm numbers).
6. Wash pellet to remove any collagenase by adding 1 ml of culture medium.
7. Gently re-suspend pellet by flicking at the tube or by pipetting.
8. Centrifuge again at between 100 and 300×g for 10 minutes.
9. Re-suspend the pellet either in remaining culture medium or add 0.2 to 0.5 ml of fresh medium.

14.5 Notes

A. Several options exist for supplies and equipment. Any routine sperm preparation medium is suitable for the preparation. In the presence of HEPES or MOPS, the medium can be incubated at 37°C with a closed cap and without CO_2. If no pH-buffering substances are in the medium, incubation is done at 37°C with an open cap at a CO_2 level of 5% to 6%. It is important to pre-incubate before use to ensure an optimal pH of the medium (for medium with HEPES, one to two hours might be enough; without HEPES, a longer pre-incubation might be necessary).
B. The use of sterile test tubes and Petri dishes is inevitable to ensure best results.

C. The centrifugation step of the DG might have to be adjusted not only to the centrifugation time and speed but maybe also to the type of semen sample. It may happen that for one sample the pellet is solid and for another one the pellet might be very soft and might detach if the supernatant is discarded by just pouring it off. Here it might be helpful to use a pipette to take the supernatant off.

D. Regarding the swim-up procedure, it might be unnecessary to incubate for one hour. If, for example, a normozoospermic sample (e.g. after failed IVF) will be used for ICSI, a decrease of incubation to 5 to 30 minutes might be enough to retrieve the best motile sperm.

References

1. Björndahl, L. and Kvist, U. Sequence of ejaculation affects the spermatozoon as a carrier and its message. *Reprod Biomed Online* 2003; 7:440–8.

2. Overstreet, J. W. et al. In-vitro capacitation of human spermatozoa after passage through a column of cervical mucus. *Fertil Steril* 1980; 34:604–6.

3. Björndahl, L., Mohammadieh, M., Pourian, M., Söderlund, I. and Kvist, U. Contamination by seminal plasma factors during sperm selection. *J Androl* 2005; 26:170–3.

4. World Health Organisation (WHO). *laboratory Manual for the Examination and Processing of Human Semen* (5th edn.) (Cambridge University Press, 2010).

5. Mortimer, D. Laboratory standards in routine clinical andrology. *Reprod Med Rev* 1994; 3:97–111.

6. Mortimer, D. *Practical Laboratory Andrology* (Oxford University Press, 1994).

7. Aitken, R. J. and Clarkson, J. S. Significance of reactive oxygen species and antioxidants in defining the efficacy of sperm preparation techniques. *J Androl* 1988; 9:367–76.

8. Ramasamy, R., Yagan, N. and Schlegel, P. N. Structural and functional changes to the testis after conventional versus microdissection testicular sperm extraction. *Urology* 2005; 65:1190–4.

15

Processing Surgically Retrieved Sperm in the IVF Laboratory

Amy E. T. Sparks

Introduction

Infertility due to azoospermia may be overcome by surgically retrieving sperm from the epididymis or testicle followed by in vitro fertilization (IVF) with intracytoplasmic sperm injection (ICSI) and embryo transfer.[1–3] The nature of the azoospermia (obstructive (OA) versus non-obstructive azoospermia (NOA)), the surgical approach (percutaneous versus open) and the timing of the sperm retrieval relative to oocyte retrieval for IVF/ICSI (fresh versus frozen sperm) contribute to the success of sperm retrieval and the number of viable sperm that will be available for the IVF/ICSI procedure.[4–7] The goal of the surgical team should be to maximize the recovery of mature, viable sperm for ICSI while minimizing patient risk and cost. The laboratory processing the samples must minimize post-recovery cell damage, preserve sample sterility and strive to optimize the efficiency of the surgery when possible by cryopreserving excess sperm for future IVF/ICSI procedures. Lastly, these teams must work together to optimize the ease of surgery coordination with the IVF procedure. It has been our experience that these goals can be achieved with excellent teamwork and communication.

A number of procedures for isolating and identifying viable sperm from surgically retrieved samples have been described and reviewed by others.[8–15] Enzymatic digestion of seminiferous tubules by collagenase[11] and eradication of erythrocyte lysing buffer[12] have been reported to enhance sperm isolation, but these methods will not be addressed by this chapter as we have not found them to be necessary for the specimens retrieved by the methods described herein (Notes A and B).

15.1 Reagents, Supplies and Equipment (Note C)

15.1.1 Epididymal Aspirate

15.1.1.1 Method of Retrieval: Microsurgical Epididymal Aspiration (MESA) (Note D)

- Human tubal fluid (HTF) HEPES (mHTF) + 7.5% protein (serum substitute supplement)
- HTF + 7.5% protein
- 1-, 5- and 10-ml sterile polystyrene serological pipettes
- PureSperm 100 sterile colloidal silica suspension for a density gradient
- Polystyrene conical 15-ml centrifuge tubes (Falcon 2095)
- Polystyrene round-bottom snap-cap tube (Falcon 2054)
- Coverslips and slides

- 20- and 200-µl pipetter with sterile tips
- 1.2-ml cryovials (Nunc)
- Sterile gloves
- Compound microscope with phase contrast and 10× or 20× and 40× objectives
- Standard Count counting chamber
- Centrifuge

15.1.2 Testicular Tissue

15.1.2.1 Method of Retrieval: Testicular Sperm Extraction (TESE) or Testicular Sperm Aspiration (TESA)

- HTF HEPES (mHTF) + 7.5% protein
- Polystyrene round-bottom snap-cap tube (Falcon 2054)
- 35-mm sterile Petri dishes approved for human embryo culture
- 60-mm sterile Petri dish approved for human embryo culture
- Two No. 5 sterile jeweler's-style forceps
- Coverslips and slides
- 20- and 200-µl pipetter with sterile tips
- 1.2-ml cryovials (Nunc)
- Sterile gloves
- Compound microscope with phase contrast and 10× or 20× and 40× objectives
- Standard Count counting chamber
- Eosin Y stain (Sigma E4382), 5 g/litre in 9 g/litre saline (NaCl) (Note E)
- 3 mM pentoxifylline (Sigma P-1784) in HTF HEPES + protein

15.2 Quality Control

1. Specimens retained for processing will be transferred to pre-labelled Nunc vials that have been filled with 0.5 ml HTF HEPES + 7.5% protein and warmed to 37°C (+1°C) in a small Dri-Bath. The temperature is monitored by a calibrated digital thermometer with an audible alarm that is set to the range of 36°C (low alarm) to 38°C (high alarm).

2. An andrology technologist will report to the operating room with the sperm retrieval cart for all epididymal sperm retrievals and testicular biopsies for men diagnosed with non-obstructive azoospermia (NOA).

   a. Epididymal aspirates will be examined for the presence of motile sperm. Patients with OA undergoing MESA are expected to have sperm in the aspirate. The percentage of sperm exhibiting motility will depend on the nature of the obstruction and the patient's health.

   b. Testicular biopsies will be examined for the presence of mature sperm. If tail movement is not observed, seminiferous tubule contents will be overlaid with an equal volume of eosin stain and examined with 40× phase contrast to assess sperm viability. Testicular sperm viability as determined by eosin stain exclusion should exceed 70% for patients with OA.

3. The presence of an andrology technologist is not required for OA TESE or TESA cases. If an andrology technologist was not present for the case, a total of five biopsies will be

sent to the laboratory – three for three IVF procedures, one for pre-cryopreservation and 1 for post-thaw viability assessment. The surgeon must be alerted immediately if no viable sperm are found in the pre-cryopreservation biopsy.

15.3 Procedure

15.3.1 Epididymal Aspirate

1. The day before aspirate preparation for IVF/ICSI, prepare 5 ml of HTF + 7.5% protein and pre-equilibrate in 5% to 6% CO_2 overnight.
2. Measure the volume of the sample with a 1-ml sterile serological pipette.
3. Determine the motile and total sperm concentration per standard semen analysis protocol.
4. Label all tubes used for the procedure with the patient's name and IVF case number.
5. Prepare the 90% density solution (2.3 ml PureSperm + 0.3 ml HTF HEPES) and 45% density solution (0.9 ml 90% density solution + 0.9 ml HTF HEPES). Create a two-layer gradient by carefully pipetting 90% density solution and then 45% density solution into a Falcon 2095 tube. The volume of each layer may be adjusted based on the total motile sperm and quality of the aspirate.

   a. >500,000 motile sperm, use 1.5-ml layers.
   b. 100,000–500,000 motile sperm, use 1.0-ml layers.
   c. <100,000 motile sperm, use 0.5- to 0.8-ml layers.

6. Layer the aspirate on the gradient. Centrifuge at 300×g (1,225 rpm) for 20 minutes.
7. Carefully remove and discard the aspirate, 45% fraction and 45% to 90% interface. Discard pipette after these layers have been aspirated from all tubes.
8. Wash the pellet by mixing it with 2 ml of pre-equilibrated HTF + 7.5% protein, and centrifuge the suspension at 300×g (1,225 rpm) for 10 minutes.
9. Remove and discard all but sperm pellet. It is important to remove the supernatant down to pellet to eliminate silica particles from the final sperm preparation.
10. Using a 200-μl pipetter with a sterile pipette tip, pre-load the pipette tip with 20 to 30 μl of HTF + 7.5% protein, and mix the culture medium with the final sperm pellet.
11. Transfer the suspension to a clean Falcon 2095 tube, and determine the motile sperm concentration in the inseminant.
12. Place the inseminant tube loosely capped in a 37°C 5% to 6% CO_2 incubator until ICSI.

15.3.2 Testicular Biopsies (Note F)

1. Warm 15 ml of HTF HEPES + 7.5% protein to 37°C.
2. Estimate the amount of time you will need to search for sperm for ICSI. If viable sperm were readily identified by the andrology technologist, start processing the biopsy 20 to 30 minutes before you wish to perform ICSI. If rare sperm were observed, two embryologists should begin searching for sperm 60 minutes before ICSI.
3. Use the lid of the 60-mm Petri dish for your ICSI dish. Label the bottom of the ICSI dish with the patient's last name and IVF procedure number. Prepare the ICSI dish (Figure 15.1), and cover the drops with culture oil.

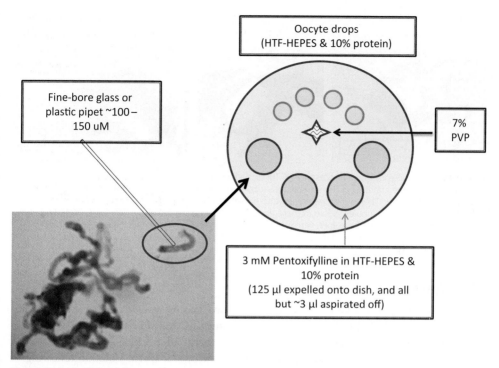

Oocyte drops
(HTF-HEPES & 10% protein)

Fine-bore glass or
plastic pipet ~100–
150 uM

7%
PVP

3 mM Pentoxifylline in HTF-HEPES &
10% protein
(125 µl expelled onto dish, and all
but ~3 µl aspirated off)

Figure 15.1 The ICSI dish for testicular sperm procedures. Seminiferous tubule contents are expelled into the large, flat drops of 3 mM pentoxifylline. The ICSI pipette is primed with 7% PVP before viable sperm are picked up and transferred to a peninsula of the PVP drop. (Method adapted from Craft and Tsirigotis.[10]) (A black and white version of this figure will appear in some formats. For the color version, please refer to the plate section.)

4. Aliquot 3 ml of HTF + 7.5% protein to each three 35-mm Petri dishes.

5. Rinse the testicular biopsy through all three dishes, moving the tissue with the jeweler's forceps.

6. Holding the tissue in the third dish, release the cells from within the seminiferous tubules by gently squeezing the cells out with the forceps (Figure 15.2). Grasping the tissue with too much pressure will cause the tubule to break. If you are working with a biopsy from a NOA patient, focus on the areas of the tubules that are the most dilated and appear to have the most cells.

7. Once the cells are released from tubules, you will want to transfer the cells to one of the 3 mM pentoxifylline drops in the ICSI dish. Gently disrupt the cell mass by pipetting. Remove any cell masses that float to the top of the drop. Limit the amount of search time for each drop to 30 minutes.

8. Transfer mature, motile sperm to a designated peninsula of the PVP drop. You may either strike the tail immediately or wait until you are ready to perform ICSI.

9. If no motile sperm are observed, but viability was confirmed by eosin dye exclusion, select sperm that have pliable tails, and transfer them to the PVP drop. Place the sperm near the edge of the drop. Touch the sperm tail with the tip of the ICSI pipette and force the tail to move. Sperm with tails that demonstrate flexibility are considered viable and suitable for ICSI in the absence of motile sperm. Sperm with rigid tails may not be used for ICSI.

10. Repeat steps 6 to 9 as needed.

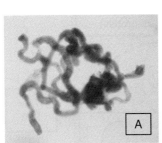
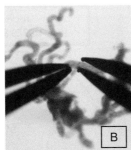
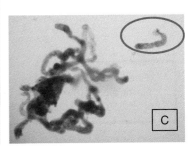

Figure 15.2 Seminiferous tubule processing. (A) Tubules are gently teased apart. (B) Two pairs of jeweler's forceps are used to release the contents of the seminiferous tubules by gentle squeezing. (C) The seminiferous tubule contents are in the circle. They will be transferred and dispersed into a drop of 3 mM pentoxifylline in the ICSI dish. (Please note that the tubules shown in these photographs are not typical of the very large, dilated tubules observed in testicular biopsies from men with OA. This specimen was selected because the narrow tubules allowed clearer images of the procedure. (A black and white version of this figure will appear in some formats. For the color version, please refer to the plate section.)

15.4 Notes

A. Laboratories that receive PESA samples may have specimens with high concentrations of red blood cells (RBCs) and therefore may find RBC lysis to be necessary.

B. Laboratories that are unable to identify mature sperm after releasing cells from seminiferous tubules by mincing have reported successful sperm isolation following enzymatic digestion with collagenase type IV (1,000 IU/ml) and 25 µg/ml DNase I.[11] It has been my experience that rare sperm may be recovered without enzymatic digestion. Using the testicular tissue-processing approach described in this chapter allows the andrology technologist or embryologist to methodically dissect the seminiferous tubule. Transferring the tubule contents directly to the ICSI dish avoids the cell loss that may occur if the cells are subjected to further processing.

C. The supplies and equipment listed are examples. Any culture medium containing a zwitterion that will maintain the aspirate or biopsy at a slightly alkaline pH may be substituted. Similarly, alternative protein sources and solutions used for the density gradient should produce similar results.

D. TESE, TESA and micro-TESE are preferred by our programme over MESA as sperm viability in the testis is superior to that of the sperm in the epididymis of an OA patient.

E. The simple and rapid viability testing by eosin alone is preferred for viability assessment in the operating room as it may be performed on a wet preparation as opposed to the eosin-nigrosin method, which requires the specimen to be dry before examination.

F. Testicular biopsies from NOA patients should be retrieved with the aid of an operating microscope, which allows the surgeon to selectively remove small biopsies with the most dilated tubules. Biopsies received by my laboratory range from 5 to 10 mg. I refer laboratories that are burdened with searching large biopsies to a quote from Esteves and Verza: 'It is far less technically demanding and labor intensive to extract spermatozoa from small volume specimens than large pieces of testicular tissue that must be dissected, red blood cells lysed and the rare spermatozoa searched for in a tedious fashion under an inverted microscope. TESE sperm processing may be incredibly labor intensive, and the search process may miss rare spermatozoa within a sea of seminiferous tubules and other cells.'[13]

References

1. Palermo, G., Joris, H., Devroey, P. and van Steirteghem, A. C. Pregnancies after intracytoplasmic sperm injection of single spermatozoan into an oocyte. *Lancet* 1992; 340:17–8.

2. Craft, I., Twirigotis, M., Bennett, V., Taranissi, M., Khalifa, Y. et al. Percutaneous epididymal sperm aspiration and intracytoplasmic sperm injection in the management of infertility due to obstructive azoospermia. *Fertil Steril* 1995; 63:1038–42.

3. Devroey, P., Liu, J., Nagy, Z. P., Goossens, A., Tournaye, H. et al. Pregnancies after testicular extraction (TESE) and intracytoplasmic sperm injection (ICSI) in non-obstructive azoospermia. *Hum Reprod* 1995; 10:1457–60.

4. Bachtell, N. E., Conaghan, J. and Turek, P. J. The relative viability of human spermatozoa from the vas deferens, epidydmis and testis before and after cryopreservation. *Hum Reprod* 1999; 14(12):3048–51.

5. Nagy, Z. P., Joris, H., Verheyen, G., Devroey, P. and Van Steirteghem. A. C. Correlation between motility of testicular spermatozoa, testicular histology and the outcomes of intracytoplasmic sperm injection. *Hum Reprod* 1998; 13:890–5.

6. Park, Y.-S., Lee, S.-H., Sang, J. S., Jun, J. H., Koong, M. K. et al. Influence of motility on the outcome of in vitro fertilization/intracytoplasmic sperm injection with fresh vs. frozen testicular sperm from men with obstructive azoospermia. *Fertil Steril* 2003; 80:526–30.

7. Ohlander, S., Hotaling, J., Kirshenbaum, E., Niederberger, C. and Eisenberg, M. L. Impact of fresh versus cryopreserved testicular sperm upon intracytoplasmic sperm injection pregnancy outcomes in men with azoospermia due to spermatogenic dysfunction: a meta-analysis. *Fertil Steril* 2014; 101:344–9.

8. Karacan, M., Alwaeely, F., Erkan, S., Cebi. Z., Berberoglugi, M. et al. Outcome of intracytoplasmic sperm injection cycles with fresh testicular spermatozoa obtained on the day of or the day before oocyte collection and with cryopreserved testicular sperm in patients with azoospermia. *Fertil Steril* 2013; 100:975–80.

9. Ord, T., Marello, E., Patrizio, P., Balmaceda, J. P., Silber, S. J. et al. The role of the laboratory in the handling of epididymal sperm for assisted reproductive technologies. *Fertil Steril* 1992; 57:1103–6.

10. Craft, I. and Tsirigotis, M. Simplified recovery, preparation and cryopreservation of testicular spermatozoa. *Hum Reprod* 1995; 10:1923–7.

11. Ramasamy, R., Reifsnyder, J. E., Bryson, C., Zaninovic. N., Liotta, D. et al. Role of tissue digestion and extensive sperm search after microdissection testicular sperm extraction. *Fertil Steril* 2011; 96(2):299–302.

12. Nagy, Z. P., Verheyen, G., Tournaye, H., Devroey, P. and Van Steirteghem, A. C. An improved treatment procedure for testicular biopsy specimens offers more efficient sperm recovery: case series. *Fertil Steril* 1997; 376–9.

13. Esteves, S. C. and Verza, S., Jr. PESA/TESA/TESE sperm processing. In *Practical Manual of In Vitro Fertilization: Advanced Methods and Novel Devices*, ed. Z. P. Nagy, Varghese and A. Agarwal (pp. 207–20) (Berlin: Springer Science + Business Media, 2012).

14. Popal, W. and Nagy, Z. P. Laboratory processing and intracytoplasmic sperm injection using epididymal and testicular spermatozoa: what can be done to improve outcomes? *Clinics* 2013; 68(S1):125–30.

15. Muller, C. H. and Pagel, E. R. Recovery, isolation, identification, and preparation of spermatozoa from human testis. In *Spermatogenesis: Methods and Protocols* (Methods in Molecular Biology 927), ed. D. T. Carrell and K. I. Ashton (pp. 227–40) (Berlin: Springer Science + Business Media, 2013).

Chapter

16

Cryopreservation of Sperm for IVF
Semen Samples and Individual Sperm

Nina Desai and Pooja Rambhia

Introduction

Cryopreservation of human spermatozoa offers male patients the option to preserve fertility prior to initiating cancer therapy, vasectomy or assisted reproductive technology (ART) treatment. Human sperm can be easily cryopreserved in liquid nitrogen and stored for years. A number of cryopreservation techniques and cryoprotectants have been investigated. To date, however, vapour-phase or programmed slow cooling using a glycerol/egg yolk buffer cryoprotectant has been the most widely applied sperm cryopreservation protocol. Sperm cryosurvival rates of 40% to 60% are generally achievable. However, in patients having low motility or low sperm number at the outset, cryopreservation and recovery of viable sperm can be more challenging. In such cases, freezing of single sperm or small numbers of sperm is emerging as a valuable tool. With this technique, intracytoplasmic sperm injection (ICSI) can be performed even in cases with only a few frozen spermatozoa.

16.1 Background

Human spermatozoa were one of the first reproductive cells to be successfully cryopreserved. In 1949, Polge et al.[1] first reported on glycerol's unique ability to protect sperm cells being cryopreserved on dry ice, heralding the beginning of a new era in reproductive medicine. In 1953, the first human births from artificial insemination with cryopreserved semen were reported.[2] Cryostorage of human spermatozoa is now an integral component in the preservation of fertility for cancer patients prior to chemotherapy or radiation therapy, elective vasectomy patients, for ART procedures and in cases of azoospermia and severe oligozoospermia.

The field of sperm cryobiology has rapidly evolved with better understanding of sperm and their interactions with different types of cryoprotectants as well as tools for measuring post-thaw sperm parameters. The methodology for freezing needs to maximize post-thaw survival and sperm DNA integrity as well as the potential to create a viable embryo after in vitro fertilization (IVF)/ICSI. Lastly, the type of storage vessel also needs consideration and perhaps optimization for the number of sperm available.

Over the years, a multitude of cryopreservation methods and cryoprotective agents have been used. Sperm cryopreservation protocols can be divided in to three general types.[3] The most common freezing techniques are (1) slow programmed freezing, where temperature is slowly decreased in a step-wise manner either manually or using a programmable cell freezer and (2) vapour freezing, where the sperm are exposed to liquid nitrogen vapour for one to two hours, followed by immersion into liquid nitrogen. The third method is vitrification, where the sperm specimen is quickly plunged into liquid nitrogen. Both the slow freeze and vapour freeze techniques yield a cryosurvival rate of around 40% to 60%, with higher cryosurvival seen in normospermic samples as opposed to compromised samples from infertile men. It is not clear whether any one method is superior. With the vapour freeze technique, the temperature drop cannot be as precisely controlled, leading to variation in cooling temperatures and reproducibility from sample to sample. However, in contrast to the slow programmed method, during vapour freezing, sperm are cooled at a faster rate with shorter duration of exposure to cryoprotective agents, which can reduce sperm damage. Vitrification for sperm cryopreservation has not been as widely applied. With this technique, cells are cryopreserved at ultra-rapid cooling rates of over 1,000°C per minute. The idea is to avoid a phase change and thus the potential for damage by ice crystal formation. Recent data suggest that vitrification results in low overall DNA damage whilst maintaining sperm membrane integrity, mitochondrial activity and post-thaw survival rates.[4-6] Nevertheless, the debate as to whether vitrification is preferable to the traditional slow freeze and vapour freeze techniques is still on-going, and pregnancy outcome data are needed to further validate this technique.

An important aspect of the cryopreservation process is the selection of appropriate cryoprotectants. During the freeze-thaw process, sperm are exposed to a number of non-physiologic environments and subjected to both osmotic and oxidative stress. This may negatively affect sperm function, ultimately impairing the sperm's fertilizing capacity and ability to generate a viable embryo. To prevent intra/extracellular ice crystal formation, cryoprotective agents are mixed in with the sperm specimen prior to freezing. To date, glycerol is one of the most successfully used permeable cryoprotectants. Glycerol easily traverses the plasma membrane and can slowly equilibrate within sperm cells to reduce intracellular fluid volume and also provide an osmotic buffer for intracellular solutes. Freeze medium containing glycerol along with egg yolk and two zwitterionic buffers TES and Tris to maintain sperm pH is one of the most widely used cryoprotectant solutions (known as TEST yolk buffer-glycerol). Egg yolk buffer included in cryoprotectant solutions protects sperm plasma membrane fluidity during exposure to extreme cold temperatures as well as acrosome integrity. Other permeating cryoprotectants commonly used include DMSO, ethylene glycol and 1,2-propanediol.

Use of permeable cryoprotectants, however, has also been associated with damage to sperm acrosomal membrane and nuclear integrity. Investigators have proposed that the high concentration of proteins/sugars and minimal fluid volume within sperm create a natural viscous intracellular matrix, eliminating the need for chemical cryoprotectants. Very promising results have been achieved with cryoprotectant-free sperm vitrification using only non-permeating sugars such as sucrose along with human serum albumin (HSA).[4-6]

16.2 Semen Cryopreservation

The first step in semen cryopreservation is assessment of sperm count, motility and morphology. Whole semen cryopreservation involves combining the semen specimen with a cryoprotectant solution before freezing.[7] However, in patients with low-quality sperm, washing the sample prior to mixing with cryoprotectant can be advantageous. Sperm washing separates out cellular debris, seminal plasma and dead sperm from viable sperm and thus improves post-thaw sperm quality parameters. The washed sperm sample is then mixed with an equal volume of cryoprotectant and then frozen. A post-thaw assessment should be performed on cryopreserved specimens to assess percent sperm recovery, survival and motility. To facilitate this evaluation, at each freezing episode, a tiny 'Test' aliquot of the initial sperm specimen should be frozen and used for the post-thaw assessment.

Popular freezing vessels for sperm cryopreservation include cryovials and insemination straws. Post-thaw sperm parameters can be influenced by volume of sperm sample loaded into the selected cryovessel. Cryovials allow aseptic filling and can accommodate larger sample volumes, but uneven heat exchange and leakage of liquid nitrogen into the specimen-containing vials can be problematic. In contrast, straws can be heat sealed, but aseptic filling requires more care so as to avoid getting sperm specimen on the outer surface of the straw.

16.3 Single-Sperm Cryopreservation

Intracytoplasmic sperm injection has radically altered the severity of male factor infertility that can be treated. Techniques such as epididymal sperm aspiration and testicular biopsies have allowed sperm recovery from azoospermic patients. In patients with severe non-obstructive azoospermia, decline in function of testicular tissue may be so extreme that it significantly limits the number of viable sperm that can be harvested. Conventional freezing methods/vessels are less than optimal as the rare sperm in the surgical specimen can often be lost during sperm processing for freeze-thaw through adherence to the cryovessel. Single-sperm cryopreservation offers the possibility of identifying and freezing individually selected sperm or even just small aliquots containing 20 to 50 sperm. Efficient cryopreservation of small numbers of sperm allows for multiple ICSI treatments to be performed from a single testicular or epididymal sperm extraction procedure, thus avoiding risks associated with repeated surgical interventions.

Numerous methodologies have been described for freezing individually selected sperm as well as small aliquots containing 10 to 100 sperm.[8,9] These techniques are collectively referred to as 'single-sperm freezing'. The first attempts used 'empty' zonae from evacuated animal or human oocytes to sequester individual sperm.[10] The method was surprisingly successful with live births, but ultimately, use of this type of biological carrier, especially if of animal origin, had its limitations. Many of the alternate techniques attempted, such as sperm storage in microdrops on a culture dish or in ICSI pipettes, were either not practical or not robust enough to allow for safe long-term storage. A novel method for cryopreservation of as few as 2 to 10 individually selected sperm in fluid suspended on a cryoloop has also been reported.[4,11] The major limitation with all these techniques is that they allow direct contact between the sperm sample and liquid nitrogen, introducing the possibility of cross-contamination and pathogen transmission. Lack of a suitable sealed vessel that allows for easy loading, long-term storage and eventual recovery of small numbers of sperm has been a major impediment in advancing single-sperm freezing methodology.

Our own laboratory has explored use of the closed High-Security Vitrification (HSV) straw, as a vessel for the aseptic storage of small numbers of sperm.[12] Sperm vitrification in 50-μl capillary tubes as well as a new type of cryovial known as the Cell Sleeper (Nipro, Japan) represent other avenues being tested for single-sperm freezing in a sealed vessel.[5,13] Freezing of single sperm or small numbers of sperm still remains a challenge, and insufficient clinical outcome data are available on any of these published methods.

16.4 Semen Cryopreservation Protocol

16.4.1 Reagents, Supplies and Equipment

- Eppendorf pipette
- Sterile serologic pipettes (1.0, 2.0 and 5 ml)
- Sterile specimen container
- TEST yolk buffer-glycerol (TYB-Gly) cryoprotectant
- Cryovials (2 ml) (Nunc)
- Aluminium cane and plastic sleeves for storage of cryovials
- Metal tabs for labelling canes
- Liquid nitrogen storage tank or chest freezer
- Warmer or incubator
- Laboratory safety goggles
- Conical 15-ml centrifuge tubes
- Eppendorf centrifuge tubes (1.5 ml)
- Density gradient, 50% and 90%
- Human serum albumin
- Human tubal fluid (HTF) supplemented with 10 mg/ml HSA (IVF medium)
- Centrifuge

16.4.2 Cryopreservation Procedure

1. Semen samples should be handled wearing gloves, using sterile technique and following universal precautions guidelines set forth for handling any bodily fluids.
2. Place the semen sample in the warm air oven for 10 to 20 minutes to liquefy. Samples collected off-site may be processed immediately. Verify that all paperwork and consent forms are completed.
3. Pre-label cryovial(s) with patient's first and last names, a unique patient identifier such as medical record number, date of collection and vial ID. Vials are labelled consecutively A, B, C, etc. Also prepare an extra vial, and designate it as 'Test'.
4. Assess sperm cell count, percent motility and type of progression before freezing. Record information on the cryolog form.
5. Slowly dilute the semen sample 1:1 with TYB-Gly cryoprotectant, mix thoroughly and allow to equilibrate at room temperature for 10 to 15 minutes. *Note:* Washed semen, epididymal aspirates and testicular biopsy homogenates are also prepared for cryopreservation in this same manner.
6. Pipette a small aliquot of the cryoprotectant-sperm mixture into the 'Test' vial (generally 25–100 µl depending on total sample volume). Distribute the remaining sample in aliquots of 0.2 to 1.0 ml amongst the other pre-labeled vials. Ideally, each vial should contain sufficient sperm for a single cycle of IVF/ICSI.
7. Load vials to be frozen onto an aluminium cane. Slide a plastic sheath over the cane to prevent vials from being inadvertently dislodged. Prepare a metal tab with the patient's name, ID number and freeze date, and affix it to the cane.
8. Hold cane in the vapour phase of a liquid nitrogen tank or liquid nitrogen chest freezer for one hour, and then plunge the cane with the samples into liquid nitrogen.

9. Record each vial frozen and its location individually on the cryolog form.
10. Thaw the 'Test' vial as described next in steps 1 to 4. This should be done well before the patient returns for a procedure.

16.4.3 Thawing Procedure

1. Locate the sample to be thawed. With the help of a second laboratory worker, verify the patient's name, unique patient identifier, vial ID and date frozen.
2. Wearing protective eye goggles, remove the sample from the storage unit. Hold the sample at room temperature for two to three minutes, loosening the cap as soon as possible to release any gas pressure from trapped liquid nitrogen.
3. Place the sample in a warmer at 37°C for 20 to 30 minutes until it is completely thawed.
4. Determine cell count, percent motility and progression in the thawed specimen.
5. Pipette 0.5 to 1.0 ml of a density gradient column such ISolate (a colloidal suspension of silica particles) into a 15-ml conical centrifuge tube. The 90% density gradient is used for sperm samples with high counts. For lower sperm counts ranging from 2 to 10 million per millilitre, the 50% density gradient is preferable, allowing for the greatest sperm recovery. The volume of density gradient used should be reduced with smaller specimen samples.
6. Carefully pipette the sperm sample over the appropriate density gradient column and spin at $250{\times}g$ (1,100–1,200 rpm) for 10 to 20 minutes to pellet sperm.
7. Remove the supernatant to just above the sperm pellet. Add 0.5 to 1.0 ml of IVF medium, and re-suspend the sperm. Wash by centrifugation for 5 minutes, and re-suspend the sperm pellet in fresh medium.
8. Perform a final assessment of sperm count, motility and progression. Record in the laboratory log. IVF sperm samples should be loosely capped and allowed to equilibrate at 37° C in the incubator with 6% CO_2.

16.4.4 Notes

- The 'Test' thaw is particularly valuable with compromised samples. It gives information on the post-thaw quality of the frozen specimen that can be helpful in case management decisions.
- With severely compromised sperm specimens, a gradient column should not be used. The specimen should instead be centrifuged to remove cryoprotectant and re-suspended in 100 to 200 μl of medium. Our laboratory uses Eppendorf tubes (1.5 ml) for preparing and washing such samples as the sperm pellets are quite small.

16.5 Cryopreservation of Single Sperm and Small Numbers of Sperm

16.5.1 Reagents, Supplies and Equipment

- Inverted microscope fitted with micro-manipulation station
- TEST yolk buffer-glycerol cryoprotectant
- Human serum albumin
- Modified HTF HEPES medium
- High Security Vitrification Straw (HSV Straw, Irvine Scientific, Irvine, CA)

- Mineral oil
- ICSI needle
- ICSI dish (Falcon 1006)
- Aluminium canes and plastic cryosleeves

16.5.2 Cryopreservation Single or Small Quantities of Sperm

1. Prepare a 50:50 cryoprotectant solution (CPA) by mixing equal volumes of TYB-Gly and mHTF with 10 mg/ml HSA.
2. Prepare ICSI dish with a 5-μl drop of mHTF/10 mg/ml HSA, a second 1-μl drop to hold isolated sperm and a 1-μl drop of the cryoprotectant solution. Overlay with oil.
3. Add a dilute aliquot of the sperm specimen to the 5-μL mHTF/HSA drop.
4. Identify motile or twitching sperm at 400× magnification using an inverted microscope and an ICSI needle move to the 1-μl medium drop.
5. After sperm isolation is completed, transfer selected sperm to the CPA drop, and equilibrate for at least 15 minutes.
6. The HSV Straw has two components – an outer straw and a thin capillary tube that contains a pre-formed gutter on the end. Place the HSV Straw on the lid of a Falcon 1006 dish so that the end is lying flat on the dish. Lightly affix in place with tape.
7. Move the dish with sperm to a dissecting scope, and observe under dark field, with the light set at maximum illumination. Sperm are easily visualized under the dissecting scope, and highly motile sperm tend to localize at the periphery of the drop.
8. Using a very finely drawn glass micropipette, draw CPA and then sperm into the tip. Deposit in the gutter closest to the open end of the capillary tube. Be careful not to blow bubbles. A nice mounded microdrop drop of cryoprotectant with sperm should be visible by eye. Be careful not to overload or else the drop will flatten.
9. Keeping the capillary tube horizontal, carefully insert it into the HSV outer straw. Close off the flared end with a heat sealer.
10. Keeping the straw containing the capillary tube horizontal, slow cool by holding it 2 to 3 inches above the vapour phase of liquid nitrogen. After three minutes, plunge it into liquid nitrogen.
11. Store HSV Straws in a goblet fitted on to an aluminium cane.

16.5.3 Thaw Procedure

1. Place a 5-μl drop of modified HTF HEPES/HSA medium into an ICSI dish.
2. Cut the HSV Straw, and bring the inner capillary tube with sperm quickly into focus under the dissecting scope.
3. Before the drop thaws, use a micropipette to push the frozen drop onto the surface of the ICSI dish (near the 5-μl drop). Aspirate any remaining fluid in the channel of the capillary rod, and add it to the sample on the ICSI dish without introducing bubbles.
4. Immediately overlay with oil, and allow the sperm 10 minutes to settle. Visualize sperm at 400× magnification. Move individual sperm from the thawed sample to the media drop using an ICSI needle.
5. Assess recovery rate and viability based on exhibition of some degree of motility or else twitching in place.

16.5.4 Note

- In cases where at least 20 sperm are observed per microlitre of specimen, it is also possible to freeze small numbers of sperm by simply mixing with equal volume of cryoprotectant and pipetting the specimen directly onto the carrier device.

References

1. Polge, C., Smith, A. U. and Parkes, A. S. Revival of spermatazoa after vitrification and dehydation at low temperatures. *Nature* 1949; 164:666.

2. Bunge, R. G. and Sherman, J. K. Fertilizing capacity of frozen human spermatozoa. *Nature* 1953; 172:767–8.

3. Di Santo, M., Tarozzi, N., Nadalini, M. and Borini, A. Human sperm cryopreservation: update on techniques, effect on DNA integrity, and implications for ART. *Adv Urol* 2012; 2012:854837.

4. Isachenko, V., Isachenko, E., Katkov, I. I., Montag, M., Dessole, S. et al. Cryoprotectant-free cryopreservation of human spermatozoa by vitrification and freezing in vapor: effect on motility, DNA integrity, and fertilization ability. *Biol Reprod* 2004; 71:1167–73.

5. Isachenko, V., Maettner, R., Petrunkina, A. M., Sterzik, K., Mallmann, P. et al. Vitrification of human ICSI/IVF spermatozoa without cryoprotectants: new capillary technology. *J Androl* 2012; 33:462–8.

6. Slabbert, M., du Plessis, S. S. and Huyser, C. Large volume cryoprotectant-free vitrification: an alternative to conventional cryopreservation for human spermatozoa. *Andrologia* 2015; 47:594–9.

7. World Health Organization (WHO). *laboratory Manual for the Examination and Processing of Human Semen* (5th edn.) Geneva: World Health Organization, 2010.

8. AbdelHafez, F., Bedaiwy, M., El-Nashar, S. A., Sabanegh, E. and Desai, N. Techniques for cryopreservation of individual or small numbers of human spermatozoa: a systematic review. *Hum Reprod Update* 2009; 15:153–64.

9. Gangrade, B. K. Cryopreservation of testicular and epididymal sperm: techniques and clinical outcomes of assisted conception. *Clinics* 2013; 68 (Suppl 1):131–40.

10. Cohen, J., Garrisi, G. J., Congedo-Ferrara, T. A., Kieck, K. A., Schimmel, T. W. et al. Cryopreservation of single human spermatozoa. *Hum Reprod* 1997; 12:994–1001.

11. Desai. N. N., Blackmon , H. and Goldfarb, J. Single sperm cryopreservation on cryoloops: an alternative to hamster zona for freezing individual spermatozoa. *Reprod Biomed Online* 2004; 9:47–53.

12. Desai, N., Goldberg, J., Austin, C., Sabanegh, E. and Falcone, T. Cryopreservation of individually selected sperm: methodology and case report of a clinical pregnancy. *J Assist Reprod & Genetics* 2012; 29:375–9.

13. Coetzee, K., Ozgur, K., Berkkanoglu, M., Bulut, H. and Isikli A. Reliable single sperm cryopreservation in Cell Sleepers for azoospermia management. *Andrologia* 2015.

Chapter

17

Oocyte Collection for IVF

Marcela Calonge

Introduction

Oocyte retrieval is the starting point of a complex laboratory process with the final objective of delivering a healthy baby at home. Meticulous attention to detail at every step of the treatment is essential for optimizing the patient´s chance of delivering a healthy baby. It is the in vitro fertilization (IVF) laboratory's responsibility to provide a stable and optimal environment for oocyte fertilization and embryo development.

Exposure of oocytes to inappropriate conditions could potentially disrupt fertilization and early development. It is well accepted that minimizing stress imposed upon gametes and embryos during their manipulation within the IVF laboratory is critical for optimizing outcomes. These potential stressors include various environmental parameters controlled within the laboratory, including pH of the culture medium[2] and temperature. Therefore, precautions must be taken to maintain adequate conditions of pH and temperature to protect zygote and embryo homeostasis.[3]

HEPES buffer medium is used for oocyte retrieval because it provides pH stability through buffering action. The recovery and processing of oocytes should be done quickly for workflow but, more importantly, to maintain optimal oocyte temperature. It is known that the meiotic spindle starts to de-polymerize at around 35°C; thus the oocytes need to be kept at body temperature (close to 37°C) as much as possible. Following temperature-induced de-polymerization, the spindle reassembles spontaneously once the temperature rises again, but errors during this process may cause aneuploidy.[1]

This chapter describes a simple and reproducible procedure for oocyte retrieval revealing the method to employ and important points to keep in mind to provide optimal conditions in oocytes care.

17.1 Equipment, Utensils and Reagents Required for Oocyte Retrieval

- Laminar flow hood with heated surface, stereo microscope, heating block for test tubes, warming oven and culture incubator
- Follicular flushing medium to be placed in the operation room, washing buffer medium, oocyte culture medium and mineral oil
- 14-ml plastic tubes, 100-mm Petri dishes, 60-mm Petri dishes, 35-mm Petri dishes, sterile Pasteur pipettes, 16G needles, 1-ml syringes (without needle), plastic bulbs, gloves and masks

17.2 Material Preparation for Oocyte Retrieval

One day before follicular aspiration, the embryologist should examine the patient's case notes and prepare the laboratory materials for the following day' oocyte retrievals. Check the patient's previous history, and study all details of any previous assisted conception treatment, including response to stimulation, number of oocytes, type of treatment, embryo quality, transfer day and any detail that may be important for the present cycle. Be attentive to laboratory procedures in the current cycle, and prepare the following laboratory materials:

Pickup and cleaning dishes/ HEPES media. Prepare 60-mm dishes containing 6 to 7 ml of HEPES medium and 6 to 8 ml of mineral oil to be used for pickup and cleaning of oocytes. These dishes must be placed inside the warming oven at 37°C the day before to oocyte retrieval. It is recommended to make between two and four dishes based on the expected number of oocytes.

Washing dishes/culture medium. Prepare 35-mm dishes containing 2 ml of culture medium and 2 ml of mineral oil to be used for washing HEPES from the oocytes. These dishes must be placed inside the incubator at 37°C and 6% CO_2 the day before oocyte retrieval.

Culture dishes/culture medium. Prepare 60-mm dishes containing three 100-µL microdrops on the top and six 50-µL microdrops in the center of the culture medium dish and 10 to 12 ml of mineral oil for incubating oocytes before to denudation or insemination time. Each 50-µl microdrop is used to incubate two oocytes. These dishes must be placed inside the incubator at 37°C and 6% CO_2 the day before to oocyte retrieval. It is recommended to make between one and five dishes based on the expected number of oocytes.

Culture tubes/follicular flushing medium. Prepare 10 ml of follicular flushing medium in a 14-ml Falcon tube to be used for the follicular aspiration in the operation room (OR). This tube must be placed inside the warming oven at 37°C the day before to oocyte retrieval.

17.3 Oocyte Retrieval Procedure

17.3.1 Prior to Oocyte Pickup

Deliver the tube with follicular flushing medium to the OR nurse. Petri dishes for scanning oocytes, collection tubes and heating blocks should be pre-warmed at 37°C.[3] Before each oocyte retrieval begins, the embryologist sets 100-mm Petri dishes over the heated surface of the laminar flow hood. Subsequently the nurse places the collection tubes in the heating block which is over the hood.

Oocyte recovery is performed with gloves and masks. The purpose of this protective measure is both to protect the laboratory staff and to ensure aseptic conditions for gametes. All body fluids should be treated as potentially contaminated.[3]

Prior to the start of the retrieval, the patient is identified in the OR by the embryologist and the doctor. All laboratory procedures must include provision for unique patient identification as well as identification of the corresponding gametes, zygotes and embryos while retaining patient confidentiality.[3] After verifying the patient's data, place the patient's dishes in the working incubator.

17.3.2 Oocyte Recovery

Oocyte retrieval is performed in the OR under intravenous sedation. Ovarian follicles are aspirated using a needle guided by trans-vaginal ultrasonography. Follicular fluids are scanned by the embryologist with a stereo microscope to locate all available oocyte-corona-cumulus complexes (OCCCs). Once the OCCCs are found, washed and placed in a special medium, they are evaluated to estimate the oocyte's maturation and quality (see Figure 17.1).

The OR must be near to the IVF laboratory, preferably adjacent with a door or pass-through window. If is not in proximity to each other, then the laboratory must ensure that the necessary conditions for embryo viability are not compromised.[4] The OR must have an electric heated block to keep retrieval tubes warm. Right after follicular pickup, the tubes must be transported to the IVF laboratory as soon as possible. When they are in the laboratory, the next steps are:

- Leave the tubes in the heating block.
- Pour the follicular fluid into pre-heated 100-mm Petri dishes.
- Evaluate the follicular fluid under the stereo microscope by systematic screening of the dishes. Use the lowest magnification to visualize a bigger field, which will improve localization of the OCCCs; if the OCCCs cannot be found, shake the dishes with the

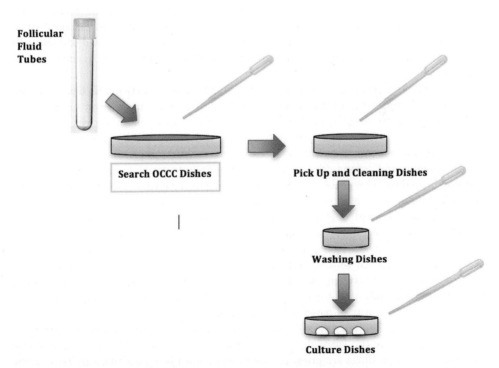

Follicular Fluid Tubes

Search OCCC Dishes

Pick Up and Cleaning Dishes

Washing Dishes

Culture Dishes

Figure 17.1 General scheme of oocyte pickup in the IVF laboratory. Tubes with follicular fluid are transported to the laboratory. OCCCs are first searched for in the follicular fluid. Once located, the OCCCs are picked up with a Pasteur pipette and transported to the cleaning dishes. Syringes and needles are used to clean the OCCCs. When they are cleaned, the OCCCs are transported to a washing dish to remove the HEPES medium. Finally, the OCCCs are transported to the tissue culture dish and stored in the culture incubator until denudation or insemination.

follicular fluid. OCCC visualization is relatively easy since they have a birefringent aspect frequently surrounded by characteristic cumulus.

- Use a Pasteur pipette to aspirate approximately 100 μl of washing buffer medium. Then pick up an OCCC with the minimum amount of follicular fluid and transfer it to the pickup and cleaning dishes.
- When oocyte retrieval is finished, move the OCCCs to a clean area (without blood) of the cleaning dish. Clean the OCCCs in the following way: hold the OCCC with the left needle (if you are right-handed), and cut, with a smooth movement, the excess of blood and cumulus cells. Once finished cutting all the OOOCs, transfer them to a washing dish, taking care to remove all the HEPES medium.
- When all oocytes are placed in a clean washing dish, proceed to distribute them into different droplets in a 60- or 35-mm culture dish. It is recommended not to put more than 10 oocytes in each dish.
- Briefly evaluate oocyte maturation, and note it in the patient's record.
- Carry the dishes to the incubator assigned to the patient (37.3°C and 6.0% CO_2) until insemination or denudation.
- Clean the laminar flow hood with detergent and distilled water.

17.4 Oocyte Grading

Mammalian follicular development is a complex process that influences the fertilizability and developmental potential of an oocyte. The morphological and functional changes in an oocyte occur in close relation with the changes in its surrounding specialized somatic cells (i.e. the cumulus and corona cells) and are influenced by the hormones in the follicular environment.[5]

A preliminary determination of oocyte maturity can be performed based on the morphological appearance of the OCCC at the time of oocyte retrieval, and it reflects the state of nuclear maturation.[6] In conventional IVF, direct evaluation of nuclear maturity is possible only 16 to 18 hours later, when the oocyte is denuded of the cumulus and corona cells before assessment of fertilization. However, in intracytoplasmic sperm injection (ICSI), cumulus and corona cells are removed routinely to facilitate handling during the injection procedure. This enables a precise assessment of the nuclear maturity of the oocyte only a few hours after retrieval. Numerous studies have shown a poor relation between OCCC morphology and oocyte nuclear maturity with this approach.[7] Therefore, it is important to keep in mind that could be a discrepancy between the assessment of the OCCC crown done by the embryologist and the real state of oocyte maturation.[8] The level of subjectivity associated with any type of morphology grading system may contribute to this lack of a relation between OCCC morphology and oocyte maturity.[7] For this reason, this assessment is only preliminary, and it does not have much relevance, especially in clinics where the majority of patients undergo ICSI.

The maturation of oocytes was graded by Veeck[9] into three states: mature (pre-ovulatory), immature (un-ripened) and degenerative (non-viable) at the time of follicular aspiration. These gradings are given on the basis of morphological characteristics of the ooplasm, corona radiation, cumulus formation and associated free membrane granulosa cells of the follicle. New classifications have subsequently emerged, all based on similar parameters. My group evaluated maturation and also classified OCCC maturation into three different grades[10] based on the degree of expansion of the corona layer (see Figure 17.2):

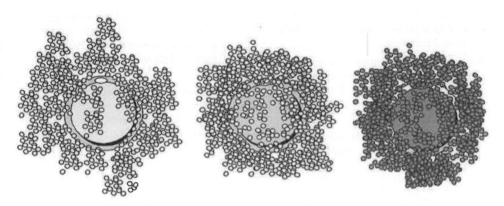

Figure 17.2 Grade 1, 2 and 3 oocytes, respectively.

- **Grade 1**. Corresponds to oocytes that have expanded and have a loose crown; they are generally metaphase II oocytes (MII). Nuclear maturation or MII stage is reached when the oocyte has reached metaphase of the second meiotic division and expelled the first polar body.[11]
- **Grade 2**. Corresponds to oocytes with cumulus cells in an intermediate state between compact and loose; it may correspond to oocytes in metaphase I (MI).
- **Grade 3**. Corresponds to oocytes with very compacted cumulus cells; there is no expansion of surrounding cells. A large nucleus is still present and may generally correspond to an oocyte in germinal vesicle state.

References

1. Pickering, S. J., Braude, P. R., Johnson, M. H., Cant, A. and Currie, J. Transient cooling to room temperature can cause irreversible disruption of the meiotic spindle in the human oocyte. *Fertil Steril* 1990; 54:102–8.

2. Swain, J. E. Optimizing the culture environment in the IVF laboratory: impact of pH and buffer capacity on gamete and embryo quality. *Reprod Biomed Online* 2010; 21:6–16.

3. Magli, M. C., Van den Abbeel, E., Lundin, K., Royere, D., Van der Elst, .J et al. Committee of the Special Interest Group on Embryology. Revised guidelines for good practice in IVF laboratories. *Hum Reprod.* 2008; 23(6):1253–62. Epub 28 March 2008. doi: 10.1093/humrep/den068

4. Practice Committee of American Society for Reproductive Medicine, Practice Committee of Society for Assisted Reproductive Technology. Revised guidelines for human embryology and andrology laboratories. *Fertil Steril* 2008; 90(5 Suppl.):S45–59. doi: 10.1016/j.fertnstert.2008.08.099.

5. Eppig, J. J., O'Brien, M. and Wigglesworth, K. Mammalian oocyte growth and development in vitro. *Mol Reprod Dev* 1996; 44:260–73.

6. Mehlmann, L. M. Stops and starts in mammalian oocytes: recent advances in understanding the regulation of meiotic arrest and oocyte maturation. *Reproduction* 2005; 130(6):791–9.

7. Rattanachaiyanont, M., Leader, A. and Léveillé, M. C. Lack of correlation between oocyte-corona-cumulus complex morphology and nuclear maturity of oocytes collected in stimulated cycles for intracytoplasmic sperm injection. *Fertil Steril* 1999; 71(5):937–40.

8. Veeck, L. L.Oocyte assessment and biological performance. *Ann NY Acad Sci* 1988; 541:259–74.

9. Veeck, L. L. The morphologic estimation of mature oocytes and their preparation for insemination. In *In Vitro Fertilization*, ed. Norfolk (p. 81). (Baltimore:Williams & Wilkins, 1986).

10. Pehlivan, T. Clasificación del complejo corona-cúmulo-ovocito. In *Manual práctico de esterilidad y reproducción Humana-Laboratorio de reproducción asistida*, ed. Remohi, Cobo, Prados, Romero, Pellicer (4th edn., pp. 115–20) 2012.

11. Trounson, A., Anderiesz, C. and Jones, G. Maturation of human oocytes in vitro and their developmental competence. *Reproduction* 2001; 121(1):51–75.

Chapter

18

In Vitro Maturation of Oocytes for IVF

Satoshi Mizuno and Aisaku Fukuda

18.1 Background

The first human baby birth attained through in vitro maturation–in vitro fertilization (IVM) was reported by Cha et al. in 1991.[1] And several authors have reported pregnancy and delivery following the transfer of embryos derived from immature oocytes.[2–4] However, the clinical outcomes from early experiences of IVM cycles were not satisfactory compared with standard IVF followed by controlled ovarian stimulation (COS). Since then, IVM protocol, including its laboratory procedures, has been developed, and nowadays IVM is one of the most important technologies for assisted reproduction.

In modern assisted reproductive technologies, ovarian stimulation is commonly carried out to increase the number of oocytes retrieved and achieve better clinical outcomes. However, use of ovarian stimulation involves higher treatment costs for the daily injection of gonadotrophins such as human menopausal gonadotrophin (hMG) or follicle-stimulating hormone (FSH) and sometimes accompanies ovarian hyper-stimulation syndrome (OHSS), which has the potential to result in a worst scenario, such as thrombosis of cerebral vessels. One of the characteristics of IVM cycles is no or very few injections of exogenous gonadotrophins. As a result, treatment cost can be reduced, and the risk of side effects also can be eliminated. There are more than several reports suggesting that IVM is beneficial, especially in patients with polycystic ovarian syndrome (PCOS) who have potential risk of developing OHSS.[5–7]

In addition, IVM could be a procedure of choice not only for infertility treatment but also for fertility preservation in cancer patients. IVM is beneficial for fertility preservation in hormone-dependent cancer patients who should avoid estradiol elevation because there is no need for ovarian stimulation. Furthermore, IVM is also favourable for the cancer patients who do not have extra time to receive ovarian stimulation due to the need for immediate chemotherapy or surgery. Recently, in the case of ovarian tissue cryopreservation for fertility preservation, IVM is required if the patients do not choose an autologous transplantation of the tissue after cancer treatment because the oocytes obtained from frozen-thawed ovarian tissue are usually immature.[5,6]

In laboratory aspects, the IVM procedure is more difficult than standard IVF with COS due to various stages of development of cumulus-oocyte complexes (COCs) from the smaller size of ovarian follicles and extra steps during culture. Major differences of IVM procedures from standard IVF are oocyte identification, maturity determination and maturation culture. Details of identification of COCs during oocyte retrieval, maturity determination before and after maturation culture and method of maturation culture are as follows. There are no differences in the procedures of intracytoplasmic sperm injection (ICSI), denuding of oocytes and embryo culture between IVM and standard IVF.

18.2 Oocyte Identification

The method of oocyte identification in IVM is the first and most critical procedure and is quite different from standard IVF with COS. The follicular fluid containing COCs collected in IVM cycles is usually contaminated with a larger number of red blood cells than standard IVF. More blood comes during oocyte retrieval in IVM because of technical difficulties in retrieving COCs from small follicles sized from 5 to 8 mm in diameter in comparison with standard IVF with 18-mm follicles.

At the same time, the COCs retrieved in IVM cycles contain fewer but more compacted cumulus cells compared with standard IVF. These conditions make it more difficult for embryologists to identify the COCs floating in the bloody follicular fluid aspirated from the ovaries in IVM cycles.

There are two options to identify and separate the COCs from follicular aspirates collected in IVM cycles. In the first approach, which we do not use any more, follicular aspirates are poured directly into tissue culture dishes, and COCs are searched for under a stereoscopic dissecting microscope. In the second approach, which we now use, the bloody follicular fluid containing COCs is initially filtered through a nylon mesh strainer to facilitate COC detection. COCs are retained on the filter in this method. We can identify the COCs in non-bloody culture medium back-flushed from the mesh strainer. Therefore, this method requires much less time, and the number of culture dishes for oocyte identification is significantly decreased.

IVM is primarily applied to patients with PCO whose ovaries have many small follicles, and many oocytes are generally collected from these patients in one cycle. Accordingly, a more efficient method of oocyte identification is required. In our facilities, the aforementioned latter method is adopted. Stepwise procedures of oocyte identification in culture medium heavily contaminated with blood are as follows:

1. Disposable products used for oocyte identification are listed in Table 18.1. All media used for the procedures are equilibrated with their desired gas conditions at 37°C until use. A syringe with a needle is filled with 20 ml of flushing medium just before the procedure. The components of flushing medium are shown in Table 18.2.
2. The cell strainer, a nylon mesh filter with 70-μm pores, is placed onto a 60-mm tissue culture dish, and the mesh of the cell strainer is soaked in the flushing medium (Figure 18.1A).
3. The cell strainer is transferred to a 100-mm tissue culture dish. Then all follicular aspirates from oocyte retrievals are poured onto the cell strainer (Figure 18.1B).
4. The remaining contents on the cell strainer are rinsed with the flushing medium (Figure 18.1C).
5. After rinsing, the cell strainer is transferred to another 60-mm tissue culture dish and set reversed. The COCs sticking on the filter are dropped onto the dish by swiftly squirting from backside of the filter with flushing medium (Figure 18.1D). This procedure is repeated twice. After recovery of COCs in the dish, the cell strainer is returned to the original 60-mm tissue culture dish prepared in step 2.
6. COCs in the flushing medium of the 60-mm tissue culture dish are located and identified under a stereoscopic dissecting microscope.
7. The rinsed cell strainer is checked again under a stereoscopic dissecting microscope to determine whether there are any remaining COCs (Figure 18.1E).
8. The COCs identified are incubated in the culture medium for the next step, which is a maturity check on the same day.

Table 18.1. Disposable Products Used for Oocyte Identification

Product	Number	Supplier	Catalog No.
Cell strainer (70 μm)	1	Corning (NY, USA)	352350
Tissue culture dish (60 mm)	3	Corning (NY, USA)	353002
Tissue culture dish (100 mm)	1	Corning (NY, USA)	353003
Syringe (20 ml)	1	NIPRO (Osaka, JP)	15D02
Needle (18G)	1	NIPRO (Osaka, JP)	15D272

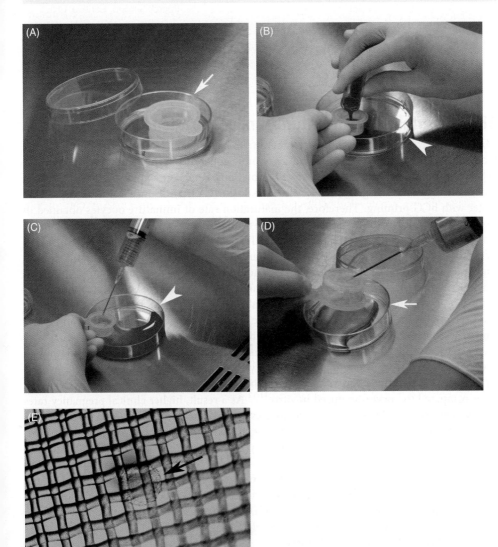

Figure 18.1 Procedures for oocyte identification. (A) Preparation of the cell strainer (arrow: 60-mm tissue culture dish). (B) The cell strainer and filtration of follicular aspirates (arrowhead: 100-mm tissue culture dish). (C) Red blood cells removed by the flushing medium. (D) Recovery of the COCs on the mesh filter. (E) A COC remaining on the cell strainer after rinsing (black arrow). A black and white version of this figure will appear in some formats. For the color version, please refer to the plate section.

Table 18.2 Components of Culture Media for IVM

Use	Basic medium	Supplement and concentration
Flushing medium[a]	Modified human tubal fluid (HTF) (Irvine Scientific, CA, USA)	14 U/ml heparin sodium (Mochida, Osaka, JP)
Maturation medium	Medicult IVM medium (Origio, Måløv, DK)	75 mIU/ml FSH: Follistim (MSD, NJ, USA)
		100 mIU/ml HCG: Profasi (Merck Serono, Geneva, CH)
		10% human serum albumin: HSA (Irvine Scientific, CA, USA)

[a] Heparin is supplemented with flushing medium to prevent blood coagulation of the follicular fluid from small follicles. A general handling medium containing HEPES is used.

18.3 Determination of Maturity and Maturation Culture

Maturity determination and maturation culture are also characteristic procedures in IVM. According to several reports, human chorionic gonadotrophin (hCG) priming before retrieval of immature oocytes is effective in obtaining better outcomes in IVM cycles.[8,9] It has been suggested that germinal vesicle breakdown (GVBD) of immature oocytes occurs faster with hCG priming. Therefore, the maturation rate of immature oocytes obtained in cycles with hCG-primed IVM is higher than with no hCG priming cycles.[8] Higher rates of implantation and pregnancy in hCG-primed IVM cycles also have been reported.[9] However, some papers have reported that there are no significant differences in the clinical outcomes between hCG-primed IVM cycles and cycles no hCG priming.[10] Thus, it remains unclear whether hCG priming in IVM cycles could improve the rates of oocyte maturation, fertilization, good-quality embryos and clinical pregnancy. In our facilities, hCG priming has been applied in most of the IVM cycles because we had higher retrieval rates and better pregnancy outcomes compared with cycles without hCG priming.

Some of the oocytes collected in hCG-primed IVM cycles are already matured, though they are collected from small follicles. The oocytes already matured in vivo in hCG-primed IVM cycles have competency to develop into better-quality embryos and higher blastocyst rates compared to oocytes matured in vitro.[11,12] As a result, higher clinical pregnancy rates can be achieved in IVM cycles in which oocytes matured in vivo are retrieved than in cycles without in vivo matured oocytes. Of course, matured oocytes should not be cultured any more. Thus, determination of oocyte maturity on the same day as oocyte retrieval is so important not only to obtain better outcomes but also to avoid over-culture for matured oocytes in hCG-primed IVM cycles. ICSI of matured oocytes has to be performed on the day of retrieval to prevent aging of those oocytes. However, it is known that cumulus cells play an important role in oocyte maturation. Therefore, maturity determination of the oocytes retrieved must be conducted without denuding them so that the immature oocytes can be cultured with cumulus cells thereafter.

Although there are a number of reports regarding human IVM, the culture duration of IVM recorded in each article is highly variable from 26 to 56 hours.[13] According to these reports, the maturation culture time in hCG-primed IVM cycles tends to be shorter than

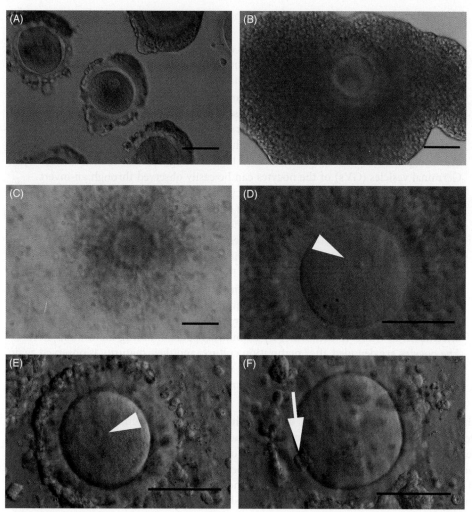

Figure 18.2 COC morphology and maturity of oocytes retrieved in IVM cycles. (A) An oocyte with sparse cumulus cells. (B) An oocyte with compacted cumulus cells. (C) An oocyte with expanded cumulus cells. (D) An oocyte with compacted cumulus cells and their GVs (arrowhead). (E) An oocytes with expanded cumulus cells and their GVs (arrowhead). (F) An oocyte with a first polar body (arrow) reflecting its maturity. Bar = 75 μm. (A black and white version of this figure will appear in some formats. For the color version, please refer to the plate section.)

that where no hCG-priming cycles are performed.[13] The duration of maturation culture in our facilities is set between 26 and 28 hours because most of our IVM cycles are performed with hCG priming. Determinations of oocyte maturity are performed twice, just after oocyte retrieval and after the maturation culture. Time tables of maturity determination and maturation culture are described below.

1. The determination of the oocyte maturity is performed within one hour of oocyte retrieval.
2. The COCs recovered in IVM cycles are roughly classified into the following three types by the morphology of corona and cumulus cells attached to the oocytes: an oocyte with sparse cumulus cells (fewer granulosa cells attached) (Figure 18.2A), an oocyte with

compacted cumulus cells (Figure 18.2B) and an oocyte with expanded cumulus cells (Figure 18.2C).

3. Maturity of the oocyte with sparse cumulus cells (Figure 18.2A) can be easily determined with an invert microscope. The immature oocytes are cultured in the maturation medium. However, ICSI is performed on mature oocytes on the day of retrieval.

4. Maturity of the oocyte with compacted cumulus cells (Figure 18.2B) or expanded cumulus cells (Figure 18.2C) should be observed by thinning the layer of aggregated cumulus cells by the following method. First, COCs are transferred into the 60-mm tissue culture dish filled with 1 to 1.5 ml of handling medium. Then the layer of cumulus cells is expanded by the surface tension of the handling medium to make a thin layer. Germinal vesicles (GVs) of the oocytes can be easily observed through an invert microscope (Figure 18.2D and E). The oocytes at GV stage are cultured in the maturation medium. However, observation of the polar body is somewhat difficult, even with the layer of cumulus cells thinned. Therefore, all the oocytes without GVs are denuded. The oocytes at GVBD are cultured in the maturation medium, but mature oocytes are fertilized with ICSI on the retrieval day.

5. The procedures for denuding oocytes and ICSI are the same as in standard IVF. The maturation of immature oocytes is performed in maturation medium for 26 to 28 hours. The components of maturation medium are shown in Table 18.2. The number of oocytes cultured in one well (1 ml of maturation medium) should be limited to prevent attachment of COCs to each other by cumulus expansion during maturation culture. The oocytes are denuded after maturation culture, and their maturity is observed again. And then the mature oocytes are fertilized with ICSI. The procedures after ICSI, including fertilization check, embryos culture and preparation for embryo transfer, are completely the same as in standard IVF.

The whole process of IVM is more laborious than standard IVF with COS because of more steps in the laboratory procedure and the requirement for more meticulous techniques to deal with COCs from small follicles. Therefore, higher skills are required not only by medical doctors at retrievals but also by embryologists in handling oocytes and embryos in IVM cycles. Their skills directly influence the clinical outcomes of IVM. In other words, only proficient physicians and embryologists should carry out IVM for better outcomes.

References

1. Cha, K. T., Koo, J. J., Ko, J. J., Choi, D. H., et al. Pregnancy after in vitro fertilization of human follicular oocytes collected from nonstimulated cycles, their culture in vitro and their transfer in a donor oocyte program. Fertil Steril 1991; 55:109–13.

2. Trounson, A., Wood, C. and Kausche, A. In vitro maturation and the fertilization and developmental competence of oocytes recovered from untreated polycystic ovarian patients. Fertil Steril 1994; 62(2):353–62.

3. Barnes, F. L., Crombie, A., Gardner, D. K. et al. Blastocyst development and birth after in-vitro maturation of human primary oocytes, intracytoplasmic sperm injection and assisted hatching. Hum Reprod 1995; 10(12):3243–7.

4. Russell, J. B., Knezevich, K. M., Fabian, K. F. and Dickson, J. A. Unstimulated immature oocyte retrieval: early versus midfollicular endometrial priming. Fertil Steril 1997; 67 (4):616–20.

5. Lin, Y. H. and Hwang, J. L. In vitro maturation of human oocytes. Taiwan J Obstet Gynecol 2006; 45(2):95–9.

6. Lim, K. S., Chae, S. J., Choo, C. W., Ku, Y. H. et al. In vitro maturation:

clinical applications. *Clin Exp Reprod Med* 2013; 40(4):143–7.

7. Farsi, M. M., Kamali, N. and Pourghasem, M. Embryological aspects of oocyte in vitro maturation. *Int J Mol Cell Med* 2013; 2(3):99–109.

8. Chian, R. C., Buckett, W. M., Tulandi, T. and Tan, S. L. Prospective randomized study of human chorionic gonadotrophin priming before immature oocyte retrieval from unstimulated women with polycystic ovarian syndrome. *Hum Replod* 2000; 15(1):165–70.

9. Son, W. Y., Yoon, S. H. and Lim, J. H. Effect of gonadotrophin priming on in-vitro maturation of oocytes collected from women at risk of OHSS. *Reprod Biomed Online* 2006; 13(3):340–8.

10. Soderstrom-Anttila, V., Makinen, S., Tuuri, T. and Suikkari AM. Favourable

pregnancy results with insemination of in vitro matured oocytes from unstimulated patients. *Hum Reprod* 2005; 20(6):1534–40.

11. Son, W. Y., Chung, J. T., Demirtas, E., Helzer, H., et al. Comparison of in-vitro maturation cycles with and without in-vivo matured oocytes retrieved. *Reprod Biomed Online* 2008; 17(1):59–67.

12. Son, W. Y., Chung, J. T., Chian, R. C., Herrero, B. et al. A 38 h interval between hCG priming and oocyte retrieval increase in vivo and in vitro oocyte maturation rate in programmed IVM cycles. *Hum Reprod* 2008; 23(9):2010–16.

13. Son W. Y. and Tan, S. L. Laboratory and embryological aspects of hCG-primed in vitro maturation cycles for patients with polycystic ovaries. *Hum Reprod Update* 2010; 16:675–89.

Chapter
19

Oocyte Grading by Morphological Evaluation

Basak Balaban

19.1 Background

Optimal oocyte morphology is defined as an oocyte with a spherical structure enclosed by a uniform zona pellucida with a uniform translucent cytoplasm that is free of inclusions and has a size-appropriate polar body.[1,2,6] However, metaphase II (MII) oocytes retrieved from patients after ovarian stimulation are known to show significant morphological variations that may affect the developmental competence and implantation potential of the derived embryo.

This chapter focuses on the morphological abnormalities of the MII oocyte, discusses briefly their correlation with clinical outcome to provide an idea about which features must be examined as a priority and proposes an oocyte grading scheme to be used in routine practice in in vitro fertilization (IVF) laboratories. Morphological abnormalities of the oocyte will be observed under two different subgroups: extracytoplasmic abnormalities and cytoplasmic abnormalities.[1–6]

19.2 Cytoplasmic Abnormalities

19.2.1 Centrally Located Granulation of the Cytoplasm (CLCG)

Condensed granulation that is centrally located within the cytoplasm with a clear border is unlike various degrees of diffused granulation, which is subtly defined in the literature due to the different modulation of the optical path in phase contrast microscopies in various laboratories. It's easily distinguishable with a significant darker appearance than normal cytoplasm, which could be clearly visible by any modulation type of the optical path in different phase contrast microscopes. It is defined as a rare morphological feature of the oocyte that is diagnosed as a large, dark, spongy granular area in the cytoplasm, and the severity is based on both the diameter of granular area and the depth of the lesion. Various studies have shown its detrimental effect on clinical outcome, with high risk of aneuploid embryos and high abortion rates. Significantly lower cryosurvival rate, blastocyst formation with poor quality and hatching deficiencies can be obtained with cryopreserved day 3 cleavage-stage embryos derived from oocytes with CLCG oocytes. CLCG oocytes, also defined as 'organelle clustering', are the only repetitive dysmorphism seen as a sign of severe intrinsic pathology in consecutive cycles and are a negative predictor of pregnancy and implantation rates in intracytoplasmic sperm injection (ICSI) cycles.[3–6]

19.2.2 Refractile Bodies

'Refractile bodies' are cytoplasmic inclusions that can be dark incorporations, fragments, spots, dense granules, lipid droplets and lipofuscin. The average diameter of a recognizable refractile body under bright-field microscopy is approximately 10 μm. Published studies show controversial results for the affect of refractile bodies in the cytoplasm on clinical outcome. It is most likely that controversial results might be correlated to the factors that are still unknown, and one possible confounding factor could be the differing diameters of refractile bodies, and the clinical outcome is detrimentally affected only if diameter is over 5 μm.[4–6]

19.2.3 Vacuoles

'Vacuoles' are membrane-bound cytoplasmic inclusions filled with fluid that is virtually identical with perivitelline space liquid. The incidence of vacuoles in MII oocytes varies from 3.1%[11] to 12.4%. However, multiple vacuolization is a less likely seen phenomenon at approximately 1% to 1.5%. A cut-off value of 14 μm for vacuole diameter for fertilization outcome is suggested, as larger vacuoles or multiple vacuoles may cause a much more detrimental effect on the oocyte than a small vacuole, since a larger portion of the cytoskeleton (e.g. microtubules) cannot function as it is supposed to. Besides the negative effect on fertilization rates, it has also been shown that blastocyst formation, quality and hatching rates, as well as percentage of euploid embryo rates, can be impaired after ICSI of vacuolated oocytes. Vacuolization in MII oocytes can also decrease cryosurvival rates and subsequent embryonic development of the derived cryopreserved embryos.[4–6]

19.3 Smooth Endoplasmic Reticulum Clusters (sERCs)

Smooth endoplasmic reticulum clusters (sERCs) can be easily distinguished from fluid-filled vacuoles because they are not separated from the rest of the ooplasmic volume by a membrane and are seen as translucent vacuoles. Even though the mechanism responsible for sERCs is still unknown, it is assumed to be correlated to some functional and structural alterations of the ER during oocyte maturation. The incidence of affected cycles with such oocytes varied from 5% to 10% as perhaps the variety in the diameters of translucent vacuoles can be missed under the conditions used in clinical embryology laboratories for examination. Studies had shown that implantation potential is detrimentally affected if the oocyte is from the cohort of oocytes where at least one oocyte has clusters. Besides the viability of the derived embryos, the most important issue with the presence of sERCs had been the neonatal safety based on evidence proof in the literature. The first report of the transfer of an affected embryo indicated that the baby was diagnosed with Beckwith-Wiedemann syndrome, whereas other studies showed a significantly lower take-home baby rate and higher miscarriage rate; in addition, two unexplained neonatal deaths were reported in the group with affected gametes. Following evidence-based data reporting multiple malformations and ventricular septal defects after the transfer of embryos originated from oocytes with sERCs, it is strongly recommended that oocytes with such feature should be precisely examined and preferably be disgarded if non-affected embryos are available for transfer.[6]

19.4 Extracytoplasmic Abnormalities

Some prominent morphological anomalies at the oocyte stage are shown in Figure 19.1.

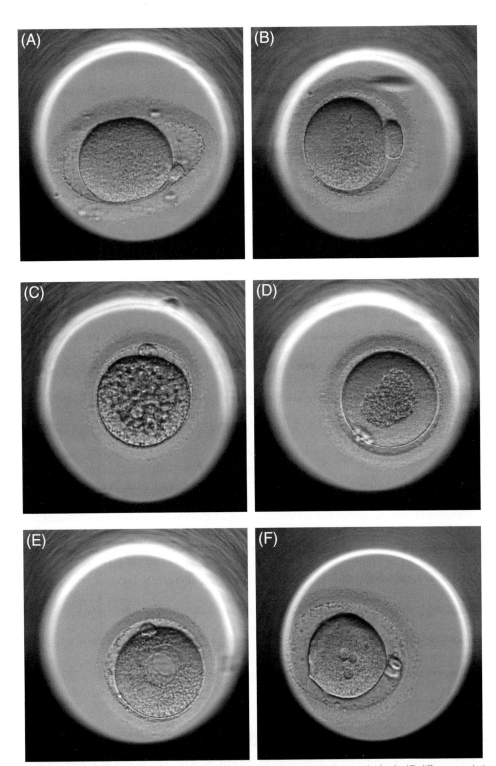

Figure 19.1 Overview of morphological anomalies: (A) zona anomaly; (B) large polar body; (C) diffuse granulation; (D) dense granulation; (E) smooth endoplasmic reticulum clusters and (F) vacuoles.

19.4.1 Dysmorphic Zona Pellucida (ZP)

Amongst the conceivable changes in oocyte performance, it is possible that the secretion/patterning of the ZP from the secondary follicle onwards could be altered or interrupted. This could result in either dysmorphism that can be seen under a light microscope or in more subtle changes of the three-dimensional structure of the ZP.

From conventional IVF, it is known that thicker zonae (e.g. >20 μm) are associated with lower fertilization rates. This has been linked to patient and stimulation parameters. In ICSI, however, a thicker zona interferes neither with subsequent fertilization nor with implantation, since assisted hatching can be applied.[6]

19.4.2 Discoloration

Irrespective of the actual thickness of the ZP, ovarian stimulation sometimes generates gametes showing a ZP that appears dark or brownish under a light microscope. In the literature, it is reported that the presence of a discoloured ZP is a common phenomenon (e.g. 9.5% to 25.7%).

It has to be kept in mind that it is not completely clear that dark or brown zonae/oocytes occur for the same reasons. Recently, these oocytes were termed 'brown eggs' because they were found to be dark with a thick ZP, a rather small perivitelline space (sometimes filled with debris) and granular cytoplasm. Studies comparing the outcome of brown gametes with that of gametes of normal appearance have shown similar fertilization, embryo quality, implantation and clinical pregnancy rates both for IVF and for ICSI cycles.[6]

19.4.3 Shape Anomalies

Even if the thickness or colour of the ZP is inconspicuous, it is not automatic that the shape of the gametes is spherical. The vast majority of ovoid ova, it can be assumed, are the result of a pre-existing anomaly generated during maturation within the follicle. Despite the fact of reports demonstrating the existence of ovoid eggs with fertilization capacity and giving rise to healthy babies, the degree of the shape anomaly was not objectively quantified.

If an objective measurement of the shape abnormality of the MII oocyte and ZP were to be performed, it would be shown that the degree of shape anomaly is neither correlated to fertilization nor to embryo quality, but interestingly, two types of cleavage pattern were observed on day 2. Either ovoid gametes cleaved normally like a tetrahedron (a crosswise arrangement of four cells with three blastomeres lying side-by-side) or, if the ovoid zona failed to exert its shaping function, a rather flat array of four blastomeres resulted. Since the abnormal pattern reduces the number of cell-to-cell contact points from six to five or four, compaction and blastulation of the corresponding embryos may be delayed.[6]

19.4.4 Perivitelline Space (PVS)

The size of PVS is closely related to the maturational phase of the oocyte, and its full size is reached only at the completion of maturation (MII). Studies show that up to 50% of all ova show a large PVS that results in a lower fertilization rate. Even though patient parameters such as female age and indication had not been reported to influence PVS performance, the ratio of estradiol to testosterone (and to progesterone) had significant influence.

Data from in vitro and in vivo matured oocytes indicate that a large PVS may be ascribed to over-mature eggs. In other words, such eggs have shrunk in relation to the ZP, resulting in a large gap between them. A large PVS would also occur if a larger portion of the cytoplasm is extruded together with the haploid chromosomal set during first polar body formation. This would result in a large first polar body and a large PVS.[6]

19.4.5 First Polar Body Morphology (1st PB)

Despite earlier reports of various groups suggesting a scoring system based on the morphological appearance of the 1st PB, use of 1st PB morphology as a diagnostic tool to assess embryo quality and implantation potential can have limited predictive value due to the dynamic formation of this structure, which is highly changeable over the hours of culture. Even though the efficiency of scoring 1st PB morphology, which is mainly based on the fragmentation level, is debatable, the appearance of a large 1st PBs should be noted, and the use of such MII oocytes should be prevented, if possible, as embryos derived from such oocytes have a high risk of chromosomal abnormality.[1-6]

19.4.6 Debris in the Perivitelline Space (PVS)

Two hypotheses have been described to explain the origin of debris in the PVS. One hypothesis is derived from ultra-structural data indicating the presence of an extracellular matrix comprised of granules and filaments in the space between the oolemma and ZP, since the matrix is identical to that found between cumulus cells and the corona radiata. Studies support the latter theory because they found a close relationship between the frequency of PVS granularity and maturation. It has been demonstrated that the presence of PVS granules is gonadotrophin dose dependent, and the incidence of oocytes with debris in the PVS significantly increased for high-dose patients. Even though fertilization rate, cleavage rate and embryo quality were found to be unaffected by the presence of coarse granules in the PVS, various studies had shown that rates of implantation and pregnancy can be decreased.[6]

19.5 Conclusion

Despite the limited value of assessing oocyte quality and viability by means of morphology, it should not be under-estimated as it is still the sole method of choice for oocyte selection until a more effective technology with long-term clinical validation can substitute in routine practice in clinical in vitro fertilization (IVF) laboratories worldwide. Beyond the predictive value of oocyte morphology, it must not be forgotten that information linking dysmorphism with genetic disorders is of great value and scarce because these disorders are directly correlated with the health of the offspring in assisted reproductive technology (ART) applications.

Based on current scientific evidence on the relative weight of various morphological abnormalities, a practical standard operating procedure (SOP) can be suggested to be used in routine practice in IVF laboratories.

19.5.1 Oocyte Grading Scheme

- Check the maturity stage of the oocyte after cumulus-corona removal.
- Morphological deviations that should be examined with high priority are in the following order:
  - Oocytes that are large in size (giant oocytes) and oocytes that have a large first polar body should not be used for insemination because of the high risk of chromosomal abnormalities. If the patient has only such oocytes, pre-implantation genetic screening (PGS) for the derived embryo can be recommended.

- Oocytes should be observed for the presence of smooth endoplasmic reticulum cluster(s) within the cytoplasm. The patient should be informed that embryos derived from such oocytes may have significantly reduced rates of healthy offspring
- Oocytes should be observed for the presence of vacuole(s) within the cytoplasm. Patients should be informed that MII oocytes with vacuole(s) that are 14 μm or greater have significantly lower chance of getting fertilized compared with oocytes with normal morphological appearance.
- Oocytes should be observed for the presence of organelle clustering/centrally located condensed granulation within the cytoplasm. Patient should be informed that embryos derived from such oocytes may have a higher risk of chromosomal abnormalities.
- Oocytes defined with other cytoplasmic deviations, such as refractile bodies/cytoplasmic inclusions, or with dark cytoplasm/dark cytoplasm–granular cytoplasm/dark cytoplasm with slight granulation/dark granular appearance of the cytoplasm/diffused cytoplasmic granularity should be documented.
- Ovoid oocytes with ovoid zona and normally shaped oolemma or ovoid zona and ovoid oolemma should be observed as the blastocyst formation rate of embryos derived from such oocytes may be detrimentally affected and delayed.
- Oocytes with an extremely large perivitelline space (PVS) may result in reduced fertilization rates and higher degeneration rates following ICSI.
- Dysmorphic zona pellucida, discoloration of the oocyte, first polar body morphology and debris in the PVS should be documented.

References

1. Alpha Scientists in Reproductive Medicine, ESHRE Special Interest Group of Embryology. The Istanbul consensus workshop on embryo assessment: proceedings of an expert meeting. *Reprod Biomed Online* 2011; 22:632–46.

2. Alpha Scientists in Reproductive Medicine and ESHRE Special Interest Group of Embryology. The Istanbul consensus workshop on embryo assessment: proceedings of an expert meeting. *Hum Reprod* 2011; 26:1270–83.

3. Rienzi, L., Balaban, B., Ebner, T. and Mandelbaum, J. The oocyte. *Hum Reprod* 2012; 27: 2–21.

4. Balaban, B. and Urman, B. Effect of oocyte morphology on embryo development and implantation. *Reprod Biomed Online* 2006; 12:608–15.

5. Ebner, T. Is oocyte morphology prognostic of embryo developmental potential after ICSI? *Reprod Biomed Online* 2006; 12:507–12.

6. Balaban, B. and Ebner, T. Morphological selection of gametes and embryos: oocyte. In *A Practical Guide to Selecting Gametes and Embryos*, ed. M Montag (pp. 81–96) (Boca Raton, FL: CRC Press, Taylor & Francis Group, 2014).

Chapter

20

Vitrification of Oocytes for IVF

Laura Rienzi, Benedetta Iussig and Filippo M. Ubaldi

Introduction

Oocyte cryopreservation is a breakthrough technique available for fertility preservation. It has been quite ignored until recently mainly because of the technical difficulties relative to cell structure and sensitivity. However, it offers valid solutions to many clinical, ethical, legal and social problems such that it is considered a precious option to embryo freezing.

Conventional slow-freezing methods have been gradually replaced by more efficient vitrification systems, and the excellent results obtained with this fine procedure indeed justify its widespread application. Initially, its effectiveness had been proven for extremely good-prognosis patients, such as egg donors; nevertheless, many current published studies validate its application even in the poorer-prognosis infertile population. In fact, the outcomes obtained with vitrified/warmed oocytes in in vitro fertilization (IVF) are similar to those of fresh counterparts and significantly contribute to the cumulative pregnancy and delivery rates. Recently, on the basis of these valuable achievements, the European Society of Human Reproduction and Embriology (ESHRE) and the American Society for Reproductive Medicine (ASRM) recognized the usefulness of the vitrification technique so that it is no longer considered 'experimental'.

20.1 Background

20.1.1 Introduction

Oocyte cryopreservation has been largely neglected for a long time as a contributor to overall implantation and pregnancy rates, mostly due to technical difficulties related to cell special structure and sensitivity. However, it may be an important opportunity, providing several valid solutions to clinical, ethical, logistical and social problems. Above all, oocyte cryopreservation offers useful options in infertility programmes in case of (1) collection of supernumerary eggs, (2) risk of ovarian hyper-stimulation syndrome, when ethical/legal concerns or restrictions limit embryo freezing, (3) in vitro fertilization (IVF) delay due to the lack of or an inadequate sperm sample and (4) reported previous implantation failures with good-quality embryos. Moreover, it represents a valid alternative to embryo freezing in case of legal issues; fertility preservation in case of systemic anti-cancer treatment that pre-figures gonadotoxic chemotherapy/radiotherapy and eventually oophorectomy; fertility preservation in case of premature menopause and cryobanking for oocyte donation or delayed motherhood.[1-4]

Unfortunately, although the first report of birth after oocyte freezing was published approximately 30 years ago,[5] the overall low efficiency of the procedure due to a defective protocol hampered widespread application. Only recently have we seen considerable improvements in the cryopreservation field, leading to the design of new, effective methods that resulted in a breakthrough for this fine procedure.

20.1.2 Cryopreservation Methods: A Survey

Currently adopted cryopreservation methods for oocytes differ considerably in the type and concentration of cryoprotectants used, cooling rates and carrier tools. Cryoprotectants (CPAs) are classified as 'permeating' (1,2-propanediol (PROH), dimethyl sulphoxide (DMSO) and ethylene glycole (EG)) and 'non-permeating' (disaccharides such as sucrose): while the first type can pass the cell membrane, replacing intracellular water, non-permeating CPAs create an osmotic gradient for cellular dehydration without entering the cell. Since CPAs may be toxic, their concentrations must be balanced with appropriate cooling rates to avoid cell stress and injury.

Traditionally, there are two main approaches to cryopreservation, namely, 'slow freezing' and 'vitrification'. Conventional slow freezing methods achieve gradual cell dehydration combining low CPA concentrations with slow cooling rates; although they have been modified over the years, the results have been somewhat disappointing such that they have been progressively abandoned. The real turning point was the advent of vitrification, consisting of exposure of the cell to a high CPA concentration immediately followed by ultra-rapid cooling in liquid nitrogen ($-196°C$), resulting in the complete elimination of ice crystal formation, which is recognized as the main cause of potential cell injury. Vitrification has been proven to increase cryopreservation efficiency in terms of survival and pregnancy rates,[2,4] and at present there is no evidence as to an increased risk of sub-cellular disorganization, altered embryonic metabolic profiles and adverse perinatal and obstetric outcomes.[6-8] As a consequence, vitrification is nowadays considered the method of choice to preserve both gametes and embryos.[2,4]

However, even among vitrification protocols, significant variations exist that make the difference. As to the types of CPAs, the many excellent results obtained so far and recently reviewed by the ASRM[2] used a combination of DMSO and EG. Moreover, vitrification methods may vary on the tools used and, consequently, may be classified as 'closed' or 'open' systems. The distinction is intuitive: whereas in closed systems the sample is physically separated from liquid nitrogen during the entire procedure, direct contact between the sample and liquid nitrogen is allowed in open systems.

Over the past few years, scientists have compared the relative advantages and disadvantages in a passionate debate. Theoretically, closed systems protect the sample from any potential contamination deriving from liquid nitrogen; as a consequence, they have been considered safe from a disease-transmission point of view and proposed as the unique applicable vitrification option. However, many embryologists underline the fact that in closed systems cooling rates may be compromised, thus resulting in impaired results. Noteworthy, the question is much more complicated.

In a recent review of the literature, Vajta et al.[9] described five different vitrification methods, of which four are traditionally classified as closed. Nevertheless, the borderline between them is not so sharp and definite, and in the end, only one is completely closed.

In this chapter we are going to describe the most commonly used technique for safe and effective oocyte cryopreservation. It is based on the method first described by Kuwayama[10] with only slight modifications. This protocol provides consistent survival, in vitro development, pregnancy and delivery rates similar to those of fresh counterparts.

20.2 Reagents, Supplies and Equipment

20.2.1 Vitrification/Warming Media

- **Basic solution (BS).** HEPES-buffered TCM-199 supplemented with 20% serum substitute supplement (SSS) or trehalose. Other protein sources containing both albumin and globulin, for example, Plasmanate (Bayer, Leverkusen, Germany), were also found suitable.
- **Equilibration solution (ES).** 7.5% EG and 7.5% DMSO dissolved in BS.
- **Vitrification solution (VS).** 15% EG, 15% DMSO and 0.5 M sucrose dissolved in BS.
- **Warming solution (WS).** 1.0 M sucrose dissolved in BS.
- **Dilution solution (DS).** 0.5 M sucrose dissolved in BS.

20.2.2 Carrier Tool and Consumables

- Open device equipped with a protective cap (It is suggested to load no more than three oocytes per device.)
- Handling 140- and 170-μm-diameter flexible polycarbonate pipettes
- 2- to 20-μl and 100- to 1,000-μl micropipettes and tips
- 60-mm polystyrene cell culture dish (and lid)
- 100-mm polystyrene cell culture dish (and lid)
- 35-mm polystyrene cell culture dish
- Polystyrene four-well dishes for IVF
- Six-well dishes (Reproplate, K1)
- Fine-tip cryomarkers for tool labelling
- Liquid nitrogen and storage tanks
- Visiotubes and goblets with different colours and diameters
- Cooling rack: sterile stainless or disposable single-use Styrofoam box
- Sterile pincers and scissors
- Heat gun
- Flexible polyethylene tubes designed for cryostorage in liquid nitrogen (LN_2)
- Stainless steel weight
- Ultraviolet (UV) LN_2 sterilization device
- Personal protective equipment required for liquid nitrogen handling
- Stopwatch or timer

20.3 Quality Control

- There should be a dedicated room to stock the liquid nitrogen tanks, far from any biological, chemical or atmospheric contamination source. Only authorized staff should be let in.
- In order to ensure vitrification safety, as requested by the European Union Tissues and Cells Directives,[11-13] tanks integrity should be regularly inspected, and liquid nitrogen should be periodically checked for contamination through standard microbiological tests. In the case of contamination, effective decontamination should be applied, as described previously, and certified.

- To avoid any potential risk of sample cross-contamination, there should be dedicated liquid nitrogen tanks in case of infective samples.
- To positively trace the materials and reagents throughout the vitrification process, all the media and plastic batch number should be certified by the manufacturer and conveniently registered in the IVF laboratory.
- To ensure the maximum efficiency of the technique, the operators should be properly instructed and trained (murine or immature oocytes), and their performances should be accurately monitored (survival rate).

20.4 Procedure

20.4.1 Vitrification Setup

1. The main equilibration and cooling procedure must be performed under a vertical flow hood without exposing the oocytes to be vitrified to a CO_2-rich atmosphere.
2. Bring BS, ES and VS to room temperature (25–27°C). It is strongly recommended to mix the CPAs containing solutions immediately prior their aliquoting during each step of the procedure in order to avoid their separating out of solution.
3. Complete all necessary paperwork and electronic archive registration.
4. Complete device and visiotube labelling, reporting patient name, unique identification (ID) number, date of vitrification, type of cryopreserved sample (MII stage oocytes) and number of oocytes per support (we suggest loading no more than three oocytes per device). This procedure must be verified by a second appropriately trained operator who witnesses the labelling accuracy and the correct identification of the patient at the beginning of cryopreservation.
5. Turn off the heat stage, as the vitrification procedure is performed at room temperature.
6. It is recommended to use a 140-μm flexible polycarbonate pipette in order to minimize the volume of solution transferred with each step without compromising oocyte integrity.
7. UV-sterilize LN_2.[14]
8. Prepare hermetical containers for safe cryostorage of the specimens.[15]

   a. Seal one end of a flexible polyethylene tube designed for LN_2 cryostorage.
   b. Cut the tube to a final length of ~25 cm.
   c. Disinfect the outer and inner surfaces of the tube, wiping it with ethanol for about five minutes.
   d. Put a stainless steel weight in the sealed tube in order to prevent it from floating in the LN_2.
   e. Put a previously sterilized appropriately labelled coloured visiotube inside the tube, and pre-cool the cryocontainer obtained, submerging it in UV-sterilized LN_2 and keeping it in a vertical position in order to avoid any LN_2 infiltration (at least 10 minutes).

20.4.2 Oocyte Equilibration, Cooling and Storage

1. Place a 20-μl BS drop on the lid of a 60-mm tissue culture dish.
2. Place a 20-μl ES drop close to the BS drop.

3. Place an oocyte in the BS drop, and then immediately merge it with the ES drop (ES to BS direction). Incubate three minutes.

4. Place another 20-μl ES drop perpendicularly close to the first ES drop, and then immediately merge it with the previously merged BS-ES drop (ES to merged BS-ES direction). Incubate three minutes.

5. Move the oocyte to a pure 20-μl ES drop, and then incubate for six to nine minutes. It is possible to equilibrate three to nine oocytes contemporaneously for a maximum of three oocytes per drop (for a maximum of three ES pure drops). If this is the case, the first set of one to three oocytes should be incubated in pure ES for six minutes; then the others follow closely behind (not more than nine minutes of incubation).

6. Before the time limit, fill the cooling rack with previously UV-sterilized liquid nitrogen on the work stage and place it in a comfortable position (e.g. on the left if the operator is right-handed).

7. Transfer a single set of oocytes (one to three contemporaneously) in 600 μl VS prepared in a four-well dish for IVF, and then incubate for one minute. Since VS differs from ES in density, oocytes should disperse on the surface of the solution, becoming difficult to trace. In order to avoid this drawback, it is recommended to slither them in the VS.

8. Within the one-minute deadline, load the single set of oocytes (one to three contemporaneously) to the tip of a previously labelled support. The procedure may be simpler if the device is laid upon a lid of a clean 100-mm cell culture dish.

9. Filmstrip the oocytes on the device in a minimum VS volume, removing the excess solution after loading.

10. Immediately submerge the device into previously UV-sterilized liquid nitrogen stored in the cooling rack with a single uninterrupted rapid movement.

11. While the device is submerged in the liquid nitrogen, fasten the protective plastic cap to the device, being helped by the use of sterile pincers.

12. Put the samples in the previously labelled cryo-container.

13. Seal the remaining open end of the cryo-container.

14. Store the hermetical cryo-container in liquid nitrogen dedicated tanks (below the temperature of $-180°C$).[16]

20.4.3 Warming Setup

1. The main warming procedure must be performed under a vertical flow hood without exposing the oocytes to be warmed to the CO_2-rich atmosphere.

2. Bring DS and BS to room temperature (25–27°C), and pre-warm WS in 35-mm cell culture dishes using a temperature incubator. It is strongly recommended to mix the cryoprotectants containing solutions immediately prior their aliquoting during each step of the procedure to avoid their separation out of solution.

3. Complete all necessary paperwork and electronic archive registration.

4. Turn off the heat stage, as also the warming procedure is performed at room temperature.

5. It is recommended to use a 170-μm-diameter flexible polycarbonate pipette in order to minimize extra stress on the warming oocytes.

6. UV-sterilize the LN_2 according to the manufacturer's indications.[14]

20.4.4 Warming and Dilution

1. Retrieve the samples from the liquid nitrogen tanks, immediately transferring the devices to a cooling rack full of previously sterilized liquid nitrogen.
2. Place the cooling rack on the work stage in a comfortable position for the operator (e.g. on the left if the operator is right-handed).
3. Drop 200 µl DS into the first well and 200 µl BS each into the second (BS1) and third wells (BS2) of a K1 ReproPlate.
4. While the cryo-container is submerged in the liquid nitrogen, open it.
5. Identify the correct side of sample loading in order to immediately recognize and remove the oocytes from the filmstrip.
6. With a rapid movement, transfer the device to warmed WS. Make sure that the tool tip is completely submerged. Incubate for one minute.
7. During the one-minute incubation, lightly tap the oocytes to remove them from the filmstrip; then carefully remove the support.
8. Delicately aspirate the oocytes in the pipette, taking an extra 2 mm of WS.
9. Blow the WS directly on the bottom of the DS well; then place the oocytes in the WS layer. Incubate for three minutes.
10. Delicately aspirate the oocytes in the pipette, taking an extra 2 mm of DS.
11. Blow the DS directly on the bottom of the first BS well (BS1); then place the oocytes in the DS layer. Incubate for five minutes.
12. Transfer the oocytes to the second BS well (BS2) with a minimal volume of BS1. Incubate for one minute.
13. Transfer the oocytes to a cell culture dish, and incubate in a temperature- and gas-controlled incubator for full recovery.
14. Wait two hours before performing ICSI.

20.5 Notes

Cryopreservation protocols have been significantly improved in recent years, especially thanks to the widespread application of vitrification, finally freed of the heavy label 'experimental'.[2] Effective cryopreservation of oocytes using vitrification is a breakthrough procedure now available for fertility preservation applicable to a great variety of cases, such as ovum donation,[17] infertility programmes[18–20] and medical and social egg freezing. An overview of outcomes is available in the document released by the Practice Committee of the American Society for Reproductive Medicine and the Society for Assisted Reproductive Technology.[2]

References

1. ESHRE Task Force on Ethics and Law, including Dondorp, W., De Wert, G., Pennings, G. et al. Oocyte cryopreservation for age-related fertility loss. *Hum Reprod* 2012; 27:1231–7.

2. Practice Committees of the American Society for Reproductive Medicine and the Society for Assisted Reproductive Technology. Mature oocyte cryopreservation: a guideline. *Fertil Steril* 2013; 99:37–43.

3. Loren, A. W., Mangu, P. B., Beck, L. N. et al. Fertility preservation for patients with cancer: American Society of Clinical Oncology clinical practice guideline update. *J Clin Oncol* 2013; 31:2500–10.

4. Glujovsky, D., Riestra, B., Sueldo, C. et al. Vitrification versus slow freezing for women undergoing oocyte cryopreservation (review). *Cochrane Database Syst Rev* 2014; 5(9):CD010047.

5. Chen, C. Pregnancy after human oocyte cryopreservation. *Lancet* 1986; 1:884–6.

6. Martinez-Burgos, M., Herrero, L., Megias, D. et al. Vitrification versus slow freezing of oocytes: effects on morphologic appearance, meiotic spindle configuration, and DNA damage. *Fertil Steril* 2011; 95:374–7.

7. Dominguez, F., Castello, D., Remohi, J. et al. Effect of vitrification on human oocytes: a metabolic profiling study. *Fertil Steril* 2013; 99:565–72.

8. Noyes, N., Porcu, E., Borini, A. et al. Over 900 oocyte cryopreservation babies born with no apparent increase in congenital anomalies. *Reprod Biomed Online* 2009; 18:769–76.

9. Vajta, G., Rienzi, L. and Ubaldi, F. Open versus closed systems for vitrification of human oocytes and embryos. *Reprod Biomed Online* 2015; 325–33.

10. Kuwayama, M. Highly efficient vitrification for cryopreservation of human oocytes and embryos: the Cryotop method. *Theriogenology* 2007; 67:73–80.

11. Directive 2004/23/EC of the European Parliament and of the Council of 31 March 2004 on Setting Standards of Quality and Safety for the Donation, Procurement, Testing, Processing, Preservation, Storage and Distribution of Human Tissues and Cells. *Official Journal of the European Union* 2004; L 102/48–58.

12. Commission Directive 2006/17/EC of 8 February 2006 Implementing Directive 2004/23/EC of the European Parliament and of the Council as Regards Certain Technical Requirements for the Donation, Procurement and Testing of Human Tissues and Cells. *Official Journal of the European Union* 2006; L 38/40–52.

13. Commission Directive 2006/86/EC of 24 October 2006 Implementing Directive 2004/23/EC of the European Parliament and of the Council as Regards Traceability Requirements, Notification of Serious Adverse Reactions and Events and Certain Technical Requirements for the Coding, Processing, Preservation, Storage and Distribution of Human Tissues and Cells. *Official Journal of the European Union* 2006; L 294/32–50.

14. Parmegiani, L., Cognigni, G. E. and Filicori, M. Ultra-violet sterilization of liquid nitrogen prior to vitrification. *Hum Reprod* 2009; 24:2969.

15. Parmegiani, L. and Rienzi, L. Hermetical goblets for cryostorage of human vitrified specimens. *Hum Reprod* 2011; 26:3204.

16. Cobo, A., Romero, J. L., de Los Santos, M. J. et al. Storage of human oocytes in the vapor phase of nitrogen. *Fertil Steril* 2010; 94:1903–7.

17. Cobo, A., Meseguer, M., Remohi, J., et al. Use of cryobanked oocytes in an ovum donation programme: a prospective, randomized, controlled, clinical trial. *Hum Reprod* 2010; 25:2239–46.

18. Rienzi, L., Romano, S., Albricci, A., et al. Embryo development of fresh versus 'vitrified' metaphase II oocytes after ICSI: a prospective randomized sibling-oocyte study. *Hum Reprod* 2010; 25:66–73.

19. Rienzi, L., Cobo, A., Paffoni, A. et al. Consistent and predictable delivery rates after oocyte vitrification: an observational longitudinal cohort multicentric study. *Hum Reprod* 2012; 27:1606–12.

20. Cobo, A., Garrido, N., Crespo, J. et al. Accumulation of oocytes: a new strategy for managing low-responder patients. *Reprod Biomed Online* 2012; 24:424–32.

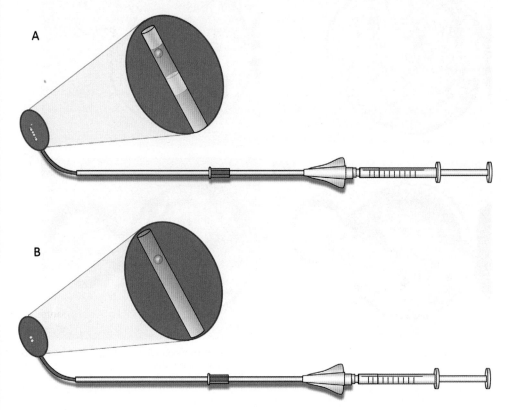

Figure 5.1

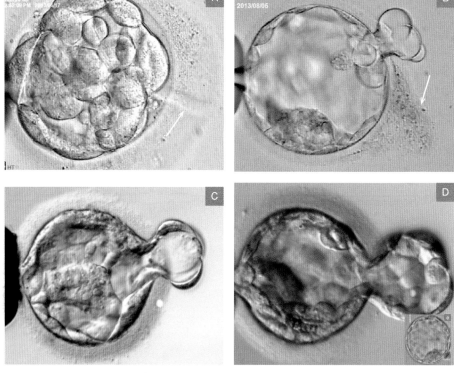

Figure 7.1 Embryos with laser-assisted hatching. (A) Day 5 embryo with abnormally thick zona pellucida, breached with the laser (arrow). (B) Day 5 embryo with trophectoderm cells protruding through the laser breach in a multi-layered abnormal zona pellucida. (C and D) Day 5 embryos hatching through a breach introduced in the zona pellucida using a laser on day 3 of development. Note the thickness of the zona pellucida compared with the day 5 embryo shown in the inset (E) with an un-manipulated zona pellucida.

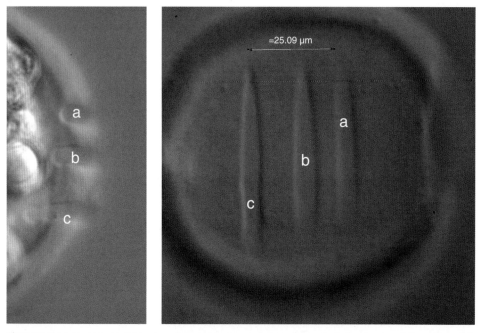

Figure 7.2 Laser-assisted hatching in a discarded human embryo to demonstrate the shape and dimensions of the opening (a–c). (A) Side view of three openings, each cutting further into the pervitelline space. (B) Top view of the same openings after removal of the cells/fragments. The deeper the cut (a–c), the longer the corresponding opening in the zona pellucida (a–c).

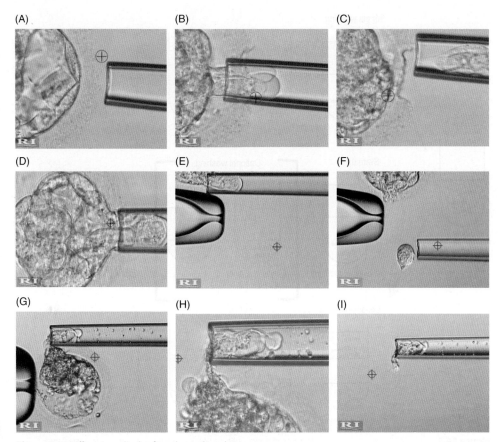

Figure 8.1 Different methods of trophectoderm biopsy.

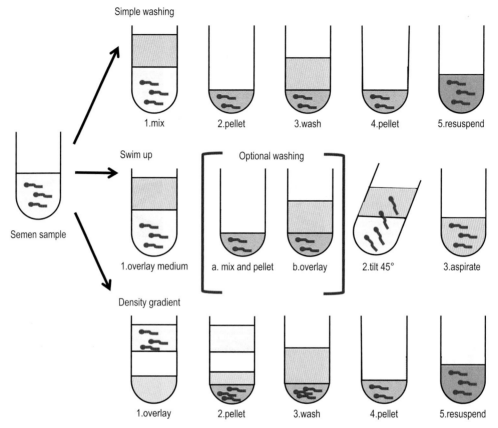

Figure 14.1 Schematic presentation of sperm preparation techniques (for exact procedure, see respective sections).

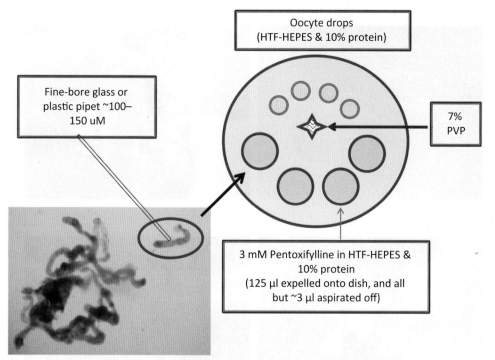

Figure 15.1 The ICSI dish for testicular sperm procedures. Seminiferous tubule contents are expelled into the large, flat drops of 3 mM pentoxifylline. The ICSI pipette is primed with 7% PVP before viable sperm are picked up and transferred to a peninsula of the PVP drop. (Method adapted from Craft and Tsirigotis.[10])

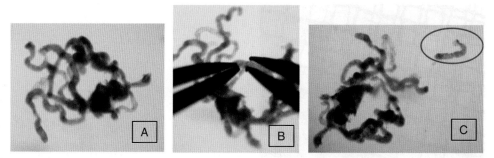

Figure 15.2 Seminiferous tubule processing. (A) Tubules are gently teased apart. (B) Two pairs of jeweler's forceps are used to release the contents of the seminiferous tubules by gentle squeezing. (C) The seminiferous tubule contents are in the circle. They will be transferred and dispersed into a drop of 3 mM pentoxifylline in the ICSI dish. (Please note that the tubules shown in these photographs are not typical of the very large, dilated tubules observed in testicular biopsies from men with OA. This specimen was selected because the narrow tubules allowed clearer images of the procedure.

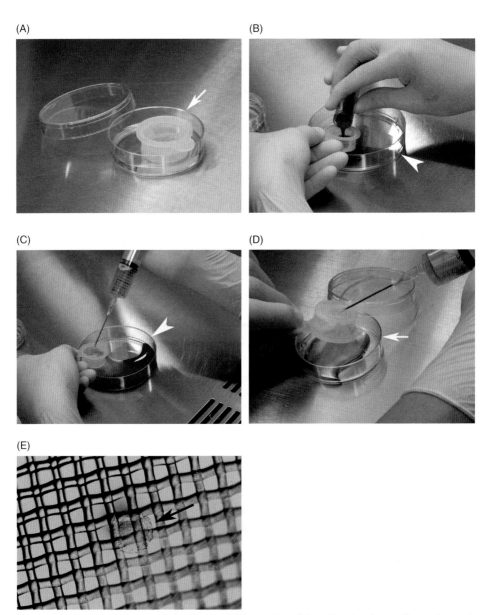

Figure 18.1 Procedures for oocyte identification. (A) Preparation of the cell strainer (arrow: 60-mm tissue culture dish). (B) The cell strainer and filtration of follicular aspirates (arrowhead: 100-mm tissue culture dish). (C) Red blood cells removed by the flushing medium. (D) Recovery of the COCs on the mesh filter. (E) A COC remaining on the cell strainer after rinsing (black arrow).

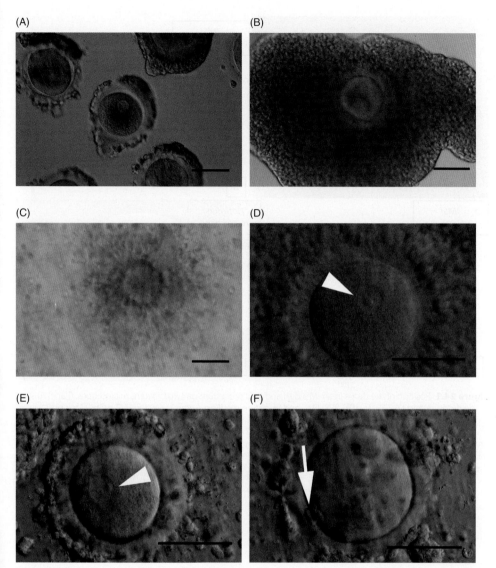

Figure 18.2 COC morphology and maturity of oocytes retrieved in IVM cycles. (A) An oocyte with sparse cumulus cells. (B) An oocyte with compacted cumulus cells. (C) An oocyte with expanded cumulus cells. (D) An oocyte with compacted cumulus cells and their GVs (arrowhead). (E) An oocytes with expanded cumulus cells and their GVs (arrowhead). (F) An oocyte with a first polar body (arrow) reflecting its maturity. Bar = 75 μm.

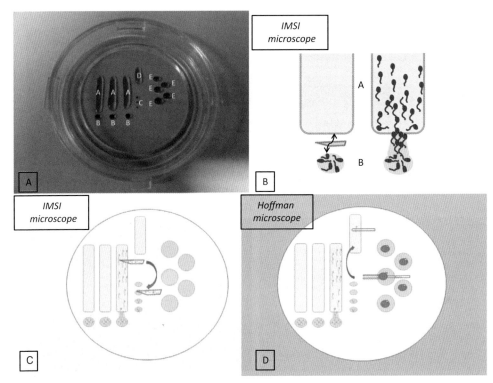

Figure 24.1 Position of the drops in an IMSI dish and IMSI procedure on two different microscopes. (Panel A) View of the drops: (A and D) 7.5% to 10% PVP; (B, C and E) culture medium. Sperm-selection PVP drops (A); sperm aliquot drops (B); host-selected spermatozoa microdrops (C); sperm immobilization drops (D); oocytes injection drops (E). (Panel B) Bridge with the selection micropipette between the sperm aliquots drops (B) and the sperm-selection PVP drops (A) (on the IMSI microscope). (Panel C) Selection of the spermatozoa in the sperm-selection PVP drops (A) and transfer to the host-selected spermatozoa microdrops (C) (on the IMSI microscope). (Panel D) Conventional ICSI on the Hoffman ICSI microscope.

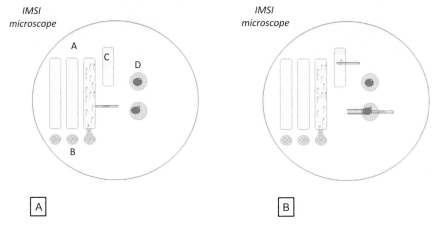

Figure 24.2 IMSI: description of the different steps for sperm selection (Panel A) and oocyte injection on the IMSI microscope (Panel B).

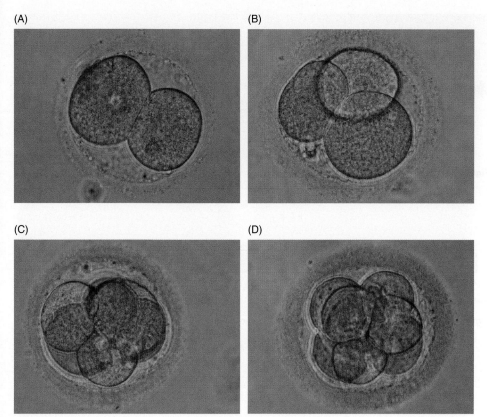

Figure 30.1 Cleavage embryo assessment. (A) Forty-three hours after insemination. Symmetrical blastomeres cleave with no fragmentation. (B) Forty-five hours after insemination. Asynchronous cleavage showing three blastomeres with no significant fragmentation. (C and D) Seventy hours after insemination. Day 3 embryos demonstrating symmetrical cleavage without significant fragmentation.

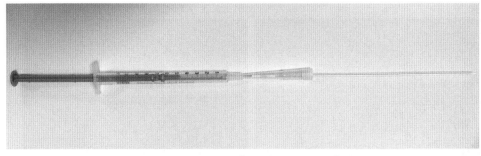

Figure 34.1 Syringe attached to pipette tip and straw for loading/expelling of straw.

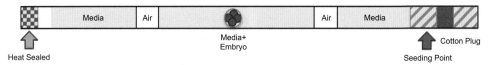

Figure 34.2 Schematic diagram of embryo loading and seeding.

(A)

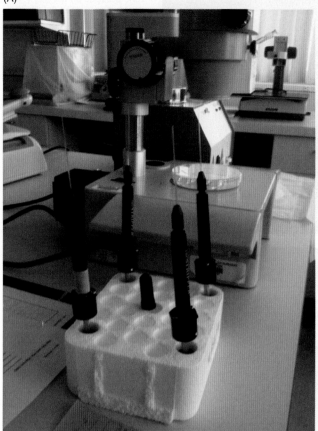

Figure 35.1 Micro-secure VTF setup includes a VTF dish (A) with distinct rows of solutions, which use three wash droplets before placement in distinct, numbered equilibration droplets. Additionally, individual pipetters with shortened VTF tips (i.e. 300-μm ID flexipettes) are secured and organized in a Styrofoam tube rack (B), which can be rotated for orderly use.

(B)

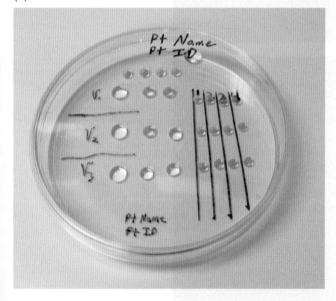

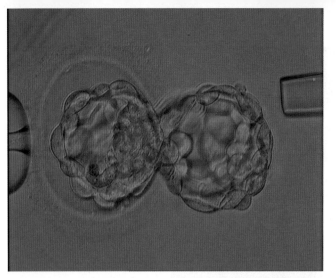

Figure 36.1 Herniating blastocyst. When opening the zona pellucida on day 3 or 4, as the blastocyst grows, it will start to herniated; that is, trophectoderm cells will begin to come out of the zona pellucida.

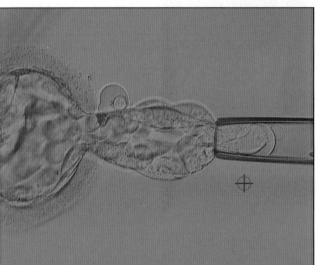

Figure 36.2 Aspiration of herniating trophectoderm cells. Tension is applied to the blastocyst by both holding and aspiration pipettes in order to stretch the blastocyst, showing a narrow bridge of trophectoderm cells between the aspirated cells and the cells still inside the zona pellucida.

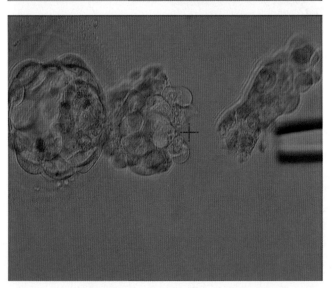

Figure 36.3 Fully detached biopsy piece. The trophectoderm biopsy piece is left in the biopsy dish (for the diagnostic laboratory), while the blastocyst is returned to the culture dish prior to vitrification, allowing time for the genetic analysis and potential transfer in a subsequent cycle.

Chapter

Insemination

21

Caroline McCaffrey, Melicia Clarke-Williams and
David H. McCulloh

Introduction

Appropriate procedures must be documented that describe all the steps performed during
an insemination of oocytes for in vitro fertilization (IVF). These procedures must be
designed to both optimize the fertilization of oocytes and prevent circumstances that
increase the risk of introduction, transmission or spread of communicable diseases through
the collection, preparation, culture and/or transfer of patients' gametes and embryos.

21.1 Background

During insemination, a sperm penetrates the oocyte's 'investments' (surrounding cumulus
cells, zona pellucida and ooplasmic membrane), depositing the contents of the sperm (its
nucleus and cytoplasm) in the cytoplasm of the oocyte. This can be accomplished either by
relying on the sperm's natural ability to insert itself into the cytoplasm of the egg (conventional insemination) or by intracytoplasmic sperm injection (ICSI).

Deciding which method of insemination to employ is complex and vitally important: in
conventional insemination, a suspension of motile sperm is co-incubated with the cumulus
oocyte complexes either for several hours or overnight. There is evidence to show that the
cumulus cells surrounding the oocyte continue to communicate with the oocyte even after
removal from the follicle and work in concert with the egg to perform, among other
functions, some 'natural selection' of the sperm that effects fertilization.[1]

With ICSI, each mature oocyte is injected with a sperm selected by the embryologist
under high-power magnification. While ICSI has been routinely employed now for more
than two decades with high success rates, it is undoubtedly more invasive than conventional
insemination, and while there appears to be no evidence that the procedure itself increases
chromosomal disorders, we believe that it should be applied only when there is a justifiable
reason to do so. In addition, while ICSI reduces the odds of complete failure of fertilization
or low fertilization, it does not provide a guarantee that it will increase the number of eggs
fertilized. This is so because (1) only eggs that are mature at time of ICSI will be injected
and therefore can be fertilized, (2) eggs appearing to have an extruded polar body but still at
the telophase stage of maturation may miss the window of fertilization following ICSI and
(3) some eggs may not survive the invasive procedure and become degenerate after ICSI
even in the most experienced hands.

It seems logical to assume that reducing the chance of failed fertilization will result in
more fertilized zygotes, leading to a high number of embryos from which to pick the best
embryo(s) for transfer. This, in turn, might be anticipated to improve the chances of
pregnancy when examined across many patient couples. However, this assumes that all

embryos, regardless of the means used to achieve fertilization, have the same probability of leading to a healthy live birth. For many years at several different facilities, we have observed that the incidence of live birth following insemination is slightly higher than the incidence of live birth following ICSI. Here at the New York University Fertility Clinic (NYUFC) between 2003 and 2013, for fresh transfers, live birth rates (live-born babies per embryo transferred) were 25.6 + 0.42% (N = 7,391 cases) for conventional insemination and 23.8 + 0.68% (N = 2,721 cases) for ICSI. Success with conventional insemination was significantly different from that with ICSI ($P \sim 0.027$). There could be several reasons for this: that sperm requiring ICSI are poorer in quality and lead to less optimal embryos with poorer potential to lead to a live birth or that the sperm injection procedure itself (or possibly the extended period outside the incubator during the procedure) may be harmful to oocytes, thereby rendering them slightly less likely to lead to a live birth. We believe that the invasive ICSI procedure is more likely to lead to irreparable harm[2] to an oocyte than is co-incubation with sperm. However, achieving fertilization using insemination is sometimes a challenge. Clearly, if ICSI is the only way to achieve fertilization, then it is the method that must be used; however, we have found that fertilization can be achieved using sperm that would be used only for ICSI in other facilities. At present, our use of ICSI is limited to roughly 25% to 30% of our cases. Typically, we use ICSI only when the sperm count and/or motility is below normal parameters (count < 20 million/ml, motility < 50% per World Health Organization edition 4 guidelines[3]), when the patient has a history of low or failed fertilization or for surgically retrieved sperm. Analysis of our own data has shown us that morphology assessment is of limited value and is not relevant when sperm counts and motility are above these normal thresholds. We found that when the total recovery of motile cells met or exceeded 2 million cells, ICSI was not necessary to effect fertilization.[4] An important adjunct to the widespread use of insemination is the widespread counselling of patients and management of their expectations by explaining that achieving fertilization is important but that ICSI does not always maximize the number of oocytes fertilized.

21.2 Equipment, Reagents, Standards and Controls

21.2.1 Equipment
- Dissecting microscope
- Inverted microscope
- Centrifuge
- Biological safety cabinet
- Sperm counting chamber
- Incubator (maintaining CO_2 at 6%, with or without low O_2 (5%))

21.2.2 Materials and Supplies
- Fertilization medium
- Protein supplement
- Sterile pipette tips
- Pasteur pipettes, 9-inch soda lime
- Pipetter
- Gloves, PVC powder free

21.2.3 Precautions

21.2.3.1 For Staff Safety

Use the necessary precautions for working with bodily fluids and tissues. Hands should be washed thoroughly before entering the laboratory, after completing a procedure and when leaving the laboratory for any period of time. Gloves and a mask should be worn during the preparation and handling of vessels containing gametes or embryos.

Sperm and oocytes as well as the medium in which they reside must be considered biohazardous and may contain pathogens that could affect your health. Sperm and oocyte specimens should be handled with care to avoid your exposure to any infectious diseases that may be in these specimens (treat them as though they are infectious).

All used supplies and solutions should be treated as biohazardous waste and disposed of accordingly in 'red bag' waste. 'Sharps' should be collected in labelled receptacles for disposal.

21.2.3.2 For the Safety of the Gametes and Embryos

Sperm and oocyte specimens should be handled with care to avoid contaminating the cultures with any pathogens (treat these cultures with sterile technique). Do not touch the fluid in the specimen.

Gametes and embryos are to be maintained at body temperature (37°C), and the pH of the medium is maintained by elevated CO_2 levels in the atmosphere surrounding the cultures. Minimize periods of handling oocytes and embryos outside the incubator in order to avoid the negative impact of temperature or pH fluctuations.

21.2.3.3 Specimens Required

1. The sperm specimen should be in a tube labelled with patient identification. Following specimen collection and processing, the final sample is re-suspended in pre-equilibrated protein-supplemented fertilization medium so that the final concentration is 10 to 20 × 10^6 sperm/ml with >90% motility. The sample is held in the CO_2 incubator pending the insemination procedure. The total motile sperm recovered is calculated using the following equation:

Sperm count (conc./ml) × volume of final suspension × percent motile/100%

   Example: Conc. $14 × 10^6$/ml, volume 0.2 ml, 93% motility $= 14 × 0.2 × 93\%/100\%$

   $= 2.6 × 10^6$ total motile

   Where the total motile sperm recovered is >2 million cells and in the absence of other factors such as prior failed or low fertilization or request by the patient, conventional insemination will be performed.

2. Oocytes should be in dishes labelled with patient identification. Following oocyte retrieval, the embryologist will have performed an assessment of the cumulus-oocyte complexes (COCs) and gently removed any blood or dark cells retained on the COCs with 1-ml tuberculin syringes fitted with 25G needles. The COCs are then rinsed with drops of pre-equilibrated culture medium and placed two per drop in 75-μl drops of pre-equilibrated, protein-supplemented culture medium that is overlaid with oil and placed in the incubator. Oocytes are inseminated approximately three to four hours after retrieval.

21.3 Procedure

Insemination is performed approximately three to four hours after retrieval, that is, approximately 40 hours after human chorionic gonadotrophin (hCG) or gonadotrophin-releasing hormone (GnRH) agonist trigger administration. The processed sperm specimen used for insemination should not be more than several hours old (time since preparation). For this procedure, only one patient couple's specimens (egg and sperm) can be removed from the incubator and handled at a workstation at any one time. Furthermore, this procedure requires two embryologists, one performing the insemination and the other performing an independent verification that the patient names and information on the appropriate tubes and dishes are correct and match. (Alternatively, the verification of identities and match can be performed electronically if the laboratory is equipped with an electronic witnessing system.)

Quality Control Check. The embryologist performing the insemination and a second embryologist must confirm that the patient information is correct and matches on the culture tube and dish, the semen analysis and sperm preparation report and the embryo tracking record.

21.4 Step-by-Step Instructions

1. A sterile Pasteur pipette is pulled using an alcohol burner to create a long, narrow bore tip and placed in the workstation where the insemination is to be performed. The pipette is fitted with a rubber bulb and checked that it allows for control of medium aspiration and displacement.

2. The semen analysis and sperm preparation report is reviewed, and the patient's name and date of birth and her partner's name are verified.

3. The dish(s) containing the oocytes is(are) removed from the incubator along with the culture tube containing the prepared sperm. A final check of all identity parameters on the oocyte dish(es) and sperm preparation tube is conducted by both embryologists to ensure that samples are correctly matched to each other.

4. Using the sterile pulled pipette, mix the sperm suspension well by pipetting it up and down in the tube. A final check of the sample quality and motility is performed by placing a small aliquot of the sperm suspension in the centre drop that contains no oocytes. This is to identify sperm samples in which motility of the processed specimen drops off dramatically, indicating a potential problem with sperm viability. When this situation occurs, the use of conventional insemination is re-evaluated. If warranted, the method of insemination will be changed to ICSI.

5. Depending on the sperm concentration and overall quality of the sperm, add a small aliquot of the sperm suspension (roughly 1–2 µl) to each of the droplets containing the oocytes. Perform this step while observing the drops under the dissecting microscope.

6. Confirm the concentration in each of the drops by assessing the density of sperm swimming along the bottom and edge of the drop using the inverted microscope in order to ensure that the appropriate concentration has been achieved. The number of motile sperm added ranges from 15,000 to 40,000/drop and is documented in the patient's records. This number of motile sperm deposited in a 75-µl drop results in a final concentration of between 200,000 and 533,000 motile sperm per millilitre.

7. Place the dishes back in the patient's designated location in the incubator and allow them to remain undisturbed overnight until fertilization assessment is performed 18 to 20 hours later.

8. Update the patient's record to document the time at which the insemination procedure was performed and the identities of the laboratory staff who performed the insemination and witnessing steps.

21.5 Calculations

Calculation of volume of sperm preparations to add to achieve the concentration in culture:

$$[\text{Sperm}]_{\text{final}} = [\text{Sperm}]_{\text{sperm\_prep.}} \times \text{Volume}_{\text{sperm\_aliquot}} / (\text{Volume}_{\text{oocyte\_drop}} + \text{Volume}_{\text{sperm\_aliquot}}) \tag{21.1}$$

where

$[\text{Sperm}]_{\text{sperm\_prep.}}$ = concentration of motile sperm (M/ml) in prepared sperm specimen

$[\text{Sperm}]_{\text{final}}$ = desired concentration of motile sperm (M/ml) in insemination drop

$\text{Volume}_{\text{oocyte\_drop}}$ = volume (μl) of insemination drop holding the oocytes

and

$$\text{Volume}_{\text{sperm\_aliquot}} = \text{volume (μl) of prepared sperm specimen to be added to insemination drop}$$

When $[\text{Sperm}]_{\text{final}} \ll [\text{Sperm}]_{\text{sperm\_prep.}}$, then $\text{Volume}_{\text{sperm\_aliquot}}$ is negligible compared to $\text{Volume}_{\text{oocyte\_drop}}$, and then the calculation simplifies to

$$[\text{Sperm}]_{\text{final}} = [\text{Sperm}]_{\text{sperm\_prep.}} \times \text{Volume}_{\text{sperm\_aliquot}} / \text{Volume}_{\text{oocyte\_drop}} \tag{21.2}$$

Since $[\text{Sperm}]_{\text{sperm\_prep}}$ is adjusted to be between 10 and 20 M/ml, and since the desired range of $[\text{Sperm}]_{\text{final}}$ is about 0.2 to 0.6 M/ml (200,000 to 600,000 sperm per millilitre), the required condition $[\text{Sperm}]_{\text{final}} \ll [\text{Sperm}]_{\text{sperm\_prep}}$ is met, and the simpler Equation (21.2) may be used. Rearrangement of Equation (21.2) yields the volume of sperm preparation to add ($\text{Volume}_{\text{sperm\_aliquot}}$) to achieve a desired $[\text{Sperm}]_{\text{final}}$:

$$\text{Volume}_{\text{sperm\_aliquot}} = \text{Volume}_{\text{oocyte\_drop}} \times [\text{Sperm}]_{\text{final}} / [\text{Sperm}]_{\text{sperm\_prep}} \tag{21.3}$$

21.6 Frequency and Tolerance of Controls

There are no controls for this procedure. The two reagents (sperm and oocytes) are unique to the patient couple. Whereas use of donor sperm with the oocytes or donor oocytes with the sperm would be a valid control, it is generally not acceptable to the patient couple.

21.7 Expected Values

We monitor fertilization rates for both conventional insemination and ICSI on an ongoing basis and conduct a review of this key performance index every three months to ensure that values are within expected parameters. Fertilization rates for conventional insemination have remained very steady for over 10 years, averaging around 70% of the mature oocytes (as identified on day 1 following fertilization check) having two pronuclei. For the three-year period between 1 January 2012 and 31 December 2014, the standard deviation of this value was 22%. Thus, we typically anticipate that any fertilization rate above 26% is within the 95% confidence limit of the mean value. If multiple occurrences of fertilization rates occur with less than a 26% fertilization rate within a small number of consecutive cases, one should consider whether there is some systemic problem.

Despite careful review of each case using the criteria described, we experienced 1.4% cases (112 of 7,844 over the 10-year period 2005–2014) with complete fertilization failure using conventional insemination. Whether these are due to an egg-related issue or a sperm parameter is difficult to determine, but the incidence of fertilization failure is much greater (8.5%) in patient couples with fewer than five mature eggs (56 of 661 cases). Following fertilization failure with conventional insemination, subsequent cycles will always be conducted using ICSI. Surprisingly, we also observed complete fertilization failure with ICSI in our practice for 1.8% of our cases (64 of 3,496 over the same 10-year period but including only ICSIs performed on day 0). We routinely review all cases that occur with 0% fertilization rate.

21.8 Procedural Notes

We believe that fertilization occurs through the chance collision of sperm with the investments surrounding the oocyte. We also believe that these investments do not 'consume' significant numbers of sperm during insemination. Therefore, we believe that the probability of sperm colliding with the investments occurs as a function of the concentration of sperm in the insemination drop (as a first-order chemical reaction, commonly referred to as 'occurring by mass action'). Hence, we use the same procedure for insemination of each drop in the dish regardless of the number of oocytes in the droplet.

21.9 Limitations

The decision whether to use conventional insemination versus ICSI is a complex and important one because complete fertilization failure means that the treatment cycle has already failed. While many laboratories have opted to perform ICSI in all or most cases to minimize the possibility of fertilization failure, we review every case individually. Factors affecting that decision include sperm count and motility on semen analysis, history of fertilization for the couple in prior IVF cycles, prior pregnancies naturally or with intrauterine insemination (IUI) cycles, patient requests, count, motility and recovery of motile sperm on the day of retrieval as well as oocyte maturity. Some eggs may benefit from the continued contact with the COC possible with conventional insemination. In cases where it is unclear whether there may be low-grade male factor infertility or egg-related issues, a good option is to perform split ICSI/insemination if an adequate number of mature eggs have been retrieved. This approach allows for a diagnosis as well as providing a safety net for the patient and laboratory.

References

1. Tanghe, S., Van Soom, A., Nauwynck, H., Coryn, M. and De Kruif, A. Minireview: functions of the cumulus oophorus during oocyte maturation, ovulation and fertilization. *Mol Reprod & Dev* 2002; 61:414–24.

2. McCulloh, D. H., Goorbarry, J., Shah, S. and Ahmad, K. Oocyte lysis following intracytoplasmic sperm injection: association with measures of oocyte quality and technician performance. *J Reprod Stem Cell Biotech* 2011; 2(1):46–54.

3. World Health Organization (WHO). *Laboratory Manual for the Examination of*

Human Semen and Sperm-Cervical Mucus Interaction (4th edn.) (Cambridge University Press, 2004).

4. Keegan, B. R., Barton, S., Sanchez, S., Berkeley, A. S., Krey, L. C. et al. Isolated teratozoospermia does not affect in vitro fertilization outcome and is not an indication for intracytoplasmic sperm injection. *Fertil Steril* 2007; 88 (6):1583–8.

5. Gianaroli, L., Magli, M. C., Ferraretti, A. P., Fiorentino, A., Tosti, E. et al. Reducing the time of sperm-oocyte interaction in human in-vitro fertilization improves the implantation rate. *Hum Reprod* 1996; 11:166–71.

6. Lin, S.-P., Lee, R. K.-K., Su, J.-T., Lin, M.-H. and Hwu, Y.-M. The effects of brief gamete co-incubation in human in vitro fertilization *J Assist Reprod Genet* 2000; 17:344–8.

Chapter 22

Conventional IVF with Short Co-Incubation

Giannoula Karagouga and Dean E. Morbeck

Introduction

Since the advent of in vitro fertilization (IVF), conventional insemination has remained essentially unchanged and for most IVF laboratories involves overnight co-incubation of sperm with oocytes despite the fact that few sperm reach the Fallopian tube or the oocyte in vivo. This fundamental difference between clinical practice and physiology has only received limited attention, even though the presence of potentially adverse reactive oxygen species (ROS) and other products of sperm metabolism are known and may be significant. Optimization of insemination methods thus may achieve better embryo quality and clinical outcomes. A short insemination protocol is one method that addresses this divergence. Studies on a short insemination protocol (1–4 hours instead of 15–20 hours) demonstrate similar fertilization rate, embryo cleavage rates and pregnancy rates.[1] Since human sperm capacitation requires only 45 minutes of contact between oocytes and spermatozoa, these observations are not unexpected. These findings and the information presented in this chapter illustrate that short insemination is an effective method for IVF that, furthermore, provides benefits for programmes using time-lapse (TL) imaging. While historically only intracytoplasmic sperm injection (ICSI) oocytes can be observed for fertilization with TL imaging, short co-incubation insemination facilitates early TL culture for all IVF cycles, making early-morning fertilization checks obsolete and freeing staff to perform other duties. Furthermore, TL imaging affords the advantage of identifying oocytes that show normal fertilization outside the standard window of time used for fertilization assessment.

22.1 Background

Fertilization is a delicately programmed process comprised of numerous cellular and molecular events in sequence. The fertilization process in humans involves sperm and oocyte binding, acrosome reaction, oocyte activation, formation of oocyte and sperm pronuclei and syngamy.[2] A beneficial effect of short exposure (one to four hours) of sperm to oocytes could be the result of reduced exposure to sperm by-products.[1] Morphologically abnormal spermatozoa and leucocytes are considered the main sources of ROS production in semen.[3] Sperm intracellular mechanisms may generate ROS and other deleterious products from sperm metabolism at the level of the plasma membrane[4] and mitochondria.[5] One adverse consequence of ROS is zona hardening, which may prevent embryos from hatching and reduce their viability.[6,7] The quantity and quality of spermatozoa present, as well as the duration of exposure to surrounding temperature and culture medium composition, can determine the harmful results of ROS.[8]

Overnight co-incubation with sperm exposes oocytes and zygotes to suboptimal culture medium due to increased levels of ROS. Shortening the co-incubation time of oocytes and sperm may improve IVF outcomes by reducing the detrimental effect of ROS on the zygotes and the quality of the embryos.[9–11]

The standard strategy for handling oocytes for short insemination involves removing the oocyte along with associated coronal and cumulus granulosa cells and placing them in a fresh drop of culture medium for overnight culture until fertilization check. In contrast, the protocol described here uses complete removal of coronal granulosa cells after the three-hour co-incubation to allow placement of inseminated oocytes in fresh drops for observation via TL imaging. While most of the studies on brief three-hour co-incubation of gametes include complete removal of coronal granulosa cells at the time of fertilization check (15–20 hours), studies on complete removal after six hours[13] as well as the wealth of experience with complete removal prior to ICSI indicate that the method presented herein is the next logical extension of embryology practice as it incorporates TL imaging.

22.2 Reagents, Supplies and Equipment

- Embryo growth medium
- Fertilization medium
- Human serum albumin (HSA)
- Mineral oil (washed)

22.3 Procedure

22.3.1 Conventional Insemination Three-Hour Co-Incubation Setup (Day −1)

1. Check clinic order for recommendation for type of insemination method.
2. Complete all necessary paperwork, and label dishes and tubes.
3. Prepare media, oil dishes and organ culture dishes according to the insemination method and number of follicles reported at time of human chorionic gonadothrphin (hCG).
4. Prepare the following media:

   a. Insemination medium (IM): fertilization medium + 5% HSA (5 mg/ml)
   b. Post-fertilization medium (GM): embryo growth medium + 10% serum protein substitute (SPS)
   c. Mineral oil

5. Prepare organ culture dishes for insemination and culture of oocytes after three-hour co-incubation with sperm stored in bench-top incubators.

   a. Prepare sperm/oocyte co-incubation organ culture dishes: 1.0 ml IM overlayed with 1.0 ml mineral oil.
   b. Prepare post-co-incubation rinse of organ culture dishes. Beneath the centre well, label consecutive drop numbers around the periphery of the well. Dishes will hold five drops of 20 µl GM in the centre well for oocyte culture and three drops of 100 µl in the moat for rinsing. Prepare drops and quickly cover with washed mineral oil, 1.0 ml in the centre well and 4.0 ml in the moat. Oil must be added immediately to avoid medium evaporation.

    c. Prepare embryo culture dish/slide as per standard protocol.

6. Place prepared dishes in incubators for overnight equilibration (pH target 7.30 in low oxygen (5%)).

22.3.2 Insemination Protocol: Day 0 (Retrieval)

1. Record temperatures and pH values of incubators and patient media.
2. Perform oocyte retrieval per standard protocol, making sure that the cumulus is clear of blood. Store oocytes in IM at 37°C and CO_2 appropriate to obtain desired pH (7.3).
3. After the aspirate searching is complete, place oocytes in organ culture dishes for standard insemination. Transfer the oocytes with a 5-inch pipette with no more than 20 µl of medium. Place two to six oocytes in each organ culture dish.
4. Calculate the correct insemination concentration (200,000 motile sperm/ml). Inseminate oocytes four hours after collection of last follicle aspirate (range of 4–6 hours).
5. Prior to insemination, verify patient identification during insemination by two different embryologists.
6. Use a 200-µl pipette tip for insemination into the organ culture dish. Volume of inseminate should be less than 20 µl.

    a. Place the tip with sperm at the bottom of the dish by the oocyte-cumulus mass when dispensing. In the first organ culture dish, perform a visual qualitative check for motile sperm with forward progression using the inverted microscope. If motile sperm with good forward progression are present and motility has not decreased since the last assessment, proceed with the addition of sperm to the remaining dishes. If sperm lack motility or forward progression appears reduced, consult the laboratory director and consider conversion to ICSI.

    b. Return insemination dish(es) to incubator.

7. After three hours of co-incubation of eggs and sperm, remove insemination dishes and rinse them. Using a 275- to 300-µM and then 150-µM flexible tips, completely denude each oocyte by vigorously pipetting to remove all coronal cells.
8. Rinse the oocytes through the remaining rinse drops, and place them into the 20-µl drops. Using the inverted microscope, determine maturity, and place germinal vesicle (GV) stage and atretic oocytes into separate microdrops.
9. If not culturing in TL, place the MII and MI oocytes in microdrops of culture medium with protein in equilibrated dishes and place them in the conventional or bench-top incubator until the next day for the fertilization check.
10. Note that if the cumulus mass is not dispersed (difficulty removing the egg from the cumulus) after three hours of co-incubation, add additional sperm to the microdrop at an amount of 1/50 of the original volume if using a 20-µl drops or 1/20 of the original volume if using 50-l drops. Keep oocytes overnight in microdrops with sperm for standard conventional insemination.

References

1. Huang, Z., Li, J., Wang, L., Yan, J., Shi, Y. et al. Brief co-incubation of sperm and oocytes for in vitro fertilization techniques. *Cochrane Database Syst Rev* 2013; 4: CD009391.

2. Oehninger, S., Mahony, M., Ozgur, K., Kolm, P., Kruger, T. et al. Clinical significance of human sperm-zona

pellucida binding. *Fertil Steril* 1997; 67:1121–7.

3. Saleh, R. A. and Agarwal, A. Oxidative stress and male infertility: from research bench to clinical practice. *J Androl* 2002; 23:737–52.

4. Aitken, R. J., Buckingham, D., West, K., Wu, F. C., Zikopoulos, K. et al. Differential contribution of leucocytes and spermatozoa to the generation of reactive oxygen species in the ejaculates of oligozoospermic patients and fertile donors. *J Reprod Fertil* 1992; 94:451–62.

5. Gavella, M. and Lipovac, V. NADH-dependent oxidoreductase (diaphorase) activity and isozyme pattern of sperm in infertile men. *Arch Androl* 1992; 28:135–41.

6. Quinn, P., Lydic,. M. L, Ho, .M, Bastuba, M., Hendee, F. et al. Confirmation of the beneficial effects of brief coincubation of gametes in human in vitro fertilization. *Fertil Steril* 1998; 69:399–402.

7. Dirnfeld, M., Bider, D., Koifman, M., Calderon, I. and Abramovici, H. Shortened exposure of oocytes to spermatozoa improves in-vitro fertilization outcome: a prospective, randomized, controlled study. *Hum Reprod* 1999; 14:2562–4.

8. Dumoulin, J. C., Bras, M., Land, J. A., Pieters, M. H., Enginsu, M. E. et al. Effect of the number of inseminated spermatozoa on subsequent human and mouse embryonic development in vitro. *Hum Reprod* 1992; 7:1010–3.

9. Coskun, S., Roca, G. L., Elnour, A. M., al Mayman, H., Hollanders, J. M. et al. Effects of reducing insemination time in human in vitro fertilization and embryo development by using sibling oocytes. *J Assist Reprod Genet* 1998; 15:605–8.

10. Dirnfeld, M., Shiloh, H., Bider, D., Harari, E., Koifman, M. et al. A prospective randomized controlled study of the effect of short coincubation of gametes during insemination on zona pellucida thickness. *Gynecol Endocrinol* 2003; 17:397–403.

11. Gianaroli, L., Cristina Magli, M., Ferraretti, A. P., Fiorentino, A., Tosti, E. et al. Reducing the time of sperm-oocyte interaction in human in-vitro fertilization improves the implantation rate. *Hum Reprod* 1996; 11:166–71.

12. Kattera, S. and Chen, C. Short coincubation of gametes in in vitro fertilization improves implantation and pregnancy rates: a prospective, randomized, controlled study. *Fertil Steril* 2003; 80:1017–21.

13. Xiong, S., Han, W., Liu, J. X., Zhang, X. D., Liu, W. W., et al. Effects of cumulus cells removal after 6 h co-incubation of gametes on the outcomes of human IVF. *J Assist Reprod Genet* 2011; 28:1205–11.

Chapter 23

Technical Aspect of ICSI for Ejaculated Spermatozoa

Gianpiero D. Palermo, Tyler Cozzubbo and Queenie V. Neri

Introduction

After the establishment of in vitro fertilization (IVF), it soon became clear that as many as 40% of the inseminated in vitro cycles were affected by fertilization failure or at best by an extremely low fertilization.[1] The early use of intracytoplasmic sperm injection (ICSI) required some adjustments to identify the best method to pierce the membrane and to identify the best location within the ooplasm in which to release the spermatozoon. It soon became apparent that this unconventional method of insemination was capable of fertilizing nearly every mature egg injected. Moreover, the ability to pinpoint the different steps of pronuclei appearance and to monitor the observation of the first embryonic cleavage without the obstructive layer of cumulus cells would facilitate tracking these relevant steps involved in the generation of the conceptus.

Because of its wide utility and reliability, ICSI has been widely adopted as the preferred insemination method in many circumstances.[2–5] According to the International Committee Monitoring Assisted Reproductive Technologies (ICMART), 'ICSI comprised 66% of all oocytes retrieved a continued increase from 60.6% in 2004 and 62.9% in 2005. The proportion of ICSI procedures varied according to region: 96% in the Middle East, 81% in Latin America, 70% in North America, 76% in Europe and 56% in Australia and New Zealand.' ICSI generated over 60% of the total assisted reproductive technologies (ART) children estimated at over 256,668 in 2004.[3] At our centre, there has been a steady and progressive increase in ICSI prevalence starting at 32% in 1993, rising to 50% in 1995 and reaching 73% by 2002.[6]

Since its introduction, ICSI has been awarded as the ultimate assisted fertilization procedure to be used for the treatment of male factor infertility and has rendered conception and parenthood possible to couples who otherwise would have remained childless.[7]

23.1 ICSI Indications

The ICSI procedure can be used successfully in patients with fertilization failure after conventional IVF and also in patients with too few morphologically normal and progressive motile spermatozoa present in the ejaculate (<500,000 sperm cells). High fertilization and pregnancy rates are achieved when a viable spermatozoon is injected, independent of its characteristics.[8] Injection of exclusively immotile spermatozoa results in a lower fertilization rate because it is impossible to distinguish the viable cells.[9]

When only non-vital sperm cells are present in the ejaculate, the use of testicular spermatozoa is indicated.[10] Semen parameters, such as concentration, morphological features and high titre of anti-sperm antibodies,[11] do not influence success rate.[12] Successful ICSI has also been described in patients with acrosomeless spermatozoa,[13,14] with the exception of globozoospermia type I,[12] where procedures such as assisted oocyte activation must be used.[15]

ICSI cannot be applied when no sperm cells are available or when no mature oocytes are retrieved. ICSI failure rates range from 1% to 3% when a lower number of eggs are injected; these failures are caused by a combination of missed fertilization, abnormal fertilization including one and three pronuclei (diagynic)[16,17] and lysis of the oocytes. Rarer still, fertilization with ICSI may fail despite an adequate number of oocytes and sufficient spermatozoa available because of missed ooplasmic maturation due to nuclear cytoplasmic asynchrony.[6]

A recurrent condition that is more difficult to address with ICSI is when few motile spermatozoa with suboptimal morphology are available. Our centre routinely treats severely oligospermic men with $\leq 1 \times 10^6$/ml of spermatozoa. Between 1993 and 2013, in 1,660 ICSI cycles using spermatozoa from these men, the average sperm concentration was $1.3 \pm 0.3 \times 10^6$/ml, with a motility of $20.6 \pm 22\%$ and normal morphology of only $1.0 \pm 2\%$. The fertilization in this group was 64.4% (10,131 of 15,738), resulting in an acceptable clinical pregnancy rate of 50.7% (842 of 1,660).

Once a couple has decided to use their own gametes, even in the face of difficulties, one option is to attempt the ART cycle with ejaculated spermatozoa, possibly supported by some trials of specimen cryopreservation to safeguard the couple from rare but feasible occurrences of azoospermia at the time of egg retrieval. If the initial semen specimen examination in the Makler chamber yields no spermatozoa, a high-speed centrifugation is often able to find scarce cells. In 244 cycles, after high-speed centrifugation, a mean density of $0.42 \pm 1.5 \times 10^6$/ml and motility of $35.9 \pm 32\%$ were reached. In this cohort, we obtained a fertilization of 60.3% (1,500 of 2,488), and replacement of an average of 2.6 embryos per patient resulted in a satisfactory intrauterine pregnancy rate of 48.4% (118 of 224).

23.2 Equipment

- Micromanipulation system
- Hydraulic microinjector, modified with a metal syringe
- Injector, air-filled
- BDH oil – for loading the injector (BDH Laboratory Supplies, Poole, Dorset, England)
- Inverted microscope with Polarized Optics CFI S Plan Fluor (20× and 40× objectives) and CFI Apo (2×, 4× and 10× objectives)
- Vibration-free table
- Custom-designed horseshoe-shaped heated stage
- Microtools

  . Injection pipette (4–6 µm ID; 30-degree bend angle)
  . Injection pipette (5–6 µm ID; 30-degree bend angle)
  . Holding pipette (120µm OD; 30-degree bend angle)

- Oocyte transfer and denudation pipettes (hand-pulled, flame-polished Pasteur pipettes)
- ICSI dish
- Stereomicroscope
- Repetitive pipette – ICSI medium dispenser
- Electronic repeating pipette – oil dispenser
- Pipette – polyvinylpyrrolidone (PVP) and sperm loading

23.3 Reagents

- ICSI hyaluronidase
- Embryo culture medium
- ICSI injection medium
- Tissue culture oil
- 7% PVP with human serum albumin (HSA)
- 0.35 mM pentoxifylline

23.4 Male Gamete Preparation

1. Semen samples are collected by masturbation after at least three days of abstinence; they are then allowed to liquefy for approximately 20 minutes at 37°C prior to analysis. Other methods of semen collection such as electro-ejaculation and retrograde ejaculation have been described elsewhere.[18]

2. Semen concentration and motility are assessed in a counting chamber. As might be expected, morphological quality of the sperm has a significant positive correlation with male infertility, and the evaluation is performed using the World Health Organization (WHO) 2010 criteria.[19] Evaluations are carried out by spreading 10 μl of semen or sperm suspension on pre-stained slides, which can provide rapid results. At least 200 spermatozoa per slide are categorized microscopically at 100× under oil immersion. Two counts are performed for both concentration and morphology. Semen quality is considered suboptimal when the sperm concentration is less than 15×10^6/ml, the progressive motility is less than 40% or the proportion of spermatozoa with normal morphology is less than 4% of the spermatozoa.[19]

3. For selection of spermatozoa, the sample is washed by centrifugation at 600×g for five minutes in human tubal fluid (HTF) medium supplemented with 0.4% HSA. Semen samples with fewer than 5×10^6/ml spermatozoa or fewer than 20% motile spermatozoa are washed in a home-brew medium by a single centrifugation at 600×g for five minutes. The re-suspended pellet is layered on a discontinuous density gradient on two layers (90% and 50%) or a single layer (90%) and then centrifuged at 300×g for 20 minutes. The sperm-rich fraction is rinsed by adding 4 ml of culture medium and centrifuged at 500 to 1,800×g for five minutes to remove silica gel particles. For spermatozoa with poor kinetic characteristics, the sperm suspension is exposed to a 0.35 mM solution of pentoxifylline. The concentration of the assessed sperm suspension is adjusted to 1 to 1.5×10^6/ml, when necessary, by the addition of HTF medium, and subsequently incubated at 37°C in 5% CO_2 in air.

23.5 Oocyte Collection

1. Superovulation is performed by administration of gonadotrophins in association with an agonist or antagonist protocol.[20,21] Human chorionic gonadotrophin (hCG) is administered when criteria for oocyte maturity are met, and oocyte retrieval by vaginal ultrasound-guided puncture is performed 35 hours later.

2. Under the inverted microscope at 100×, the cumulus corona cell complexes are scored as mature, slightly immature, completely immature or slightly over-mature. Thereafter, the oocytes are incubated for three to four hours.

3. Immediately prior to micromanipulation, the cumulus corona cells are removed by exposure to HTF-HEPES-buffered medium containing 40 IU/ml of hyaluronidase. The removal is necessary for observation of the oocyte and effective use of the holding and/or injecting pipette during micromanipulation. For final removal of the residual corona cells, the oocytes are repeatedly aspirated in and out of a hand-drawn Pasteur pipette with an inner diameter of ~200 µm. Each oocyte is then examined under the microscope to assess the maturation stage and its integrity, metaphase II (MII) being assessed according to the absence of the germinal vesicle and the presence of an extruded polar body. ICSI is performed only in oocytes that have reached this level of maturity.

23.6 Intracytoplasmic Sperm Injection (ICSI)

23.6.1 Tool Settings

1. The holding and injection pipettes are inserted into the respective micromanipulation tool holders mounted on an inverted microscope. The controllers are pneumatic for the holding pipette and oil filled for the injection pipette.
2. Using the coarse motorized controllers, the pipettes are positioned in the centre of the microscopic field at 20×, and then the magnification is gradually increased while maintaining the tools in focus by adjusting the hydraulic controllers. Under the highest magnification (400×), correct pipette positioning is achieved only by use of the hydraulic joysticks, and both pipettes should be able to course through the entire optical field. With regards to tool tip angles, the distal bent portions of both microtools should be slightly above parallel to avoid the elbows touching the bottom of the dish and interfering with the control. This also allows prompt immobilization and visual control of the spermatozoon inside the injection pipette.
3. Once properly aligned, the pipettes are raised by means of the coarse motorized controllers to allow placement of the ICSI dish on the microscope stage.

23.6.2 ICSI Dish Preparation

1. Nine drops containing 8 µl of injection medium are placed in a Petri dish, with one in the centre radially surrounded by the other eight. The drops should be as close together as possible to allow full visualization within the 20-mm opening on the heated stage.[22]
2. The drops should then be gently overlaid with culture oil (4 ml) to prevent evaporation.
3. Using a red non-embryo-toxic wax pencil, the 12 o'clock position is marked, a circle is drawn around the central drop and the drops are sequentially numbered starting from the 12 o'clock position, moving counter-clockwise. This allows easy navigation between droplets during ICSI.
4. The ICSI dishes are stored at 37°C until use.

23.6.3 Loading Gametes into the ICSI Dish

1. Immediately prior to injection under a stereomicroscope, the central drop is removed and replaced with 1 µl of sperm suspension diluted in 4 µl of 7% PVP.
2. Using a hand-pulled Pasteur pipette, MII oocytes are aspirated from the culture dish, and a single oocyte is placed in each drop.

23.6.4 Sperm Immobilization

1. Position the spermatozoon at 90 degrees with respect to the pipette's tip, and gently lower the cylindrical tip to compress the principal piece of the tail by rolling the posterior flagellum over the bottom of the Petri dish. If initially unsuccessful, the procedure is repeated until the tail is clearly kinked, looped or convoluted.[23] It is important to note, however, that a misshapen tail may adhere to the dish or to the inner surface of the pipette.

2. The spermatozoon is aspirated tail first. The injection needle is lifted slightly via the two control knobs of the joystick to avoid damaging the needle spike. The microscope stage is then repositioned until the injection needle enters the oocyte drop. It is important to note that the difference in media consistency (PVP versus culture medium) may allow the sperm to move distally into the pipette and become loose.

23.6.5 Injection

1. To find the egg, the magnification is briefly lowered to 200×, and once the egg is centrally in the field, the magnification is brought back to 400×.

2. The oocyte is held in place by suction through the holding pipette, and using both tools, the oocyte is rotated slowly to locate the polar body and the area of cortical rarefraction (or polar granularity). When the equatorial plane of the oocyte is located, the depth of the holding pipette is adjusted to have its internal opening in the same plane. It is ideal to have the inferior pole of the oocyte touching the bottom of the dish as it affords a better grip on the egg during the injection procedure.

3. The injection pipette is lowered and focused via the outer right border of the oolemma on the equatorial plane at 3 o'clock. Bring the spermatozoon close to the bevelled opening of the injection pipette, and then bring the pipette to the zona, press against it to begin penetration and thrust forward to the inner surface of the oolemma at 9 o'clock. At this point, a break in the membrane should occur at the approximate centre of the egg. Such a break is indicated by a sudden quivering of the convexities of the oolemma (at the site of invagination) above and below the penetration point, as well as by the proximal flow of cytoplasmic organelles and the spermatozoon back into the pipette.

4. The spermatozoon is then ejected with the cytoplasmic component. To optimize its interaction with the cytoplasm, the sperm should be ejected past the tip of the pipette to ensure a close intermingling with the ooplasmic lattices, which helps to maintain the sperm in place while withdrawing the pipette. To induce oocyte activation, additional ooplasm is gently aspirated back and forth with the injection pipette. It is paramount to avoid leaving behind residual medium with the spermatozoon as well as closing the breach of penetration. This is accomplished by generating a mild suction while removing the pipette. To do this, when the pipette is at the approximate centre of the egg, some surplus medium is re-aspirated so that the cytoplasmic structures can envelop the sperm, thereby reducing the size of the breach. This also expedites closure of the terminal part of the funnel-shaped opening at 3 o'clock.

5. Once the pipette is extracted, the edges of the entry point should maintain a funnel shape with the tip towards the centre of the egg. If the border of the oolemma becomes everted, the cytoplasmic organelles can leak out and the oocyte may lyse. The average time required to accomplish a single oocyte injection is about 30 to 40 seconds.

References

1. Cohen, J., Edwards, R. G., Fehilly, C. B., Fishel, S. B., Hewitt, J. et al. Treatment of male infertility by in vitro fertilization: factors affecting fertilization and pregnancy. *Acta Eur Fertil* 1984; 15:455–65.

2. Nyboe Andersen, A., Carlsen, E. and Loft, A. Trends in the use of intracytoplasmatic sperm injection marked variability between countries. *Hum Reprod Update* 2008; 14:593–604.

3. Mansour, R., Ishihara, O., Adamson, G. D., Dyer, S., de Mouzon, J. et al. International Committee for Monitoring Assisted Reproductive Technologies world report: assisted reproductive technology 2006. *Hum Reprod* 2014; 29:1536–51.

4. Fishel, S., Aslam, I., Lisi, F., Rinaldi, L., Timson, J. et al. Should ICSI be the treatment of choice for all cases of in-vitro conception? *Hum Reprod* 2000; 15:1278–83.

5. Aboulghar, M. A., Mansour, R. T., Serour, G. I., Sattar, M. A. and Amin, Y. M. Intracytoplasmic sperm injection and conventional in vitro fertilization for sibling oocytes in cases of unexplained infertility and borderline semen. *J Assist Reprod Genet* 1996; 13:38–42.

6. Palermo, G. D., Neri, Q. V., Monahan, D., Kocent, J. and Rosenwaks, Z. Development and current applications of assisted fertilization. *Fertil Steril* 2012; 97:248–59.

7. Moomjy, M., Sills, E. S., Rosenwaks, Z. and Palermo, G. D. Implications of complete fertilization failure after intracytoplasmic sperm injection for subsequent fertilization and reproductive outcome. *Hum Reprod* 1998; 13:2212–6.

8. Van Steirteghem, A. C., Nagy, Z., Joris, H., Liu, J., Staessen, C. et al. High fertilization and implantation rates after intracytoplasmic sperm injection. *Hum Reprod* 1993; 8:1061–6.

9. Nagy, Z. P., Liu, J., Joris, H., Verheyen, G., Tournaye, H. et al. The result of intracytoplasmic sperm injection is not related to any of the three basic sperm parameters. *Hum Reprod* 1995; 10:1123–9.

10. Tournaye, H., Liu, J., Nagy, Z., Verheyen, G., Van Steirteghem, A. et al. The use of testicular sperm for intracytoplasmic sperm injection in patients with necrozoospermia. *Fertil Steril* 1996; 66:331–4.

11. Nagy, Z. P., Verheyen, G., Liu, J., Joris, H., Janssenswillen, C. et al. Results of 55 intracytoplasmic sperm injection cycles in the treatment of male-immunological infertility. *Hum Reprod* 1995; 10:1775–80.

12. Liu, J., Nagy, Z., Joris, H., Tournaye, H., Devroey, P. et al. Successful fertilization and establishment of pregnancies after intracytoplasmic sperm injection in patients with globozoospermia. *Hum Reprod* 1995; 10:626–9.

13. Lundin, K., Sjogren, A., Nilsson, L. and Hamberger, L. Fertilization and pregnancy after intracytoplasmic microinjection of acrosomeless spermatozoa. *Fertil Steril* 1994; 62:1266–7.

14. Bourne, H., Richings, N., Harari, O., Watkins, W., Speirs, A. L. et al. The use of intracytoplasmic sperm injection for the treatment of severe and extreme male infertility. *Reprod Fertil & Dev* 1995; 7:237–45.

15. Neri, Q. V., Lee, B., Rosenwaks, Z., Machaca, K. and Palermo, G. D. Understanding fertilization through intracytoplasmic sperm injection (ICSI). *Cell Calcium* 2014; 55:24–37.

16. Moomjy, M., Colombero, L. T., Veeck, L. L., Rosenwaks, Z. and Palermo, G. D. Sperm integrity is critical for normal mitotic division and early embryonic development. *Mol Hum Reprod* 1999; 5:836–44.

17. Maggiulli, R., Neri, Q. V., Monahan, D., Hu, J., Takeuchi, T. et al. What to do when ICSI fails. *Syst Biol Reprod Med* 2010; 56:376–87.

18. Palermo, G. D., Cohen, J., Alikani, M., Adler, A. and Rosenwaks, Z. Intracytoplasmic sperm injection: a novel treatment for all forms of male factor infertility. *Fertil Steril* 1995; 63:1231–40.

19. World Health Organization (WHO). *Laboratory Manual for the Examination and Processing of Human Semen* (5th edn.) (Cambridge University Press, 2010).

20. Pereira, N., Reichman, D. E., Goldschlag, D. E., Lekovich, J. P. and Rosenwaks, Z. Impact of elevated peak serum estradiol levels during controlled ovarian hyperstimulation on the birth weight of term singletons from fresh IVF-ET cycles. *J Assist Reprod Genet* 2015; 32:527–32.

21. Huang, J. Y. and Rosenwaks, Z. In vitro fertilisation treatment and factors affecting success. *Best Pract Res Clin Obstet Gynaecol* 2012; 26:777–88.

22. Palermo, G. D., Neri, Q. V., Schlegel, P. N. and Rosenwaks, Z. Intracytoplasmic sperm injection (ICSI) in extreme cases of male infertility. *PLoS One* 2014; 9:e113671.

23. Palermo, G. D., Schlegel, P. N., Colombero, L. T., Zaninovic, N., Moy, F. et al. Aggressive sperm immobilization prior to intracytoplasmic sperm injection with immature spermatozoa improves fertilization and pregnancy rates. *Hum Reprod* 1996; 11:1023–9.

Chapter

24

Sperm Selection for ICSI by Morphology

Sabine Vanderzwalmen, David Jareno, Pierre Vanderzwalmen, Romain Imber, Maximilian Murtinger and Barbara Wirleitner

24.1 Background

A new innovative non-invasive technique for a more precise morphological evaluation of motile spermatozoa (Sp) was introduced by Bartoov in 2001.[1] An improved and more in-depth evaluation of living Sp cells at high magnification was brought into practice by using Nomarski differential interference contrast (DIC) optics instead of standard bright-field (BF) or Hoffman modulation contrast (HMC) optics. With the DIC optical microscopy, the technique of motile-sperm organelle-morphology examination (MSOME) was initiated either to analyze in real time Sp morphology for diagnostic purpose or as an approach of Sp selection before intracytoplasmic morphologically selected sperm injection (IMSI).

Even though the indications for MSOME and the usefulness of IMSI are still under debate in some in vitro fertilization (IVF) laboratories, the importance of selecting normal Sp becomes obvious when comparing the reproductive outcomes in terms of fertilization, blastocyst formation, pregnancy and abortion rates when oocyte injections are done with morphologically normal sperm and Sp exhibiting different sub-cellular defects.[2,3]

Undeniably, Sp carrying specific nuclear deficiencies defined as 'vacuole-like structures' were found to be related to DNA integrity, failures of chromatin condensation, aneuploidy and differences in DNA methylation levels.[4–7] It is advised that the presence of these structures makes the sperm nucleus more vulnerable to attacks by reactive oxygen species (ROS) in the sperm environment. The objective of this chapter is to describe our usual protocols and approaches to perform IMSI without impairing the oocyte and Sp viability.

24.2 General Equipment, Reagents and Supplies

In this chapter there will be no mention of specific brand names for equipment, reagents and supplies. Indeed, several companies offer equipment, reagents and supplies for assisted reproductive technology (ART) all over the world. Routinely used products from IVF laboratory-specific brands can be used for the protocols. An overview of the equipment, reagents and supplies to perform IMSI is presented in Table 24.1.

24.3 Sperm Preparation for Morphological Observation and Selection before IMSI

The isolation of motile Sp is performed according to the specific product instructions provided by the companies and standard operating procedures (SOPs) applied in each ART laboratory. In general, the semen sample is washed on two or three layers of discontinuous density gradient centrifugation followed by a swim-up when enough motile Sp are present.

Table 24.1 Equipment, Media, Oil and Supplies for MSOME and IMSI

	MSOME	IMSI	IMSI
	MSOME sperm selection for diagnostic and before oocyte injection	**Sp Selection and injection on different microscopes**	**Sp selection and injection on the same microscope**
Equipment			
Microscope:			
Inverted light microscope with DIC Hoffman modulation contrast (HMC)	Yes	Yes Yes	Yes
Objectives:			
DIC 40× DIC 63× DIC 100× dry lens	Yes	Yes	Yes
DIC 100× immersion lens	Yes	Yes	Yes
HMC 20× or 40× lens	Yes, for microchannel capture	Yes, for sperm injection	Yes, for sperm injection
5× or 10× lens: Adjust injection needle Adjust holding pipette	Yes	Yes Yes	Yes Yes Yes
Additionnal equipment:			
Variable zoom lens	Yes (magnification 6,600× 12,000×)	Optional	Optional
High-definition digital video camera	yes	Optional	Optional
Computer with video-software	Yes	Optional	Optional
High-resolution monitor screen	Yes, for photo library or morphometric analysis	Optional	Optional
Micromanipulators Injectors	Yes, for microchannel capture	Yes Yes	Yes Yes
Media and oil			
HTF-HEPES or sperm wash medium	Yes	Yes	Yes
Polyvinylpyrrolidone (PVP) 7% to 10%	Yes	Yes	Yes

Table 24.1 (cont.)

	MSOME	IMSI	IMSI
	MSOME sperm selection for diagnostic and before oocyte injection	Sp Selection and injection on different microscopes	Sp selection and injection on the same microscope
Immersion oil (100× immersion objective)	Optional	Optional	Optional
Mineral oil for covering the dish	Yes	Yes	Yes
Supplies			
Microscope cover glass (24 × 60 mm)	Yes		
WillCo glass-bottom Petri dish	Yes	Optional	Optional
FluoroDish	Optional	Yes	Yes
Sterile tubes (5–13 ml) (sperm preparation)	Yes	Yes	Yes
Sterile pipettes (1–5 ml, 10 ml) (handling of the semen)	Yes	Yes	Yes
Pipetting system + tips (2–200 µl) (handling of the semen)	Yes	Yes	Yes
Stripper (140 and 200 µm) (handling of the semen)	Yes	Yes	Yes
Microneedles: Injection pipette	Yes	Yes	Yes
Holding pipettes		Yes	Yes

DIC, differential interference contrast optics – Nomarski optic.

24.4 MSOME

A rapid morphological assessment and large nuclear vacuoles evaluation are performed:

- Generally in case the physician wants a fast diagnostic response about sperm morphology during consultation with a patient
- When we have to decide after the oocyte pickup whether conventional IVF or ICSI/IMSI has to be performed

This fast morphological assessment of the semen sample is performed after loading an aliquot of fresh or prepared semen in elongated PVP drops that were previously deposited on a microscope cover glass or in a glass-bottom Petri dish.[8] According to the initial concentration, 50 to 100 Sp are evaluated, classified and recorded in a specific file.[8] The evaluation of the morphology of motile Sp is done in real time.

24.5 IMSI

24.5.1 What Do We Have to Circumvent during IMSI?

The process of IMSI has to be planned to

- Restrict the time that oocytes are left outside the incubator to a minimum
- Restrict the time between oocyte pickup and Sp injection to two to three hours to avoid aging of oocytes (calculate enough time for sperm selection in a patient with severe OAT)
- Include accommodating sperm selection time in the laboratory when several IMSIs are planned

As a consequence, to fulfil these objectives, two strategies are applied: (1) the standard IMSI procedure employs two microscopes, one for Sp selection (Nomarski optics) and one for injection (Hoffman optics), and (2) selection and injection are done on the IMSI microscope but with a maximum of two oocytes at once.

24.5.2 Quality Management: Informed Consent and Safety Measures

Before starting an IMSI procedure, confirm that informed consent for IMSI therapy is signed by the couple. Safety measures during the entire procedure have to be applied:

- Under sterile conditions in the laminar flow hood, prepare the IMSI dishes, washing and handling the Sp and oocytes.
- According to your own identification procedure, label the dishes prior starting. For example, write the name of the patient or an identification number on the cover of the dish and on the side or underside of the dish.
- Double-checking should be applied at various stages of the procedure.
- Prior to depositing the Sp suspension in the dish, ask a second embryologist to double-check. Verify that the patient's name on the sperm tube corresponds to the one that is written on the IMSI dish.
- Prior to loading the ooyctes in the IMSI dish, ask a second embryologist to verify that the name on the dish after denudation is the same as the one written on the injection dish.
- After IMSI, perform double-checking before placing the injected oocyte in the long-term culture dish.

24.5.3 Usual IMSI Procedure: Sperm Selection and oocytes Injection on Two Different Microscopes

24.5.3.1 Principle and Advantages

In a first step, the Sp are selected using the inverted microscope with the DIC optic, and subsequently, the intracytoplasmic sperm injection is done on another microscope equipped with conventional BF or HMC optics.

Separating the process of MSOME and IMSI on two different microscopes permits us to achieve our objectives as described in Section 24.5.1:

- The oocytes are removed from the incubator only for the injection step. They are not present in the dish during selection of the Sp, which could take some time, especially in the case of severe teratozoospermia and/or oligozoospermia.
- After selection, the temperature of the glass-bottom dish is stabilized for 15 to 30 minutes before placing the oocytes for the injection step.
- To avoid oocyte aging in cases of poor sperm quantity, the Sp selection step may be scheduled at least around the time of oocyte pickup (OPU). With such a policy, oocyte injection can be performed two to three hours after OPU (38–40 hours after hCG administration) on the ICSI station.
- This avoids congestion at the IMSI station in the case of several IMSIs. The IMSI microscope is only occupied for the selection process and not for the injection phase.

24.5.3.2 Technical Aspects

Preparation and labelling of the dishes and oocytes and Sp loading are accomplished according to the safety measures guidelines in Section 24.5.2.

Preparation of the Glass-Bottom Dish for Sp Selection and Injection

For materials, reagents and supplies, refer to Table 24.1. Prepare a minimum of two dishes if more than 4 oocytes have to be injected. Prepare a maximum of two at once to avoid excess evaporation. As shown in Figure 24.1A, the IMSI dish is composed of five different drops:

1. Sperm selection PVP drops (A). On the left side of the dish, deposit one to three elongated drops of 7.5% to 10% PVP (~5 to 10 µl). In this drop, selection of the Sp with an injection needle will be performed.

   The number of drops depends on the quality of the semen that is assessed in a previous MSOME analysis and also on the number of MII oocytes. The purpose is that the Sp in the PVP drop must stay for a period that does not exceed 15 minutes. Moreover, according to this rule, several elongated drops and even IMSI dishes should be prepared if many MII oocytes are present.
2. Sperm aliquots drops (B). Under each sperm selection drop (A), a drop of ~10 µl of human tubal fluid (HTF)–HEPES–human serum albumin (HSA) is deposited. The drops will contain a suspension of washed Sp.
3. Host selected Sp microdrops (C). Adjacent to the elongated drops of PVP (A), very small drops (less than ~1 µl) of HTF-HEPES-HSA are created with a small stripper pipette. The microdrops will host morphologically selected normal motile Sp until oocyte injection.
4. Sperm immobilization drops (D). A small drop of 7.5% to 10% PVP in which sperm immobilization will take place is deposited in the upper part of the dish.
5. Oocytes injection drops (E). The right side of the dish contains five drops of HTF-HEPES-HSA in which oocyte injection will take place.

All drops are covered with sterile mineral oil. Then the Petri dish is covered with a lid. Place the dish on a 37°C heating stage for temperature recovery (minimum of 30 minutes).

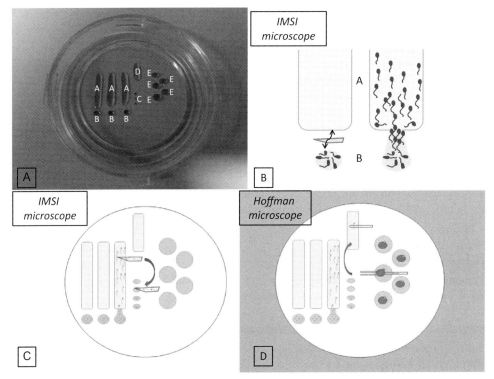

Figure 24.1 Position of the drops in an IMSI dish and IMSI procedure on two different microscopes. (Panel A) View of the drops: (A and D) 7.5% to 10% PVP; (B, C and E) culture medium. Sperm-selection PVP drops (A); sperm aliquot drops (B); host-selected spermatozoa microdrops (C); sperm immobilization drops (D); oocytes injection drops (E). (Panel B) Bridge with the selection micropipette between the sperm aliquots drops (B) and the sperm-selection PVP drops (A) (on the IMSI microscope). (Panel C) Selection of the spermatozoa in the sperm-selection PVP drops (A) and transfer to the host-selected spermatozoa microdrops (C) (on the IMSI microscope). (Panel D) Conventional ICSI on the Hoffman ICSI microscope. (A black and white version of this figure will appear in some formats. For the color version, please refer to the plate section.)

Procedure for Sp Selection on the Microscope Equipped with Nomarski DIC Microscopy (IMSI Microscope)

1. Turn on the IMSI microscope.
2. Turn on the heating stage of the microscope (Sp selection may be performed at room temperature).
3. Turn on the computer and monitor screen (if include in the IMSI platform).
4. Fix the ICSI needle for Sp selection.
5. With a micropipette (stripper) or an Eppendorf pipette, deposit a small aliquot of washed sperm (1 to 10 μl according to semen sample quality) into the drops B.
6. Place the dish on the stage of the IMSI microscope (use objective 20× or 40×).
7. Bring the ICSI needle in the elongated PVP drop (A) close to the drop that contains the sperm suspension (B).
8. With the ICSI needle, create a small bridge between drop B and drop A (Figure 24.1B).
9. Wait until you observe Sp swimming to the border of the PVP drop.
10. Place the condenser in the DIC position, and use DIC objectives 63× or 100× dry or immersion. If the 100× immersion oil objective is used, before starting, place a small

drop of oil on the objective lens. Then under the glass-bottom dish, locate the area of interest (border of drop A), and place a small drop.

11. Bring the ICSI needle close to the edge of the PVP drop.

12. At a magnification of 1,000×, aspirate the morphologically best Sp according to the standard classification.[2,8]

13. After aspirating several Sp, move the dish (manually or with the automatic system that records drop position) in order to bring the needle into drop C (Figure 24.1C).

14. Slowly release the motile Sp into the microdrop. Ensure that Sp remain motile during this step.

15. Remove the tip of the pipette from the drop, and move the plate of the microscope in order to bring the PVP drop (A) that contains the Sp close to the tip of the ICSI pipette.

16. Repeat the procedure until you have collected enough motile Sp in microdrop C. (1.5 times the number of oocytes to inject).

17. Remove the dish from the IMSI station, and place it with the lid on a 37°C heating stage for temperature recovery (~30 minutes).

Remark: If after 15 minutes you do not select enough Sp in drop A, repeat steps 8 to 17.

Method of Sp Injection on the Microscope Equipped with BF or HMC Optics (ICSI Microscope)

1. After selecting the Sp, perform denudation of the oocytes according to your own SOP.

2. Turn on the inverted microscope equipped with BF or HMC optics (Figure 24.1D).

3. Turn on the heating stage of the microscope at 37°C.

4. Turn on the computer and monitor (if include in the IMSI platform).

5. Install the holding and injection pipettes as for a classical ICSI procedure 15 to 30 minutes after sperm selection on the IMSI microscope.

7. Approximately 30 minutes after denudation, the oocytes are placed into drop (E) for injection.

8. ICSI is performed at 400× magnification (Figure 24.1D).

9. With the injection needle, motile Sp are aspirated from the pre-selected host drop (C) and immobilized in the PVP drop (D) before injection.

25.5.4 Second Approach: Sperm Selection and Oocyte Injection Using the IMSI Station

25.5.4.1 Principle

The entire procedure is performed at 37°C, and spermatozoa injection is performed directly after Sp selection and immobilization in the same dish. Before considering such a procedure, the quality of the semen sample should be assessed in order to be sure that the time spent to select a good-quality Sp will not exceed five minutes. In addition, when the purpose of the study is to follow individually the outcome of embryo development in relation to the type of injected spermatozoon (photographic documentation of the injected spermatozoon), a maximum of two oocytes are placed directly in the IMSI dish (Figure 24.2). After IMSI, each oocyte is cultured separately in small drops (in a Petri dish or with the in time-lapse incubator).

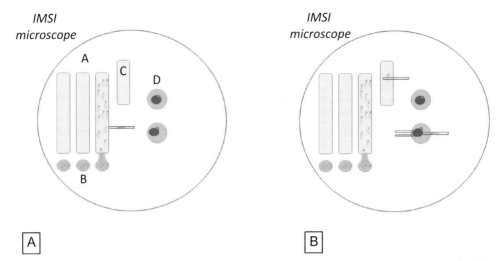

Figure 24.2 IMSI: description of the different steps for sperm selection (Panel A) and oocyte injection on the IMSI microscope (Panel B). (A black and white version of this figure will appear in some formats. For the color version, please refer to the plate section.)

24.5.4.2 Technical Aspects

Preparation and labelling of the dishes, oocytes and Sp loading should be done according to the safety measures guidelines in Section 24.5.2.

Preparation of the Dish

For materials, reagents and supplies, refer to Table 24.1. A minimum of two dishes are prepared, as mentioned previously, except that there are no host sperm drops (Figure 24.2A) The other drops are prepared similarly, as described earlier.

Method of Sp Selection and Injection on the IMSI Microscope

1. Turn on the heating stage of the microscope at 37°C.
2. Install the ICSI and holding pipettes.
3. Aspirate and select several Sp with good morphology from drop A, and bring the pipette to the immobilization PVP drop (C).
4. Slowly release several motile Sp into the PVP microdrop.
5. With the injection needle, perform immobilization of several Sp.
6. If available, use of a variable zoom lens allows you to re-evaluate (after immobilization) themorphology on the monitor at magnifications ranging between 6,600× and 12,000×.
7. For study purposes, perform photographic documentation for a subsequent analysis before aspiration of the spermatozoon in the injection pipette.
8. Bring the pipette into drop D, and perform the conventional ICSI procedure.
9. After oocyte injection, place the oocytes one by one in single culture drops in a conventional Petri dish or in a special dish for time-lapse recording.
10. The first IMSI dish is then placed on a heating stage at 37°C until the next selection and injection step is finished.
11. The next two oocytes are then placed in a new IMSI dish pre-warmed on the heating stage. Repeat steps 3 to 9.

24.6 Conclusion

One of the most essential questions is not under which technical conditions the selection of Sp should be recommended but rather whether we have to consider selecting the best Sp and, if possible, excluding those carrying defects. For this reason, MSOME and IMSI were developed. It is increasingly obvious that large vacuoles reflect a pathological situation, most probably correlated with sperm chromatin immaturity and chromosomal abnormalities. The full benefit of using MSOME as an additional tool to the ICSI procedure manifests when the procedure is performed in combination with day 5 embryo culture of all fertilized oocytes.

In addition, we have to be aware that this technique is challenging and has to be performed very carefully. The final goal for the gynecologist, the biologist, and the entire team of an IVF unit is to achieve a pregnancy and birth of a healthy baby. The prevalence of birth defects after ART is discussed controversially. Cassuto et al.[9] recently showed that babies born after ICSI presented significantly more often with de novo abnormalities than babies born after IMSI. This follow-up study emphasizes the importance of de-selecting morphological abnormal spermatozoa, seeing that the IMSI procedure is performed under optimal conditions so as not to impair the quality of oocytes, which seem to provide fewer malformations in the newborn.

References

1. Bartoov, B., Berkovitz, A. and Eltes, F. Selection of spermatozoa with normal nuclei to improve the pregnancy rate with intracytoplasmic sperm injection. *N Engl J Med* 2001; 345:1067–8.

2. Vanderzwalmen, P., Hiemer, A., Rubner, P., Bach, M., Neyer, A. et al. Blastocyst development after sperm selection at high magnification is associated with size and number of nuclear vacuoles. *Reprod Biomed Online* 2008; 17:617–27.

3. Neyer, A., Zintz, M., Stecher, A., Bach, M., Wirleitner, B. et al. The impact of paternal factors on cleavage stage and blastocyst development analyzed by time-lapse imaging: a retrospective observational study *J Assist Reprod Genet* 2015; 32:1607–14.

4. Boitrelle, F., Albert, M., Petit, J.-M., Ferfouri, F., Wainer, R. et al. Small human sperm vacuoles observed under high magnification are pocket-like nuclear concavities linked to chromatin condensation failure. *Reprod Biomed Online* 2013; 27:201–11.

5. Cassuto, N. G., Hazout, A., Hammoud, I., Balet, R., Bouret, D. et al. Correlation between DNA defect and sperm-head morphology. *Reprod Biomed Online* 2012; 24, 211–18.

6. Garolla, A., Sartini, B., Cosci, I., Pizzol, D., Ghezzi, M. et al. Molecular karyotyping of single sperm with nuclear vacuoles identifies more chromosomal abnormalities in patients with testiculopathy than fertile controls: implications for ICSI. *Hum Reprod* 2015; 30:2493–500.

7. Cassuto, G., Montjean, D., Siffroi, J. P., Bouret, D., Marzouk, F. et al. Different levels of DNA methylation detected in human sperms after morphological selection using high magnification microscopy. *Biomed Res Int* 2016; article ID 6372171, 1–7.

8. Vanderzwalmen, P., Bach, M., Gaspard, O., Lejeune, B., Neyer, A. et al. Motile-sperm organelle-morphology examination and intracytoplasmic morphologically selected sperm injection: clinical and technical aspects. In *A Practical Guide to Selecting Gametes and Embryos*, ed. M. Montag (pp. 59–80) (Boca Raton, FL: CRC Press, 2014).

9. Cassuto, G., Hazout, A., Bouret, D., Balet, R., Larue, L. et al. Low birth defects by deselecting abnormal spermatozoa before ICSI. *Reprod Biomed Online* 2014; 28:47–53.

Chapter 25

Sperm Selection for ICSI by Viability

Markus H. M. Montag

Introduction

Sperm motility is an important factor for successful fertilization and embryo development. If a patient presents only immotile sperm in the ejaculate or in a testicular sample, a viability test can help to identify among the immotile sperm those that are viable and suitable for intracytoplasmic sperm injection (ICSI). Different sperm viability tests have been introduced, and if they are applied properly, there is a good chance for successful treatment.

25.1 Background

Sperm viability is a prerequisite for fertilization of the oocyte and subsequent embryo development. The primary sign for sperm viability is motility, and any sperm that shows even the slightest movement is still alive and in principle capable for fertilizing an oocyte. In assisted reproduction, the andrology and embryology laboratory is occasionally confronted with patients who present only immotile spermatozoa in the ejaculate. The same situation may be encountered after surgical retrieval of sperm from the testis or the epididymis. Immotile sperm are not necessarily non-viable. Identifying among immotile sperm those that are still viable is mandatory. Only viable immotile sperm are capable of initiating fertilization, embryo development and eventual pregnancy. Several procedures to identify sperm viability in an ICSI treatment cycle have been described in the literature and were applied successfully in clinical routine. These include the sperm tail flexibility test,[1] the hypo-osmotic swelling (HOS) test,[2-4] laser assessment[5-7] and chemical testing by pentoxifylline[8] and theophylline.[9]

25.2 Reagents, Supplies and Equipment

- HOS swelling solution can be prepared by mixing 50% culture medium (preferably HEPES- or MOPS-buffered) with 50% de-ionized water.
- Ready-to-use commercially available theophylline solution.
- A 1.48-μm diode laser for laser-assisted viability testing.
- Culture dishes.
- ICSI microinjection needle.
- Culture medium.
- Inverted microscope equipped with micromanipulators as for ICSI.

25.3 Quality Control

- Use of commercial medium is recommended for sperm viability testing, as preparation of one's own solutions is prone to error that may result in a negative outcome.

- Check all commercial solutions for expiry date.
- Perform a regular check of the appropriate laser pulse length and laser alignment/positioning of the laser focus spot.
- Perform regular service on the laser.

25.4 Procedure

25.4.1 Sperm Tail Flexibility Test

The sperm tail flexibility test is mostly applied to testicular sperm preparations and is based on the experience that stiff sperm tails are usually characteristic of dead sperm.

1. Dispense sperm preparation/testicular preparation in a droplet of HEPES- or MOPS-buffered culture medium in an ICSI dish. The same dish should hold a droplet for collecting the sperm after testing.
2. Work at an ICSI microscope with an ICSI microinjection needle.
3. Locate sperm that have a bent and presumably flexible sperm tail.
4. Touch the sperm tail gently with the ICSI needle to see whether the sperm is moving in total or if the tail will bend and appear flexible after the capillary touch.
5. Sperm with a flexible and bending tail are more likely to be viable compared to sperm with a stiff tail/a tail that does not bend on its own.

25.4.2 HOS Test

The HOS test has been used for immotile ejaculated sperm. Currently, there is no ready-to-use commercial HOS medium available.

1. Prepare the HOS medium as described, mix thoroughly and pipette a droplet of the HOS medium into a culture dish.
2. In the same dish, pipette several droplets with HEPES- or MOPS-buffered culture medium for sperm dispersion and for sperm washing and one smaller droplet for sperm collection.
3. Dispense an aliquot of the sperm preparation into a culture medium droplet.
4. Aspirate a sperm cell with the head first into the ICSI capillary, and release the sperm tail slowly into the HOS medium.
5. A curling of the sperm tail identifies a positive HOS reaction. Other reactions may occur and can best be identified by comparing these to the different types that are illustrated in the relevant publications.[2]
6. As soon as curling is visible, aspirate the sperm cell into the ICSI needle, and transfer it into a washing droplet with culture medium.
7. After washing off the HOS medium, deposit the sperm in a collection droplet.
8. Continue until sufficient sperm are collected for ICSI.

25.4.3 Sperm Viability Assessment by Laser

1. Prepare a dish with several droplets of HEPES- or MOPS-buffered culture medium for sperm dispersion and for sperm washing and one smaller droplet for sperm collection.
2. Dispense an aliquot of the sperm preparation into the culture medium droplet.

3. Adjust the laser intensity to approximately half the pulse length that is required for drilling a 15- to 17-μm opening into the zona pellucida.
4. Place the laser focus spot close to the sperm tail, approximately in the last third from the tip of the tail. Keep a distance of approximately 5 μm to the sperm tail.
5. Apply a single laser shot, and observe the sperm tail.
6. Viable sperm will show a curling or bending that will remain in place.
7. Aspirate viable sperm with the head first, and transfer it in a collection droplet.
8. Continue until sufficient sperm are collected for ICSI.

25.4.4 Pentoxifylline/Theophylline

Theophylline-induced sperm motility will last for a limited time only. Therefore, the procedure has to be repeated if insufficient motile spermatozoa are recovered during the first round.

1. Prepare a dish with several droplets of HEPES- or MOPS-buffered culture medium for sperm dispersion and washing and one smaller droplet for sperm collection. The droplets for sperm suspension should have a defined volume (e.g. 25 or 50 μl).
2. Dispense an aliquot of the sperm preparation into the culture medium droplet.
3. Add 10% v/v of ready-to-use theophylline solution, and mix gently.
4. Start searching for motile sperm within the next 5 to 10 minutes and up to 30 minutes.
5. Aspirate motile sperm with the head first, wash in culture medium and transfer in a collection droplet.
6. After 30 minutes, add to another, new droplet an aliquot of the sperm suspension and theophylline, as described earlier, and continue searching for sperm.
7. Repeat the preceding steps until sufficient sperm have been collected for subsequent ICSI.

25.5 Notes

A. Prior to initiation of the ICSI treatment cycle, a regular eosin staining test should be performed on the patient's diagnostic sperm sample. This will give an estimate of the percentage of viable sperm that can be expected during the therapeutic cycle.
B. The sperm tail flexibility test is the least reliable test as it is based on a subjective assessment method.
C. Do not release sperm completely into the HOS medium or pipette sperm suspension into the HOS medium as due to the reduced serum/albumin content, sperm will become very sticky.
D. Pentoxifylline is not available as a ready-to-use product for sperm immobilization testing and thus needs to be prepared.
E. Carry-over of pentoxifylline into oocytes has been shown to be toxic in animal experiments. Careful washing of sperm prior to ICSI is thus mandatory.
F. Theophylline is available as a ready-to-use product.[9]
G. Theophylline can also be used in cases where only few sperm with a flickering tail are available. These are usually difficult to spot at first sight. Addition of theophylline can eventually result in forward motility and facilitate finding sperm and reduce the time needed to collect sufficient sperm.

H. For laser viability, assessment of the proper laser energy, expressed by the laser pulse length, must be determined before application. For this, a 15- to 17-µm opening should be drilled into the zona pellucida of an unfertilized or immature oocyte, and the pulse length should be noted. Taking half this value will give a good starting point.

I. During laser viability assessment, care should be taken not to shoot too close to the sperm, as this may cause permanent damage to the sperm membrane, which may be unfavourable in case the ICSI procedure is undertaken at a later time.[5]

J. In case sperm must be collected over a longer time period, it is advisable to handle sperm during collection and transfer very gently. This will help to avoid damage to the sperm membrane, as this could eventually result in a loss of the oocyte activation capacity. Gentle sperm handling involves aspiration of the head first.

K. Sperm collection will require some time, and temperature will drop slightly in the collection dish over time. Therefore, it is advised to prepare a separate dish for ICSI and to transfer the collected spermatozoa into the ICSI dish just before ICSI.

L. Before injection of the immotile sperm into the oocyte proper, immobilization must be carried out, no matter whether sperm are totally immotile or slow moving.

References

1. Oliveira, N. M., Sanchez, R. V., Fiesta, S. R. et al. Pregnancy with frozen-thawed and fresh testicular biopsy after motile and immotile sperm microinjection, using the mechanical touch technique to assess viability. *Hum Reprod* 2004; **19**:262–5.

2. Jeyendran, R. S., van der Ven, H. H., Perez-Pelaez, M., Crabo, B. G. and Zaneveld, L. J. Development of an assay to assess the functional integrity of the human sperm membrane and its relationship to others emen characteristics. *J Reprod Fertil* 1984; **70**:219–28.

3. Ved, S., Montag, M., Schmutzler, A., Prietl, G., Haidl, G. et al. Pregnancy following intracytoplasmic sperm injection of immotile spermatozoa selected by the hypo-osmotic swelling-test: a case report. *Andrologia* 1997; **29**:241–2.

4. Sallam, H., Farrag, A., Agameya, A., Ezzeldin, F., Eid, A. et al. The use of a modified hypo-osmotic swelling test for the selection of viable ejaculated and testicular immotile spermatozoa in ICSI. *Hum Reprod* 2001; **16**:272–6.

5. Montag, M., Rink, K., Delacrétaz, G. and van der Ven, H. Laser-induced immobilization and plasma membrane permeabilization in human spermatozoa. *Hum Reprod* 2000; **15**:846–52.

6. Aktan, T. M., Montag, M., Duman, S., Gorkemli, H., Rink K, Yurdakul T. Use of a laser to detect viable but immotile spermatozoa. *Andrologia* 2004; **36**:366–9.

7. Nordhoff, V., Schüring, A. N., Krallmann, C., Zitzmann, M., Schlatt, S. et al. Optimizing TESE-ICSI by laser-assisted selection of immotile spermatozoa and polarization microscopy for selection of oocytes. *Andrology* 2013; **1**:67–74.

8. Yovich, J. L. Pentoxifylline: actions and applications in assisted reproduction. *Hum Reprod* 1993; **8**:1786–91.

9. Ebner, T., Tews, G., Mayer, R. B., Ziehr, S., Arzt, W. et al. Pharmacological stimulation of sperm motility in frozen and thawed testicular sperm using the dimethylxanthine theophylline. *Fertil Steril* 2011; **96**:1331–6.

Chapter

26

Artificial Oocyte Activation for IVF

Thomas Ebner

26.1 Background

The introduction and implementation of intracytoplasmic sperm injection (ICSI) in the field of assisted reproduction has been a milestone in the treatment of male factor and unexplained infertility. This breakthrough has also allowed fertilization in couples with previous fertilization failure after conventional in vitro fertilization (IVF). This is all the more interesting as depositing a single sperm directly into the ooplasm bypasses several anatomical structures and physiological events.

In vivo, a sperm-derived enzyme called 'phospholipase C zeta' (PLCζ) has been identi-fied as the physiological stimulus of oocyte activation.[1] This factor is released after sperm–oocyte fusion whereupon it cleaves membrane-bound phosphatidylinositol bisphosphate, yielding diacylglycerol (which, in turn, initiates zona reaction) and inositol triphosphate. The latter molecule subsequently binds to its receptors located at the endoplasmic reticu-lum, causing calcium release from these internal storages.[2] The resulting Ca^{2+} influx presents in an oscillatory mode, and its effectiveness depends on number, frequency, temporal modulation and amplitude.[3] The spatio-temporal Ca^{2+} pattern ceases after pro-nuclear formation, and there are no further changes to Ca^{2+} until the cell prepares for the first mitotic division, when a spontaneous Ca^{2+} peak arises driving cleavage to the two-cell stage.

Considering the complexity of the oocyte activation process just described, it is hardly surprising that even with ICSI some oocytes cannot be activated. Indeed, complete fertiliza-tion failure after ICSI shows a prevalence of up to 3%. Moreover, low or moderate fertilization (<30%) can be observed for some patients, not uncommonly in repeated ICSI cycles.[4] In such cycles of bad prognosis, the underlying problem is most likely related to a reduction of intracellular calcium, particularly the absence of Ca^{2+} oscillations, caused by either a sperm- or an oocyte-borne deficiency.[5] Any such internal calcium shortage will have a profound impact on cell physiology, affecting either ICSI fertilization rate[4,6,7] or mitotic behaviour.[8]

This obvious drawback can be compensated by several artificial oocyte activation (AOA) techniques, all of which aim for an increase in internal Ca^{2+}. This can be achieved by depletion of internal storage and/or by influx of extracellular Ca^{2+}. One of the first approaches was to modify the ICSI technique itself. Switching to a more invasive manipu-lation; for example, doing the cytoplasmic aspiration at the opposite oolemma not only helps to recruit internal calcium from the endoplasmic reticulum but also provides more energy in the form of metabolically active mitochondria.[9] Others introduced an electrical mode of activation that acts via rearrangement of cell membrane proteins (caused by direct-current voltage), leading to the formation of pores that allow for the influx of Ca^{2+} ions.[10] More commonly, activation problems after ICSI are circumvented using a variety of chemical agents,[11] such as 6-dimethylaminopurine, puromycin, phorbol esters, thimerosal, strontium chloride or calcium ionophores (e.g. ionomycin or calcimycin (A23187)). Although the latter molecules do not result in physiological Ca^{2+} oscillations, they are more effective than those causing repetitive Ca^{2+} spikes.

So far there is only one flaw with the use of Ca^{2+} ionophores, namely, the absence of a universally applicable protocol. Vanden Meerschaut et al.[5] emphasized disparities in type, exposure time, concentration or mode of application. In particular, the latter parameter is all but standardized. The wide variety of application modes reaches from single-ionophore exposure (ionomycin or calcimycin) for 10 minutes to twofold exposure for an overall 20 minutes. The most stimulating impetus is a combination of an adapted ICSI (in which the spermatozoon is injected along with 0.1 mol/litre of $CaCl_2$ solution) and a double exposure to ionomycin, 10 and 30 minutes after injection.[12] Obviously, mammalian oocytes can respond to a variety of intracellular Ca^{2+} signals and have a high degree of tolerance for prolonged changes in cytosolic Ca^{2+}. The observed oscillations of CaMKII in temporal synchrony with Ca^{2+} peaks indicates that artificial Ca^{2+} recruitment does result in a proper biological downstream response.[13] The said enzyme activity is associated with the initial Ca^{2+} transient in a directly proportional manner,[13] thus reflecting the situation commonly found in AOA (presence of a single calcium rise). Despite this biological evidence of efficacy currently in literature, there is an intensive discussion about the safety of AOA.[14-17] This is all the more surprising since AOA is only applied with the proper indication and not as a routine method. The lack of standardized AOA methodologies led to the development and launch of a commercially available ready-to-use A23187 product (GM508 CultActive, Gynemed, Lensahn, Germany). Since GM508 CultActive is a CE marked product, the number of publications dealing with it is constantly increasing. The healthy birth of more than 250 babies and the ease of application and implementation in the routine IVF laboratory are further arguments that focus on this A23187 agent in this chapter.

26.2 Quality Control

It is important to repeat that ionophores (e.g. A23187) do not cause a physiological Ca^{2+} pattern but much rather result in a single Ca^{2+} transient. As such, it is still being considered 'experimental', and one should be forewarned of the imminent scenario of using Ca^{2+} ionophores as a routine procedure. Consequently, before application of any type of Ca^{2+} ionophore, one should thoroughly consider whether a proper indication is present at all. So far severe male factor infertility,[6] fertilization problems after ICSI,[4,7] oocyte maturation deficiency[18] and developmental arrest/delay[8] have been identified as potential conditions in which ionophore treatment might be of help. In other words, A23187 application in the first treatment cycle is an uncommon scenario.

The question remains whether the previously observed activation failure is attributed to a sperm- or an oocyte-related deficiency. This information is crucial for both the clinician and the patient while discussing prognosis, future treatment options and potential consequences for the offspring. One reliable diagnostic test available for couples suffering from ICSI activation failure is the so-called mouse oocyte activation test (MOAT), which is a heterologous ICSI model that evaluates the capacity of human spermatozoa to activate mouse oocytes.[5] Based on their percentage of heterologous egg activation, patients are then subdivided into low ($\leq$20%), intermediate (21–84%) and high activation groups ($\geq$85%). In the cohort showing the lowest activation, a sperm-related deficiency is likely to be the cause of previous fertilization failure(s), whereas in the MOAT high activation group, a sperm-related deficiency can more or less be ruled out. The intermediate class, however, remains inconclusive, although a major contribution of the sperm is expected since MOAT results below 85% exceed the lower activation limit of the positive control (donor spermatozoa with proven activation capacity).

26.3 Reagents, Supplies and Equipment

- 1 ml ready-to-use oocyte activation solution: GM508 CultActive (Gynemed) (Note A)
- Culture medium or alternative washing medium
- Mineral oil or alternative mineral oil
- Nunc four-well dish (or alternative multi-well dish)
- Pipetting microtools

26.4 Procedure

1. Determine the correct indication, for which the patient should be counselled. If oocyte activation treatment is part of a case study (e.g., ionophore treatment in the first cycle), obtain informed consent of the patient. In this case it is recommended to split the sibling oocytes.
2. Gently shake the bottle of ready-to-use activation solution before use (Note A).
3. Place a 30- to 60-μl drop of activation solution into a four-well dish.
4. Place ~200 to 300 μl of washing medium into the other three wells of the four-well dish.
5. Overlay all four wells with mineral oil.
6. For equilibration, incubate the prepared four-well dish for at least two hours in an incubator with a CO_2 atmosphere.
7. Perform ICSI as usual.
8. Immediately after ICSI, transfer injected MII oocytes to the equilibrated activation solution drop (Note B).
9. Incubate for 15 minutes (setting an alarm clock or timer is recommended).
10. Transfer the ionophore-treated oocytes to the next well containing washing medium.
11. During this first washing step, aspirate the oocytes repeatedly.
12. Repeat this washing step twice using the rest of the wells.
13. Transfer the oocytes to the routinely used culture dishes for in vitro culture.

26.5 Troubleshooting

1. If no fertilization is observed on day 1, do not dispose of the 'unfertilized' gametes because the course of fertilization events could be delayed or accelerated.
2. If no cleavage happened in the treatment cycle, oocyte activation can be adapted to the Gent protocol in the following stimulation cycle.[5] In detail, this would require two exposures to activation solution for 15 minutes, the first stimulus still immediately after ICSI and the second one after a 30-minute rest.
3. If this more excessive stimulus also results in fertilization failure, the ultimate approach would be gamete donation (optimally based on MOAT results).

26.6 Notes

A. There is only one commercial activation solution on the market (GM508 CultActive, Gynemed). The activation solution has a shelf life of six months from production and should be stored in the refrigerator at 2 to 8°C. Once a bottle is opened, it should not be used for longer than two weeks.

B. If the number of oocytes or the quality of sperm leads to prolonged ICSI (>30 minutes), the gametes should be treated sequentially with GM508 CultActive, that is, ICSI dish to ICSI dish.

References

1. Saunders, C. M., Larman, M. G., Parrington, J., Cox, L. J., Royse, J. et al. PLC zeta: a sperm-specific trigger of Ca(2+) oscillations in eggs and embryo development. *Development* 2002; 129:3533–44.

2. Berridge, M. J. Inositol trisphosphate and calcium signalling mechanisms. *Biochim Biophys Acta* 2009; 1793:933–40.

3. Ozil, J. P. and Huneau, D. Activation of rabbit oocytes: the impact of the Ca^{2+} signal regime on development. *Development* 2001; 128:917–28.

4. Montag, M., Köster, M., van der Ven, K., Bohlen, U. and van der Ven, H. The benefit of artificial oocyte activation is dependent on the fertilization rate in a previous treatment cycle. *Reprod Biomed Online* 2012; 24:521–6.

5. Vanden Meerschaut, F., Nikiforaki, D., Heindryckx, B. and De Sutter, P. Assisted oocyte activation following ICSI fertilization failure. *Reprod Biomed Online* 2014; 28:560–71.

6. Ebner, T., Köster, M., Shebl, O., Moser, M., Van der Ven, H. et al. Application of a ready-to-use calcium ionophore increases rates of fertilization and pregnancy in severe male factor infertility. *Fertil Steril* 2012; 98:1432–7.

7. Ebner, T. and Montag, M. Oocyte Activation Study Group. Live birth after artificial oocyte activation using a ready-to-use ionophore: a prospective multicentre study. *Reprod Biomed Online* 2015; 30:359–65.

8. Ebner, T., Oppelt, P., Wöber, M., Staples, P., Mayer, R. B. et al. Treatment with Ca^{2+} ionophore improves embryo development and outcome in cases with previous developmental problems: a prospective multicenter study. *Hum Reprod* 2015; 30:97–102.

9. Ebner, T., Moser, M., Sommergruber, M., Jesacher, K. and Tews, G. Complete oocyte activation failure after ICSI can be overcome by a modified injection technique. *Hum Reprod* 2004; 19: 1837–41.

10. Baltaci, V., Ayvaz, O. U., Unsal, E., Aktaş, Y., Baltaci, A. et al. The effectiveness of intracytoplasmic sperm injection combined with piezoelectric stimulation in infertile couples with total fertilization failure. *Fertil Steril* 2010; 94: 900–4.

11. Kashir, J., Heindryckx, B., Jones, C., De Sutter, P., Parrington, J. et al. Oocyte activation, phospholipase C zeta and human infertility. *Hum Reprod Update* 2010; 16:690–703.

12. Heindryckx, B., De Gheselle, S., Gerris, J., Dhont, M. and De Sutter, P. Efficiency of assisted oocyte activation as a solution for failed intracytoplasmic sperm injection. *Reprod Biomed Online* 2008; 17:662–8.

13. Markoulaki, S., Matson, S., Abbott, A. L. and Ducibella, T. Oscillatory CaMKII activity in mouse egg activation. *Dev Biol* 2003; 258:464–74.

14. Ebner, T. and Montag, M. Artificial oocyte activation: evidence for clinical readiness. *Reprod Biomed Online* 2016; 32:271–3.

15. Ebner, T., Shebl, O. and Parmegiani, L. Oldie but goldie or opening Pandora's box? *Curr Trends Clin Embryol* 2015; 2:149–52.

16. Santella, L. and Dale, B. Assisted yes, but where do we draw the line? *Reprod Biomed Online* 2015; 31:476–8.

17. van Blerkom, J., Cohen, J. and Johnson, M. A plea for caution and more research in the 'experimental' use of ionophores in ICSI. *Reprod Biomed Online* 2015; 30:323–4.

18. Kim, J. W., Yang, S. H., Yoon, S. H., Kim, S. D., Jung, J. H. et al. Successful pregnancy and delivery after ICSI with artificial oocyte activation by calcium ionophore in in-vitro matured oocytes: a case report. *Reprod Biomed Online* 2015; 30:373–7.

Section 5 **Fertilization Assessment**

Chapter

27

Fertilization Assessment in IVF and ICSI

Dara S. Berger and Heather S. Hoff

27.1 Background

Selection of the best embryo to transfer, that is, the one that will have the highest potential to result in a live birth, is one of the most important decisions in an in vitro fertilization (IVF) laboratory. A zygote forms with the amalgamation of the female and male gametes, and much information about the viability of an embryo can be gained within 16 to 20 hours after insemination.[1] Interaction of the oocyte and sperm should first be examined with an accurate assessment of fertilization.[2]

A systematic review by Nicoli et al.[3] in 2013 analyzed 40 studies on the correlation of zygote morphology with biological and clinical outcomes, including embryo quality, development to cleavage stage, progression to blastocyst stage, embryonic chromosomal status, implantation rate, clinical pregnancy and live birth rate.

A total of 15 different zygote scoring algorithms were included, many based on modifications of the original systems proposed by Scott and Smith[4] and Tesarik and Greco.[5] Scott and Smith evaluated the zygote by both size and position of pronuclei, number and alignment of nucleoli and appearance of the cytoplasm. Tesarik and Greco advocated for six categories based on number, size and polarization of the nucleolar precursor bodies (NPBs). Essentially all systems include components for grading the number and size of nucleoli, in addition to symmetrical distribution. In 2011, the Istanbul Consensus Workshop on Embryo Assessment by the Alpha Scientists in Reproductive Medicine and the European Society of Human Reproduction and Embryology (ESHRE) Special Interest Group in Embryology simplified pronuclear scoring by assigning one of three classifications: symmetrical, asymmetrical and abnormal.[6]

A correlation with zygote morphology and biological outcomes including progression to cleavage (15 of 20 studies, 75%) and blastocyst stage (7 of 8 studies, 87.5%) and embryonic chromosomal status (6 of 6 studies, 100%) was noted in the majority of studies. However, many would argue more importantly, most of the studies evaluating pregnancy and live birth rate did not find a significant difference in these clinical outcomes based on the zygote morphology of the transferred embryo. A statistically significant relationship was found in 12 of 25 studies analyzing pregnancy percentages and 1 of 4 papers examining live birth rates.[3]

Evidence suggests that these systems may not have the clinical utility once envisioned. These scoring methods are also often time-consuming and difficult to implement in large laboratories, especially when group culture is employed. Application of such zygote grading might be more practical in laboratories with time-lapse imaging and available personnel.

This chapter will discuss the techniques for fertilization verification for oocytes fertilized both conventionally and by intracytoplasmic sperm injection (ICSI). The formation of the pronuclei is the first indication of the fusion of male and female gametes. Therefore, an essential criterion for a normally fertilized zygote is visualization of two pronuclei, one representing each parent's genetic contribution. A system for grading zygote morphology based on NPBs is not outlined, but many examples are outlined in the references cited above. Practical considerations and laboratory protocols are detailed in the following sections.

27.2 Practical Considerations

Embryo assessment begins with careful observation of the respective gametes. Oocyte abnormalities such as dusky zona pellucida, enlarged perivitelline space and presence of vacuoles or dark or grainy cytoplasm may give insight into poor fertilization prognosis.[2]

Assessment of zygotes should occur 16 to 20 hours after insemination. A normal zygote fertilized by ICSI should consist of two pronuclei with two polar bodies (Figure 27.1). For conventional insemination, one or two pronuclei with two polar bodies is considered acceptable, as a single pronuclei may represent a delay in timing of one or more of the events of fertilization after the sperm penetrated the zona pellucida, which would not occur if ICSI is performed.[1] It is important to note that not all laboratories will consider single-pronuclei zygotes derived from conventional insemination normal. Up to 40% of unfertilized oocytes may appear morphologically to be normal embryos the next day, with comparable division kinetics to zygotes judged to be normally fertilized on the previous day. Up to a third of these with have arrest of further development on day 2.[7] A zygote with three or more pronuclei is always considered abnormal fertilization and may indicate failure to extrude the second polar body or polyspermic fertilization. Fluorescence in situ hybridization (FISH) analysis of these embryos reveals mosaicism of 80% to 90% after cleavage.[1]

Training for technical staff and reagents and culture conditions described previously apply with this procedure as well. It is important that zygotes are assessed within the appropriate time window as to document the number of pronuclei before they fade. If analysis is performed too late, pronuclei will fuse (syngamy will occur), and abnormal fertilization will be unable to be detected. It is also important to assess zygotes in a timely manner. The goal for any technician is to quickly and accurately record normal and abnormal fertilization and separate normal and abnormal zygotes in order to return the zygotes to the optimal environment in the incubator in which they are cultured and not remain in ambient air for long periods of time.

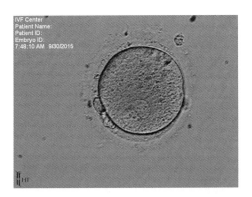

Figure 27.1 Normal zygote with 2 pronuclei and two polar bodies.

27.2.1 Identification

As with any procedure or evaluation in the IVF laboratory, care must be taken to verify patient identity. Also, time since insemination must be confirmed, ideally 16 to 20 hours after insemination, to increase the likelihood of optimal visualization of the pronuclei. Typically, dishes inseminated by ICSI are evaluated for fertilization first, as the time of sperm introduction to the egg is known precisely. Conventional insemination is generally performed approximately five hours after retrieval, and stripping is performed the following day, on day 1, immediately before fertilization evaluation.

Conventionally inseminated oocytes are covered with cumulus cells that must be removed to assess the pronuclei and polar bodies. An expedient and gentle technique must be employed, ideally while the specimen remains at 37°C and a stable pH. Denuding may be accomplished by narrow-gauge pipetting, needle dissection or rolling.[1] Pipetting the cumulous or zygote up and down slowly through the pipette will sluff the cumulous cells away from the zona pellucida. Needle dissection involves two 26-gauge needles with a 1-ml syringe attached. Use cross-motion or anchor an area of corona/cumulus mass and slice cells away from oocyte. And rolling can be performed using a 23-gauge needle on a glass probe with magnification at 12× by creating lines in the droplet with the needle and then increasing magnification to 25× and using a glass probe to remove cells by gently moving over the indents. Zygotes derived from ICSI insemination will not need to be denuded because this would have been performed prior to sperm injection.

With stripping either before or after insemination, care must be taken to keep the oolemma intact and not to over-squeeze the oocyte or zygote. If the oolemma is punctured or fractured from distension, contents of the oocyte or zygote may escape through this compromised area. The oocyte or zygote will also be at an increased risk of degenerating. If the zona pellucida and/or oolemma is fragile and appears stressed with slight manipulation, it is advised to not proceed with removal of cells with the pipetting technique but instead try to 'pop' the zygote out of the cumulous cells using needle dissection. This is achieved by cutting and spreading the cumulous cells very close to the oocyte or zygote with needles.

All dishes should be handled sterilely, and fertilization verification should occur as quickly as possible. Ideally, specimens remain at 37°C throughout the assessment.

27.3 Protocols

27.3.1 Equipment

- Culture media, oil and dishes
- Polished glass pipette with rubber bulb for macropipetting
- 'Stripper' pipette with variously sized pipette tips (i.e. 135, 150, 200 µm) for micropipetting
- Isolette or hood with heated stage and bell jar (to control environment)
- Stereoscopic and inverted microscopes
- Incubator with selected gas concentrations

27.3.2 Setup

- Ensure that all quality control testing has been performed on the necessary equipment.
- Isolette and incubators should be maintained at 37°C.

- Oxygen and carbon dioxide concentrations in incubator, bell jar or isolette should be at appropriate levels.
- Dissecting scope with functioning illumination and inverted microscope with heated stage are required.
- Clean all surfaces with distilled water.
- Have all culture dishes prepared and labelled.

27.3.3 Assessment of Zygotes Derived from ICSI

1. Remove the culture dish from the incubator.
2. Place the dish on a heated surface or isolette with microscope visualization.
3. Verify that the dish and paperwork have matching names and medical record numbers.
4. Assess fertilization status using an inverted microscope.
5. Start with the microscope at 25× magnification; increase magnification if needed. Assess fertilization by counting the number of pronuclei and polar bodies. Not all laboratories record the number of polar bodies observed.
6. It may be necessary to roll the zygotes by gently shaking the microscope stage. This is done very carefully and only when needed to improve poor visualization of pronuclei. This is required most often when the cytoplasm is dark or grainy.
7. Record the results.
8. Remove unfertilized and abnormally fertilized zygotes from normally fertilized zygotes.
9. Double-check the dish with the normally fertilized zygotes, and do a final count to ensure that all zygotes are accounted for.
10. If applicable, rinse normally fertilized zygotes through fresh culture medium. Place dish back into the incubator.
11. Dispose of or discard all unfertilized oocytes and abnormally fertilized zygotes.

27.3.4 Notes

In contrast to conventionally fertilized dishes, an oocyte fertilized by ICSI with one pronucleus should always be considered abnormally fertilized and sequestered among the zygotes with three or more pronuclei. If both ICSI and conventional insemination were performed for one patient, separate zygotes that were conventionally fertilized versus those inseminated by ICSI to properly track fertilization, cleavage and blastulation rates.

27.3.5 Assessment of Zygotes Derived from Conventional Insemination

1. Remove the insemination dish from the incubator.
2. Place the dish on a heated surface or isolette with microscope visualization.
3. Verify that the dish and paperwork have matching names and medical record numbers.
4. Under the stereo microscope, begin stripping cumulous cells away from each zygote. Using stripper tips (inner diameter slightly larger than the zygote), manipulate the zygote up and down to remove cumulous cells. Depending on the amount of cumulous

and size of the zygote, start with a 200-μm stripper tip and work down in diameter until all cells are removed from the zona pellucida.

5. Strip one to two zygotes at a time.

6. If cumulous cells are still attached firmly to the zona pellucida, denuding zygotes can be accomplished by needle dissection or the rolling method.

7. After all oocytes are denuded (or after cumulus cells have been removed from several oocytes), rinse these zygotes through fresh drops of culture medium. Place into the culture dish.

8. Assess fertilization status using an inverted microscope.

9. Start with the microscope at 25× magnification; increase magnification as needed. Assess fertilization by counting the number of pronuclei and polar bodies.

10. Normally fertilized embryos will have two polar bodies and two pronuclei. The absence of pronuclei indicates an unfertilized oocyte. One pronucleus may be considered an abnormally fertilized zygote but may represent unknown timing of sperm entering the oocyte for a conventionally inseminated oocyte, and consideration may be given to transfer it if no other acceptable embryos appear in culture or to freeze for a future cycle if no other embryos are available.

11. More than two pronuclei are always associated with abnormal fertilization and should be discarded.

12. If there is no fertilization or low fertilization, evaluate the motility of the sperm in the culture dish. Observe and document whether sperm is motile and/or whether sperm is bound to the zona pellucida.

13. Record observations. If applicable to laboratory policy, record the number of polar bodies seen along with pronuclei observations.

14. Remove unfertilized and abnormally fertilized zygotes from normally fertilized zygotes.

15. Distribute normally fertilized zygotes into drops within the culture dish, sequestering any one-pronucleus zygotes.

16. Double-check the dish with the normally fertilized zygotes, and do a final count to ensure that all zygotes are accounted for.

17. If applicable, rinse normally fertilized zygotes through fresh culture medium. Place the dish back into the incubator.

18. Dispose of or discard all unfertilized oocytes and abnormally fertilized zygotes.

References

1. Elder, K. and Dale, B. *In-Vitro Fertilization* (3rd edn.) (p. 277) (Cambridge University Press, 2011).

2. Nasiri, N. and Eftekhari-Yazdi, P. An overview of the available methods for morphological scoring of pre-implantation embryos in in vitro fertilization. *Cell J* 2015; 16(4):392–405.

3. Nicoli, A. et al. Pronuclear morphology evaluation for fresh in vitro fertilization (IVF) and intracytoplasmic sperm injection (ICSI) cycles: a systematic review. *J Ovarian Res* 2013; 6(1):64.

4. Scott, L. Pronuclear scoring as a predictor of embryo development. *Reprod Biomed Online* 2003; 6(2):201–14.

5. Tesarik, J. and Greco, E. The probability of abnormal preimplantation development can be predicted by a single static observation on pronuclear stage morphology. *Hum Reprod* 1999; 14(5):1318–23.

6. Alpha Scientists in Reproductive Medicine and European Society of Human Reproduction and Embryology. Istanbul consensus workshop on embryo assessment: proceedings of an expert meeting. *Reprod Biomed Online* 2011; 22(6):632–46.

7. Plachot, M. et al. Co-culture with granulosa cells does not increase the fertilization rate in couples with previous fertilization failures. *Hum Reprod* 1993; 8(9):1455–8.

Polar Body Biopsy for IVF

Markus H. M. Montag

Introduction

Preimplantation genetic diagnosis (PGD) and screening (PGS) involve the analyses of the genetic or chromosomal contents of the developing embryo. A direct reflection of the genetic/chromosomal status can be obtained after biopsy of blastomeres or trophectoderm cells. Biopsy of the first and second polar bodies followed by genetic analysis allows indirect assessment of the maternal contribution. Polar body biopsy requires some modification and adaption compared to the more established embryo biopsy procedures.

28.1 Background

Polar body biopsy was introduced in 1990 for genetic diagnosis.[1] It was later adapted for aneuploidy screening in different patient groups.[2] Polar bodies (PBs) are an indirect reflection of the genetic/chromosomal status of the corresponding oocyte. Polar body diagnosis can only detect the maternal contribution to the developing embryo. Most aneuploidies in human embryos are derived from the maternal side and are predominantly due to premature chromatid segregation.[3] Polar bodies can be easily removed at a very early stage after insemination and analyzed prior to formation of the embryo.[4,5] Although the first and second PBs are each single cells, whole-genome amplification followed by array-comparative genomic hybridization has been shown to be feasible for aneuploidy diagnosis.[6,7] Mosaicism is not an issue in PBs. These advantages are counter-balanced by some clear disadvantages.[8,9] Both PBs must be analyzed to achieve a complete diagnosis, and the costs are even exaggerated, as not all diagnosed oocytes may reach the blastocyst stage. Polar body biopsy requires an opening of the zona pellucida to gain access to the perivitelline space. The different biopsy methods will be described here.

28.2 Reagents, Supplies and Equipment

- Inverted microscope with heated plate and micromanipulators
- 1.48-μm diode laser
- Holding capillary
- Polar body biopsy capillary with an inner diameter of approximately 18 to 20 μm
- HEPES- or MOPS-buffered culture medium
- Oil for covering medium in the dish
- Culture dish suitable for micromanipulation

28.3 Quality Control

1. The heated table of the inverted microscope has to be checked for proper temperature in the culture medium droplet in the biopsy dish.
2. The laser requires regular service.
3. The focus area of the laser beam has to be adjusted from time to time. Especially after a longer period without using the laser, the size and shape of a laser-induced opening in the zona pellucida should be tested prior to routine biopsy application.
4. Single-cell (PB) analysis based on whole-genome amplification can be contaminated by other cells if care is not taken.
   a. Dish preparation should follow good laboratory practice for sterile work.
   b. Contamination-free environment must be regularly checked by negative control samples.

28.4 Procedures

For all procedures, the required biopsy dishes with buffered culture medium and oil overlay have to be prepared in advance and kept warm at 37°C. The heated stage of the microscope has to be switched on well in advance to achieve the correct warming temperature. For procedures requiring micromanipulation equipment, the capillaries (holding/aspiration) must be fitted before starting the manipulation.

28.4.1 Opening of the Zona Pellucida by Zona Drilling

1. Fix the oocyte to the holding capillary in an orientation whereby PBs are on top of the oocyte and at an angle of 90 degrees away from the 11 to 13 o'clock position.
2. Insert a capillary for zona drilling through the zona pellucida, starting at the 13 o'clock position and pushing through to the 11 o'clock position.[10]
3. The drilling needle should have completely penetrated the zona on both sides.
4. Release the oocyte from the holding capillary.
5. Move the drilling capillary with the pierced zona under the holding capillary, and rub the part of the zona that is between the needle penetration point back and forth at the side of the holding capillary.
6. As soon as the drilling capillary has sliced off the zona, turn the oocyte by 90 degrees so that the initial slit is facing from the bottom of the dish to the lid – the PBs are now either in the 9 o'clock position or the 3 o'clock position.
7. Fix the oocyte in this position, and push the drilling capillary again from the 13 o'clock position to the 11 o'clock position.
8. Release the oocyte from the holding capillary, and repeat the rubbing step in order to create a criss-cross zona slit opening.
9. As soon as both slits are made, release the oocyte, and position the PBs at 11 to 12 o'clock position and the middle part of the crossing slits at the 3 to 2 o'clock position.
10. Insert the aspiration needle, and proceed with simultaneous or sequential biopsy as described below.

28.4.2 Laser-Assisted Opening of the Zona Pellucida

1. Laser-assisted zona opening is the easiest method for subsequent PB biopsy.[4,5]
2. The size of the drilled opening is usually in the range of 20 μm or less.
3. If needed, the size of the opening can be easily adjusted to the diameter of the aspiration capillary.
4. The capillary can be introduced through the laser-drilled opening, and a sharp aspiration needle is not needed.
5. The opening allows the use of flame-polished blunt-ended aspiration needles, which greatly reduce the risk of damaging the PB or the remaining oocyte.

28.4.3 Timing of Polar Body Biopsy

1. For PB biopsy, timing is a crucial point.
2. The first PB degenerates with time, and doing a biopsy later than 10 hours after ICSI may already result in lower hybridization efficiency.
3. The second PB is formed around two to four hours after ICSI, but because it is firmly attached to the oolemma with a cytoplasmic strand and spindle remnants up to six hours after ICSI,[8] the optimal time for biopsy is at 8 to 16 hours after ICSI.
4. Recent data show that for testing of the second PB in array comparative genomic hybridization (CGH), the amplification efficiency of the isolated DNA is lower if biopsy is done before eight hours after ICSI.[6]
5. Based on this, one may conclude that the optimal timing for sequential biopsy is 4 to 10 hours after ICSI for the first and 8 to 16 hours after ICSI for the second PB.
6. For simultaneous biopsy of the first and second PBs, an optimal time window is at 8 to 10 hours after ICSI.

28.4.5 Simultaneous Polar Body Biopsy

1. Use a holding capillary to fix the oocyte in the proper orientation.
2. Simultaneous removal of the first and second PBs is best accomplished if the oocyte is positioned to the holding capillary with the first PB at the 12 o'clock position and the second PB located on the right side of the first one in the same focal plane.
3. An opening is drilled at between 1 and 3 o'clock.
4. The biopsy capillary is moved into the perivitelline space and pushed gently over the PBs.
5. Only minimal aspiration is required during this process.
6. While pushing the capillary further over the PBs, cytoplasmic bridging between the second PB and the oocyte will be trimmed off by the first PB, which will push the second PB into the biopsy capillary.

28.4.6 Sequential Polar Body Biopsy

1. Use a holding capillary to fix the oocyte in the proper orientation.
2. Easy removal of the first PB is best accomplished if the oocyte is positioned to the holding capillary with the first PB at the 12 o'clock position.

3. If the second PB is not yet visible, the opening can be drilled at any position that allows easy access to the first polar body. If possible, a position should be chosen where the perivitelline space shows a large gap between the zona pellucida and the oolemma.
4. If the second PB is already extruded, the opening must be located at a position that enables easy access to the first PB and later easy access to the second PB through the same opening.
5. Removal of the second PB is done at seven to nine hours after ICSI. Sufficient place should be available between the position of the second PB and the holding capillary in case the cytoplasmic bridge between the second PB and the oocyte is strong and the second PB must be pushed towards the side with the holding capillary.

28.5 Notes

A. Acidic tyrode solution as a chemical means to open the zona pellucida for subsequent biopsy cannot be used as it has a negative impact on further development if applied at the oocyte stage.
B. Following zona drilling, polar body biopsy can be performed with simple glass tools. However, multiple steps including dissection, release and rotation of the oocyte are needed, and the procedure definitely requires skill and more time.
C. It is important to drill only one opening when opening the zona pellucida. Two openings, for example, to retrieve both PBs through separate openings, may cause problems at the time of hatching. The embryo could hatch through both openings simultaneously and may get trapped within the zona.
D. It is important to generate a sufficiently large opening that allows consecutive hatching at the blastocyst stage. Smaller openings (<15 μm) may also cause trapping of the embryo followed by degeneration.

1. The laser beam generates a three-dimensional opening. Placing small openings by single laser shots side by side will finally give a sufficiently large opening in x-y direction, but the opening may be too narrow in z direction.

E. Laser-drilled openings will stay permanently in the zona, and therefore, gentle handling is recommended during subsequent transfer of oocytes to other media droplets and even during embryo transfer.
F. Cumulus cells are of the same size as PBs. Therefore, oocytes for subsequent PB biopsy must be properly denuded.
G. Strong aspiration during biopsy of the second PB may result in the formation and release of cytoplasmic fragments from the oocyte. These may contain the chromatid material that is located close to the second PB.

References

1. Verlinsky, Y., Ginsberg, N., Lifchez, A. et al. Analysis of the first polar body: preconception genetic diagnosis. *Hum Reprod* 1990; **5**:826–9.

2. Munne, S., Dailey, T., Sultan, K. M. et al. The use of first polar bodies for preimplantation diagnosis of aneuploidy. *Mol Hum Reprod* 1995; **10**:1014–20.

3. Handyside, A. H., Montag, M., Magli, M. C. et al. Multiple meiotic errors caused by predivision of chromatids in woman of advanced maternal age undergoing in vitro fertilisation. *Eur J Hum Genet* 2012; 20:742–7.

4. Montag, M., van der Ven, K., Delacrétaz, G. et al. Laser assisted microdissection of zona pellucida facilitates polar body biopsy. *Fertil Steril* 1998; **69**:539–42.

5. Harton, G. L., Magli, M. C., Lundin, K. et al. ESHRE PGD Consortium/ Embryology Special Interest Group: best practice guidelines for polar body and embryo biopsy for preimplantation genetic diagnosis/screening (PGD/PGS). *Hum Reprod* 2011; **26**:41–6.

6. Magli, C., Montag, M., Köster, M. et al. Polar body array CGH for prediction of the status of the corresponding oocyte: I. Technical aspects. *Hum Reprod* 2011; **26**:3181–5.

7. Geraedts, J., Montag, M., Magli, M. C. et al. Polar body array CGH for prediction of the status of the corresponding oocyte: I. Clinical results. *Hum Reprod* 2011; **26**:3173–80.

8. Montag, M., Köster, M.. Strowitzki, T. and Toth, B. Polar body biopsy. *Fertil Steril* 2013; **100**:603–7.

9. Capalbo, A., Bono, S., Spizzichino, L., Biricik, A., Baldi, M. et al. Sequential comprehensive chromosome analysis on polar bodies, blastomeres and trophoblast: insight into female meiotic errors and chromosomal segregation in the preimplantation window of embryo development. *Hum Reprod* 2013; **28**:509–18.

10. Cieslak, J., Ivakhenko, V., Wolf, G. et al. Three-dimensional partial zona dissection for preimplantation genetic diagnosis and assisted hatching. *Fertil Steril* 1999; **71**:308–13.

Zygote Cryopreservation for IVF

Dean E. Morbeck

Introduction

While vitrification of blastocysts is becoming the primary method to cryopreserve embryos, zygote cryopreservation remains an important option for many clinical laboratories. When coupled with controlled-rate freezing, cryopreservation of gametes can be highly effective while also promoting laboratory efficiency. Of the many advantages to freezing embryos at this stage, perhaps the most important is the ability to preserve the potential of an entire cohort of embryos for patients undergoing fertility preservation versus risking loss of potential during extended culture. A controlled-rate zygote freezing programme can improve laboratory efficiency by both decreasing the time needed to freeze a large cohort of zygotes relative to the time required for vitrification, as well as decreasing the amount of laboratory/incubator time required after oocyte retrieval if embryos were cultured to the blastocyst stage and frozen.

29.1 Background

An efficient method for human zygote freezing using propanediol was first reported in 1986 by Jacques Testart and colleagues,[1] a method used by many groups[2,3] and used extensively at the Mayo Clinic. Our own experience using this method for more than 20 years has yielded high rates of survival (>90% survival with cell division) for both in vitro fertilization (IVF) and intracytoplasmic sperm injection (ICSI) zygotes.[4,5] Though some investigators report better outcomes with vitrification (reviewed by Edgar and Gook[6]), none of these reported results similar to our experience of survival rates of greater than 90%.

In addition to legislation in some countries that limits embryo cryopreservation to the zygote stage, there are several other clinical settings where zygote freezing could be advantageous. One example is for patients with the risk of ovarian hyperstimulation syndrome (OHSS) requiring a freeze-all cycle. With an optimized zygote freezing programme, development to the blastocyst stage and implantation are equivalent to fresh blastocysts,[7] allowing the laboratory flexibility to thaw zygotes as needed for frozen embryo transfers. By slow freezing at the zygote stage, a large number of embryos can be cryopreserved at one time in a manner that is more efficient for the laboratory than performing vitrification on 10, 20 or more zygotes. This is also more effective use of laboratory time than culturing all zygotes to the blastocyst stage and vitrifying a large number of blastocysts on days 5 and 6.

A robust zygote freezing programme's biggest beneficiary may be patients who wish to preserve their fertility. It is well known that blastocyst conversion rates vary by laboratory[8] and can be influenced by variation in the quality of product used for embryo culture,[9,10] making it possible that no blastocysts develop as a result of suboptimal conditions. This effectively defeats the purpose of fertility 'preservation'. Zygote cryopreservation, particularly when there are a large number of embryos, allows incremental use of embryos and limits exposure of the whole cohort at one time. Furthermore, culture conditions should continue to improve as the field of IVF matures, making it possible that embryos that fail to develop to blastocysts with today's media and conditions may develop in the future.

The timing of pronuclear embryo freezing is critical. Freezing should be carried out after completion of pronuclear migration and before the onset of syngamy. Only 10% of early zygotes implanted compared with 28% of older zygotes show pronuclei (PNs) in close contact and display equatorially distributed nucleoli, suggesting a role for the cytoskeleton in cryodamage.[11]

The optimal time to freeze PN embryos is 20 to 22 hours after insemination when the embryo is entering G_2 phase of cell cycle. The PNs in embryos resulting from ICSI insemination develop one to two hours earlier[5]; therefore, the time for cryopreservation occurs between 18 and 20 hours after ICSI.

29.2 Reagents, Supplies and Equipment (Note A)

- HTF-HEPES (mHTF)
- Sucrose (Sigma S1888)
- 1,2-Propanediol (Sigma 398039)
- Serum substitute supplement (SSS) (Irvine Scientific 99193)
- Human serum albumin
- Mineral oil
- Cryopreserved one-cell murine embryos
- Four-well dish
- 0.25-ml[3] straws or 1.2 ml cryovials (Note B)
- Thermometer with thermocouple
- Sterile scissors
- Straw sealer

29.3 Quality Control

The controlled-rate freezing system should be tested for proper function biannually. If system includes a solenoid valve for nitrogen injection, annual replacement of the valve can be considered.

1. Between 12 and 24 hours prior to murine embryo thawing, prepare
   a. Cryopreservation and thawing solutions.
   b. Culture medium.

2. Thaw murine embryos according to standard protocol. Approximately 20 embryos (one straw) are needed.

3. After 10 minutes of rehydration, cryopreserve one-cell embryos and then thaw according to procedure outlined below. Load one to two embryos per straw or vial.

4. Allow murine embryos to remain immersed in liquid nitrogen for at least 15 minutes before beginning the thaw procedure. Thaw one or two straws/vials at a time. Continue to thaw in groups of one or two until all embryos are thawed.

5. Incubate embryos for 96 hours, and evaluate development every 24 hours. Acceptable embryo development is greater than 70% expanded blastocysts at 96 hours.

29.4 Procedure

29.4.1 Cryopreservation Setup

1. Complete all necessary paperwork and labelling of straws/vials prior to starting. Embryos are frozen in straws containing one or two embryos.
2. Prior to loading embryos into straws, a second embryologist verifies patient name and unique identifier number on the freeze dish. The second embryologist verifies straw identification with the patient dish at the time of straw filling with cryoprotectant. To ensure accuracy of the straw labels, a second embryologist verifies the straw labels for each patient regardless of the number of patients being cryopreserved and records his or her initials on cryo-form.
3. When the freezing programme is complete, transfer the straws to a Styrofoam container filled with liquid nitrogen. Remove the cane from the pre-cooling location and place it in the same container. Be sure that there is enough liquid nitrogen to cover both the straws and the cane completely. Place straws *embryo end first* (coloured rings up) in a goblet, and quickly transfer the cane back to the storage canister.
4. Working solutions are prepared at least 12 hours in advance of freeze and store at 4 to 6°C and have a shelf-life of 7 days. Bring to room temperature prior to use.

   a. Freeze solutions (FS1–FS3):

      i.   FS1: mHTF + 20% SSS
      ii. FS2: mHTF + 20% SSS + 1.5 M 1,2-propanediol
      iii. FS3: mHTF + 20% SSS + 1.5 M 1,2-propanediol + 0.1 M sucrose

   b. Thaw solutions (TS1–TS4):

      i.   TS1: mHTF + 20% SSS + 1.0 M 1,2-propanediol + 0.2 M sucrose
      ii. TS2: mHTF + 20% SSS + 0.5 M 1,2-propanediol + 0.2 M sucrose
      iii. TS3: mHTF + 20% SSS + 0.2 M sucrose
      iv. TS4: mHTF + 20% SSS

29.4.2 Embryo Equilibration

1. Turn off the heat stage, and allow enough time for the stage to reach room temperature.
2. Set up one four-well dish. Pipette 1.0 ml FS1 into the first well, 1.0 ml of FS2 into the second well and 1.0 ml FS3 into the third well. Always mix solutions with cryoprotectants immediately prior to aliquoting into dishes as cryoprotectants can separate out of solution.
3. Transfer embryo(s) into the first well containing FS1 for one minute. Place the embryos into the medium, check to make sure that all embryos are present, start the timer, gently swirl and cover for the remainder of incubation time.
4. Transfer embryo(s) into a second well containing FS2 for 15 minutes. Gently swirl dish to mix embryo with the new solution and at five-minute intervals during incubation.

Embryos should be kept at room temperature and air atmosphere during this 15 minute. *Do not* place cells to be frozen in CO_2; gas trapped in an embryo expands during cryopreservation, resulting in cellular damage.

5. During the 15-minute incubation in FS2, prepare straws according to Section 29.4.3.
6. Transfer embryos into FS3 for 10 minutes. Gently swirl dish to mix embryo(s) with the new solution.
7. After 10 minutes, complete filling of straws with FS3 and loading of embryo(s) according to Section 29.4.3. Embryos are placed into straws according to quality, with the best-quality embryo placed into straw 1.
8. Transport straws containing the embryos to the controlled-rate freezer. *Keep straws horizontal during transport.* Place straws in the freezer, making note of the location of the embryo end for purposes of seeding. Connect embryo freeze thermocouple, if available, to outlet in freezing chamber.

29.4.3 Straw Filling Method (0.25-ml³ Straw)

1. Place desired number of cryostraws on clean work surface (Note C). Handle the straws carefully by touching only the tip of the plugged end.
2. Mark each straw 20 and 40 mm from the non-plugged end with a cryomarker. Code straw with coloured rings or marks, if desired.
3. Mark each straw with patient name, ID number and straw number in the centre of the straw two times (once on each side of straw) and place in a 15-ml tube. A second technician will verify the straw identifications and document it on the cryo-form.
4. Place final cryoprotectant (FS3: 1.5 M propylene glycol with 0.1 M sucrose and 20% SSS) into a 15-ml tube. Volume calculation: 0.15 ml/straw + an extra 0.15 ml (Note D).
5. One straw is marked as a control and filled with cryoprotectant:
   a. Attach a clean, sterile 5-inch glass Pasteur pipette to a 1-ml³ syringe with a Nalgene tubing adapter.
   b. Pick up the straw by the plugged end and insert the 5-inch glass pipette into opposite end.
   c. With IVF scissors, clip the plugged end. Place clipped end into final cryoprotectant, and draw up to first mark on straw with syringe. Be certain not to touch the medium on the coloured rings.
   d. Remove and aspirate air until solution reaches second mark (20 mm from open end attached to 5-inch Pasteur pipette. Seal clipped end.
   e. Remove from 5-inch pipette, and carefully secure thermocouple to straw with tape so the end is centred between the 20- and 40-mm marks. Be sure that there are no bubbles in the 20- to 40-mm area, and tape to completely seal end of straw.

6. After embryos have been in the final cryoprotectant for 10 minutes, fill straws with solution as described in Step 5. Then
   a. Quickly locate the embryo and transfer it to a straw with a small-diameter embryo handling pipette so that it is centred between the 20- and 40-mm marks.
   b. Seal the other end of the straw. Keep the straw horizontal at all times to prevent migration of the embryo to a different region of the fluid column. Do not touch the area where the embryos are placed (between the 20- and 40-mm marks).

c. Check for proper seal with the stereomicroscope.

d. Place straws with embryos on a rack so that the embryos are aligned with the thermocouple in the control straw.

29.4.4 Controlled-Rate Freeze

1. If cryofreezer has the ability to monitor sample temperature, connect the embryo freeze thermocouple to the outlet in the freezing chamber.

2. Freeze straws with the following programme and steps:

   a. 20°C/room-temperature start. Cool at 2.0°C/minute to −7°C.

   b. −7°C hold:

      i. When sample temperature (via thermocouple) has been at the target temperature (−7°C) for five minutes, perform seeding.

      ii. Seed each straw (including control) at the halfway point between the meniscus opposite the embryo and the second mark on the straw. It is extremely important to not seed too close to the embryos; seeding too close to the embryos results in cellular damage and embryonic death. It should take approximately 30 minutes from placement in freezer to seeding.

      iii. Watch the LED sample temperature, and observe for the freezing point of the cryoprotectant (should be −4 or −5°C). The sample should take 4 to 10 minutes to return to −7°C.

      iv. After LED sample temperature has stabilized at −7°C, set timer for five minutes. After exactly five minutes, advance the programme to continue cooling.

      v. Cool at 0.3°C/minute to −30°C.

   c. −30°C final temperature:

      i. The straw temperature will reach −30°C in approximately one hour and 15 minutes. Set a timer to return to freezer at the appropriate time.

      ii. Plunge straws quickly into liquid nitrogen from freeze chamber, remove rack and plunge into Styrofoam container with liquid nitrogem.

      iii. Immediately transfer straws to storage location in storage tank.

29.4.5 Embryo Thaw

1. Review the thaw consent.

2. Working in liquid nitrogen, remove straws, and place in one cane containing liquid nitrogen. Prior to the thaw, a second embryologist verifies that the straws match the patient record and thaw consent. Keep straws in a Stryofoam container containing LN2 next to the microscope.

3. Turn off heat stage to stereomicroscope. Prepare the following:

   a. Empty dish for embryo(s) to be thawed – room temperature.

   b. One four-well dish for the thawing solutions.

4. Bring a 15-ml conical tube containing Dulbecco's phosphate-buffered saline (DPBS) to 30 ± 0.5°C by placing it in hot water or in a 37°C heat block for 20 to 25 minutes; measure the temperature of the DPBS with a sterilized (80% Ethanol) thermometer. The tube of DPBS will be used for thawing/washing outside the straw(s). The maximum

number of 0.25-ml^3 straws immersed in a tube of DPBS is three. To coordinate the thawing, a second technologist may be required when two tubes of DPBS are needed.

5. Remix TS1, and pipette 1.0 ml into the first well of the four-well dish. Repeat with TS2 through TS4 into wells 2 to 4.

6. Remove straws from the liquid nitrogen. Place horizontally on test tube rack at room temperature for 40 seconds (Note E); then, holding the non-embryo end of the straw (opposite the 20- to 40-mm marks), dip the end with the embryo (area of the 20- to 40-mm marks) into DPBS in a Falcon 2095 tube so that entire fluid column in the straw is immersed. Swirl for two to five seconds, just until the last ice disappears, and then quickly wipe dry and cut the embryo end of straw with IVF scissors, keeping the straw horizontal to prevent movement of the embryo(s). Place the cut end of the straw over an empty dish, and carefully cut the distal end of the straw, allowing the fluid column to flow into the dish. Check the dish quickly for embryo(s). If embryos are not in the droplet, proceed with flushing the straw as described below (Note F).

7. Quickly transfer the embryo(s) from the drop to the first well containing TS1 for five minutes (Note G).

8. Transfer embryo(s) to the second well containing TS2 for five minutes and swirl.

9. Transfer embryo(s) to the third well containing TS3 for five minutes and swirl.

10. Transfer embryo(s) to the fourth well containing TS4 for one minute and swirl.

11. Turn on the heat stage of the stereomicroscope. Transfer the embryos to the first drop of culture medium. Once all the embryos are in the drop, expel the remaining medium from the pipette into the well containing TS4. Gently swirl embryos in the first drop of culture medium with the pipette and transfer to the second. Rinse the pipette in the first drop. Gently swirl the embryos in the second drop. Transfer to the third drop of culture medium for incubation. Embryos should be transferred between the drops in small volumes of culture medium to provide a thorough wash. Do not aspirate the embryos up and down in the pipette for rinsing; rather, use the pipette to move them around within the drops. The aspiration and expulsion motion puts a lot of pressure on the embryos.

12. After three minutes, transfer the embryos to the fourth drop of culture medium, and swirl with the pipette. Transfer to the fifth drop for incubation. After one minute, rinse embryos through the sixth drop, and place the embryos in a microdrop for extended culture. Observe and record postthaw quality. Place the dish in the incubator.

29.5 Notes

A. Several options exist for supplies and equipment. Any routine human embryo culture medium containing a zwitterion is suitable in place of mHTF. The presence of HEPES or MOPS is critical to maintain proper pH during the freezing process. Protein supplementation is generally higher than that used for embryo culture. The amount of albumin present in the medium containing 20% SSS is equivalent to 10% HSA v/v. Straws or vials are equally effective for cryostorage. Volume of culture medium in a vial is typically 0.6 ml.

B. The thermometer thermocouple should be small enough to fit inside of a straw or to the bottom of a cryovial. If used with a cryovial, a small hole should be made in the lid of the vial in order to place the thermocouple at the bottom of the control vial.

C. When loading embryos into straws/vials, (1) place single embryos into the first straws and (2) load embryos into straws according to quality, with the best quality in the first straw and poorest in the last. Discretion is used, and the best embryos may be placed into the first and second double-loaded straws. Note whether embryos go into syngamy (breakdown of pronuclear membrane) prior to cryopreservation. If possible, these embryos should be transferred in the fresh cycle rather than frozen.

D. When embryos are placed in FS3, the entire embryonic mass shrinks away from the zona pellucida. Make a general observation of the embryos to be sure that they respond osmotically. If 75% of the embryos do not respond, make a note, as this may affect survival rate.

E. The embryo should be removed from the straw immediately upon disappearance of the last ice (internal temperature −2°C) to maximize survival rates. *The timing of the 40 seconds begins once the straws are removed from the liquid nitrogen and ends with the immersion into the 30°C DPBS. The straws are removed from the liquid nitrogen, and the 40 seconds begins. The straws are positioned on a test tube rack with the portion containing the embryos hanging over the edge. As the end of the 40 seconds approaches, pick up, invert and then loosely cap the tube of DPBS, and immerse the straws at exactly 40 seconds.*

F. In the event an embryo does not come out of a straw, the recovered embryo(s) are transferred into TS1 and transferred through TS2 to TS4 per protocol. During the intervals of equilibration, gently tap the straw in a clean area of the dish two to three times. If the embryo is not in the droplets, flush the straw with TS1. Attach a 5-inch Pasteur pipette to a 1-ml^3 syringe, and aspirate 0.5 to 1.0 ml of TS1. The pipette is attached to the distal end of the straw, and TS1 is slowly expelled through the straw into an empty dish while viewing through the stereomicroscope. The recovered embryo is placed into TS1 along with the other embryos. If the embryo was recovered quickly enough (less than one minute), there is no need to delay the transfer of all embryos to TS2. If it takes longer to recover the embryo, delay the transfer of that embryo to TS2. The late recovered embryo will be out of sync with the other embryo(s) and will be cultured separately. A second technologist is called to assist. If after an exhaustive search the embryo is not found, the laboratory director should be notified and the event documented.

G. As embryos are transferred to each solution, they are swirled within the new solution; specifically, when embryos are placed into TS1, they float to the top. When all embryos have come out of the pipette, the remaining medium within the pipette should be expelled into the centre well. Do not touch the medium in the centre well with the pipette. Expel the medium and allow the drop from the pipette to adhere to the outside of the well near the top. Rinse the pipette with TS1 and expel into the centre well. The embryos are picked up and placed in the middle of the well, and the solution is swirled using the pipette. Cover the dish and start the five-minute timer; the embryos fall to the bottom of the well during this time. At the end of five minutes, the embryos are transferred into TS2 with as little medium as possible. As the embryos are placed into TS2, there is a 'trail' of TS1. Once the embryos are in the dish, draw this 'trail' into the pipette and expel into the centre well. Rinse the pipette with TS2 and expel into the centre well. Draw the embryos into the pipette, and expel them into the centre of the well; then use the pipette to swirl the medium. Cover for five minutes. Repeat with solutions TS3 and TS4, with a five-minute incubation in TS3 and a one-minute incubation in TS4.

References

1. Testart, J., Lassalle, B., Belaisch-Allart, J., Hazout, A., Forman, R. et al. High pregnancy rate after early human embryo freezing. *Fertil Steril* 1986; 46:268–72.

2. Demoulin, A., Jouan, C., Gerday, C. and Dubois, M. Pregnancy rates after transfer of embryos obtained from different stimulation protocols and frozen at either pronucleate or multicellular stages. *Hum Reprod* 1991; 6:799–804.

3. Veeck, L. L., Amundson, C. H., Brothman, L. J., DeScisciolo, C., Maloney, M. K. et al. Significantly enhanced pregnancy rates per cycle through cryopreservation and thaw of pronuclear stage oocytes. *Fertil Steril* 1993; 59:1202–7.

4. Damario, M., Hammitt, D., Session, D. and Dumesic, D. Embryo cryopreservation at the pronuclear stage and efficient embryo use optimizes the chance for a liveborn infant from a single oocyte retrieval. *Fertil Steril* 2000; 73:767–73.

5. Damario, M. A., Hammitt, D. G., Galanits, T. M., Session, D. R. and Dumesic, D. A. Pronuclear stage cryopreservation after intracytoplasmic sperm injection and conventional IVF: implications for timing of the freeze. *Fertil Steril* 1999; 72:1049–54.

6. Edgar, D. H. and Gook, D. A. A critical appraisal of cryopreservation (slow cooling versus vitrification) of human oocytes and embryos. *Hum Reprod Update* 2012; 18:536–54.

7. Shapiro, B. S., Daneshmand, S. T., Garner, F. C., Aguirre, M., Hudson, C. et al. Similar ongoing pregnancy rates after blastocyst transfer in fresh donor cycles and autologous cycles using cryopreserved bipronuclear oocytes suggest similar viability of transferred blastocysts. *Fertil Steril* 2010; 93:319–21.

8. Glujovsky, D., Blake, D., Farquhar, C. and Bardach, A. Cleavage stage versus blastocyst stage embryo transfer in assisted reproductive technology. *Cochrane Database Syst Rev* 2012; 7:CD002118.

9. Morbeck, D. E. Importance of supply integrity for in vitro fertilization and embryo culture. *Semin Reprod Med* 2012; 30:182–90.

10. Wolff, H. S., Fredrickson, J. R., Walker, D. L. and Morbeck, D. E. Advances in quality control: mouse embryo morphokinetics are sensitive markers of in vitro stress. *Hum Reprod* 2013; 28:1776–82.

11. Wright, G., Wiker, S., Elsner, C., Kort, H., Massey, J. et al. Observations on the morphology of pronuclei and nucleoli in human zygotes and implications for cryopreservation. *Hum Reprod* 1990; 5:109–15.

Embryo Assessment at the Pre-Compaction Stage in the IVF Laboratory

Shunping Wang and Tiencheng Arthur Chang

Introduction

Historically, embryo transfer was performed during the cleavage stage, either on day 2 or day 3. With advancements in embryo culture, many in vitro fertilization (IVF) programmes have moved towards blastocyst transfer. The recent development of pre-implantation genetic screening (PGS), metabolic profiling of conditioned media and time-lapse microscopy provide additional information on embryo selection. However, the assessment of cleavage-stage embryos remains crucial in that the information provides embryologists with a preview of embryo implantation potential. This is especially critical for patients with a limited number of embryos, who do not have the luxury to carry on to blastocyst culture for transfer. At this point, embryo morphology remains the sole selection criterion for choosing embryo(s) for transfer. This chapter discusses embryo assessment with the intention of being a quick guideline for embryo selection/grading with respect to symmetry, multi-nucleation and degree of fragmentation.

30.1 Background

Embryo morphology is widely used by many embryologists as the sole selection criterion for choosing embryos for transfer. It provides a safe, non-invasive approach for embryo selection. Many features have been suggested in the past two decades to accurately assess the implantation potential of cleavage-stage embryos. Quality assessment of the zygote is discussed elsewhere in this book. In this chapter we will focus on the quality of cleavage-stage embryos, day 2 and day 3, roughly 48 and 72 hours after insemination, respectively. Several features, such as cell number, symmetry, multi-nucleation and fragmentation, are often considered to be important features when judging embryo quality.

30.2 Cell Number/Cleavage Rate

Embryo growth rate has been considered to be one of the most important characteristics when evaluating embryo quality. Sequential observations for normal embryo growth rate and developmental patterns during cleavage stages are commonly practiced by embryologists.[1] For normal development, human embryos are expected to have four to six cells 48 hours after insemination and six to ten cells after 72 hours. There are several studies indicating that abnormal developmental rates have a negative association with pregnancy rates.

30.3 Uneven Cleavage

'Uneven cleavage' is defined as the uneven distribution of cytoplasmic materials when cells divide, leading to the uneven size of blastomeres. Several studies have indicated that unevenly cleaved embryos have reduced implantation potential, probably due to chromo-somal aberrations and uneven distribution of proteins, messenger RNA (mRNA) and mitochondria. In addition, uneven cleavage of blastomeres may disturb the polarized allocation of certain proteins and genes in both oocytes and embryos, leading to reduced implantation potential.[2]

30.4 Multi-Nucleation

The definition of 'multi-nucleation' in embryos is the presence of more than one nucleus within a blastomere. The cause of multi-nucleation is largely unknown, but studies sug-gested that improper temperature control during oocyte retrieval and the effect of the culture medium may be possible reasons. Multi-nucleation is shown to have a negative association with implantation rate.[3] Also, studies have indicated that multi-nucleation is correlated with excessive chromosomal aberration and a higher degree of fragmentation.[4] When more than one nucleus in each blastomere is observed in day 2 or day 3 embryos, these embryos are considered to be multi-nucleated embryos (multi-nucleation) and are suggested to have lower implantation rates. Multi-nucleation is easily identified in day 2 embryos because fewer blastomeres are present. Multi-nucleation identification in day 3 embryos can be tricky due to increasing blastomere number. Embryologists may have to roll the embryos to have better visualization of multi-nucleation within blastomeres. The presence of multinucleated blastomeres is a predictive factor of poor embryo develop-ment and lower implantation rates.

30.5 Fragmentation

'Fragments' in human embryos are defined as anuclear membrane-bounded extra-cellular cytoplasmic structures. Fragmentation is quite common in human embryo culture, but sometimes it can be difficult to differentiate fragments from blastomeres. Some embryolo-gists have proposed that fragments be defined as less than 45 μm in diameter for day 2 embryos and less than 40 μm in diameter for day 3 embryos.[5]

Several studies suggest that fragmentation in human embryos is related to programmed cell death or abnormalities in cell chromosomal segregation.[6] The grading system for fragmentation varies among different laboratories, but many embryologists consider embryos with less than 10% fragmentation to be grade A embryos and 10% to 25% to be grade B, or of average quality. Embryos with 25% to 50% fragmentation are considered to be of sub-optimal quality, and embryos with greater than 50% fragmentation are poor quality. For easy assessment of fragmentation, percent values can be based on cell equiva-lents. For example, if the area of fragmentation is approximately equivalent to the size of a blastomere on a four-cell embryo, then it can be estimated that the degree of fragmentation is about 25%. By the same token, if the fragmentation occupies the area of one blastomere in an eight-cell embryo, the fragmentation is estimated at 12.5%.

It is proposed that highly fragmented embryos are linked to a higher degree of chromosome abnormalities, in particular, mosaicism. In addition to degree of fragmenta-tion, it is also suggested that the location and distribution of the fragments relative to the embryo are indicative of embryo implantation potential.[7] Some studies indicated that removal of these fragments using microsurgical techniques significantly improves the embryo's implantation potential.[8]

30.6 Other Parameters

Other parameters often used to judge the quality of embryos include cytoplasmic granularity on the blastomeres and thickness/color of the zona pellucida. The cytoplasmic surface of a blastomere is considered to be smooth without excessive granularity, although the association between blastomere cytoplasmic granularity and implantation potential has never been definitively established. The thickness of the zona pellucida is also used by some programmes as one of the embryo selection criteria. Assisted hatching (AH), artificial disruption of the zona pellucida, either by laser ablation or acid, is a common practice among many IVF laboratories on embryos with a thick zona pellucida.

30.7 Standardization of Embryo Assessment

Embryo assessment in cleavage-stage embryos involves many characteristics, as mentioned earlier, thus often making the assessment a complicated and daunting task. Therefore, standardization of embryo assessment is critical to avoid intra- and inter-embryologist variation. Easy adoption and standardization are keys to accurate embryo assessments. Many scoring systems have been proposed over the past years with the intention of simplifying the embryo evaluation process. In general, these scoring systems attempt to combine various parameters and establish a grade or score for ranking embryos. Some of these studies used complicated formulas and algorithms with either multiple logistic regression models or evidence-based embryo quality criteria.[9] Most of these studies were able to, at least to some degree, establish a positive association between the embryo scoring system and implantation/pregnancy success, although there is no consensus as to whether these embryo grading systems are significantly superior in assessing embryo quality when compared with a single-stage evaluation. Another limitation preventing these embryo scoring systems from being widely practiced in many IVF laboratories is that these evaluation methods are quite time-consuming for embryologists to adopt into their busy daily routine work.

30.8 Conclusions

In order to simplify the process and establish standardization for embryo assessment, a three-point grading system was developed by the Society of Assisted Reproductive Technology (SART) Embryo Morphology Subcommittee with the intention of establishing an easy protocol for embryologists to follow.[10] With this standard, cleaved embryos can be classified with an overall grade of good, fair or poor using several characteristics including cell number, ranging from one to eight; fragmentation, with 0, less than 10%, 11% to 25% and greater than 25%; and symmetry, which be categorized as perfect, moderately asymmetrical or severely asymmetrical. These parameters are now collected into the SART National Registry (SART Clinical Outcomes Reporting System (SART CORS)) by the participating SART members. The results have been validated by several studies indicating the positive association between day 3 morphology grade and live birth outcome.

Another attempt to standardize the embryo grading system has been established by the Alpha Executive and European Society of Human Reproduction and Embryology (ESHRE) Special Interest Group on Embryology.[11] For cleavage-stage embryos, several stages of development according to specific time points after insemination were proposed. For day

2 embryos, the embryo assessment should be performed 44 ± 1 hours after insemination and 68 ± 1 hours for day 3 embryos. According to this timeline, the optimal numbers of blastomeres should be four and eight cells for day 2 and day 3 embryos, respectively. The degree of fragmentation is categorized as mild (<10%), moderate (10% to 25%) and severe (>25%). Although in contrast to some previous studies, there is no consensus on the significance of fragment location within the embryos as the members feel this can be a dynamic phenomenon, and these fragments can move freely within the embryo.

As for cleavage, consensus is that all blastomeres should have similar size. Multi-nucleation assessment should be performed on day 2, and observation of multi-nucleation in a single cell is sufficient for the embryo to be considered multi-nucleated. In comparison, multi-nucleation assessment on day 3 would be technically more challenging due to smaller cell size.

Overall, cleavage-stage embryo assessment is essential in selecting embryos with high implantation potential. Even for IVF laboratories that have shifted the majority of their transfer to blastocysts, day 2 and day 3 embryo evaluation provides useful information, such as growth rate and the presence of multi-nucleation, though care must be taken to find balance between gathering enough information and avoiding the interruption of embryo culture.

(A) (B)

(C) (D)

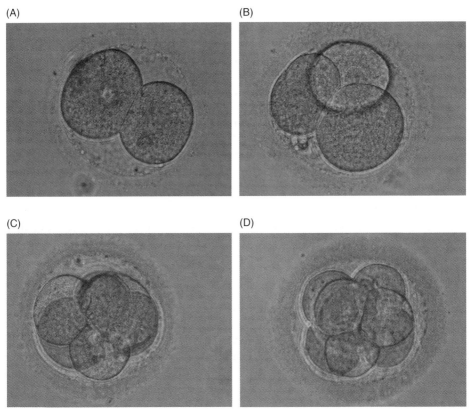

Figure 30.1 Cleavage embryo assessment. (A) Forty-three hours after insemination. Symmetrical blastomeres cleave with no fragmentation. (B) Forty-five hours after insemination. Asynchronous cleavage showing three blastomeres with no significant fragmentation. (C and D) Seventy hours after insemination. Day 3 embryos demonstrating symmetrical cleavage without significant fragmentation. (A black and white version of this figure will appear in some formats. For the color version, please refer to the plate section.)

30.9 Protocol for Cleavage-Stage Embryo Assessment

30.9.1 Principle

Cleavage-stage embryos, day 2 and day 3 after insemination, must be assessed to determine their development and quality at a specified time using the criteria defined in this protocol.

30.9.1 Responsibility

- Embryologist

30.9.2 Specimen

- Human embryos 25 to 68 hours after insemination.

30.9.3 Procedure

30.9.3.1 Equipment and Reagents

- Pipetter
- Stripper tips (150–300 μl)
- Mineral oil
- Culture medium
- Protein substitute (PS)
- Culture dishes: four-well plates
- Dissecting microscope
- Inverted microscope

30.9.3.2 Embryo Grading

1. Cleavage-stage embryos should be assessed at 200× to 400×. The embryos should be assessed for cell number, degree of fragmentation, blastomere symmetry and the presence/absence of multi-nucleation. The fragmentation, symmetry and multinucleation are scored using the following scoring system:

Fragmentation	Score	Symmetry	Score	Multi-nucleation	Score
0%	F4	Symmetrical	1	Present	1
<10%	F3	Asymmetrical	0	Absent	0
10–25%	F2	Grossly asymmetrical	−1		
26–50%	F1				
>50%	F0				

2. Timing for embryos assessments after insemination are as follows:
   - Day 1: 14 to 18.5 to 25 hours
   - Day 2: 42 to 44 hours
   - Day 3: 66 to 68 hours

3. Many IVF programmes may decide to perform day 3 transfer if the overall embryo quality is less than optimal. In Women and Infants Hospital (WIH), the algorithm for determining day of transfer is indicated as follows:

   - Day 3 transfer. On Day 2, there are fewer than four embryos with the quality of four-cell embryos, grades 3 to 4.
   - Day 5 transfer. On Day 2, there are more than four embryos with the quality of four-cell embryos, grades 3 to 4, no multi-nucleation.

4. Algorithm for selecting embryos for transfer on day 3 if possible:

   - Two PNs observed on day 1
   - Highest WIH embryo score
   - Appropriate progression day 2 to day 3 (four- to eight-cell)
   - No multi-nucleation

References

1. Hill, G. A., Freeman, M., Bastias, M. C., Rogers, B. J., Herbert, C. M., 3rd et al. The influence of oocyte maturity and embryo quality on pregnancy rate in a program for in vitro fertilization-embryo transfer. *Fertil Steril* 1989; 52:801–6.

2. Hardarson, T., Hanson, C., Sjogren, A. and Lundin, K. Human embryos with unevenly sized blastomeres have lower pregnancy and implantation rates: indications for aneuploidy and multinucleation. *Hum Reprod* 2001; 16:313–8.

3. Jackson, K. V., Ginsburg, E. S., Hornstein, M. D., Rein, M. S. and Clarke, R. N. Multinucleation in normally fertilized embryos is associated with an accelerated ovulation induction response and lower implantation and pregnancy rates in in vitro fertilization-embryo transfer cycles. *Fertil Steril* 1998; 70:60–6.

4. Munne, S. Chromosome abnormalities and their relationship to morphology and development of human embryos. *Reprod Biomed Online* 2006; 12:234–53.

5. Prados, F. J., Debrock, S., Lemmen, J. G. and Agerholm, I. The cleavage stage embryo. *Hum Reprod* 2012; 27(Suppl. 1): i50–71.

6. Perez, G. I., Tao, X. J. and Tilly, J. L. Fragmentation and death (aka apoptosis) of ovulated oocytes. *Mol Hum Reprod* 1999; 5:414–20.

7. Alikani, M., Cohen, J., Tomkin, G., Garrisi, G. J., Mack, C. et al. Human embryo fragmentation in vitro and its implications for pregnancy and implantation. *Fertil Steril* 1999; 71:836–42.

8. Chi, H. J., Koo, J. J., Choi, S. Y., Jeong, H. J. and Roh, S. I. Fragmentation of embryos is associated with both necrosis and apoptosis. *Fertil Steril* 2011; 96:187–92.

9. Steer, C. V., Mills, C. L., Tan, . S.L, Campbell, S. and Edwards, R. G. The cumulative embryo score: a predictive embryo scoring technique to select the optimal number of embryos to transfer in an in-vitro fertilization and embryo transfer programme. *Hum Reprod* 1992; 7:117–9.

10. Racowsky, C., Vernon, M., Mayer, J., Ball, G. D., Behr, B. et al. Standardization of grading embryo morphology. *Fertil Steril* 2010; 94:1152–3.

11. Alpha Scientists in Reproductive M, Embryology ESIGo. The Istanbul Consensus Workshop on Embryo Assessment: proceedings of an expert meeting. *Hum Reprod* 2011; 26:1270–83.

Chapter

31

Embryo Assessment at the Post-Compaction Stage in the IVF Laboratory

Michael L. Reed and Jun Tao

31.1 Background

Limitations to embryo culture techniques in the early years of human in vitro fertilization (IVF) required transfer and/or cryopreservation of early cleavage-stage embryos on day 2 (e.g. two to four cells) and day 3 (e.g. six to eight cells) (day of oocyte retrieval = day 0); significant translation of technology and information from non-human mammalian embryo culture had not yet occurred. Embryo quality scoring systems for these early cleavage-stage embryos were simplistic as the number of blastomeres, evenness of blastomere size, placement of blastomeres and extent of fragmentation were very evident.

As culture techniques improved, laboratories extended culture of embryos to the blastocyst stage, effectively doubling the time these embryos were maintained in vitro. Observations were commonly made at fertilization determination, mid-culture (day 3) and again at the end of the culture period (days 5 and 6). Using sequential media, it was convenient to evaluate embryos on the day that the transition was made from the first to the second medium, typically on day 3. Evaluations of embryos on days 2 and 4 were then skipped in many laboratories.

Unlike other stages of development, qualitative selection protocols for morula-stage embryos rely on metrics associated with timing of compaction, extent of compaction, morphology of blastomeres and nuclei, extent of fragmentation and cavitation, if present.

From a practical standpoint, chapters of this book are designed to provide evidence-based, clear guides or protocols for all things IVF; however, the process for grading morula-stage embryos requires a slightly different approach, in that a detailed understanding of this seldom-visited stage of development is critical to the process of assigning a quality score to an embryo. Therefore, this chapter will depart somewhat from a simple, step-by-step approach and touch on developmental details integrated into the suggested grading protocol, as well as providing evidence that morulae are overlooked as a viable clinical choice for transfer and for cryopreservation.

31.2 Developmental Biology

Blastomere compaction typically begins on day 3 after fertilization, at eight or more cells, and usually beyond the time interval when embryos are routinely observed in the laboratory – but compaction is most evident on day 4. Differentiation of human blastomeres is pronounced after genomic activation at the four- to eight-cell stage; up to this point, separated blastomeres may be potent, independently able to develop into blastocysts.[1] Transcription and translation events after genomic transition affect, among many other functions, the cell cytoskeleton, promoting formation of junctional complexes and cell adhesion processes that play critical roles during compaction of the blastomeres. For example, E-cadherin-mediated adhesion, a trans-membrane glycoprotein event, a Ca^{2+}-dependent cell-to-cell process, initiates at the eight-cell stage and is regulated post-translationally via protein kinase C and other signalling molecules; for an excellent review, see Sozen et al.[2]

Embryo compaction, a requisite for blastocoel formation, represents one of the earliest *visible* cell differentiation events; blastomere division results in cytoplasmic compartmentalization, but this is an event not readily viewed by light microscopy. During compaction, cells undergo dramatic morphological changes. Electron microscopy reveals cell surface structural alterations: density of the membrane microvilli increases compared to early cleavage stages, and these microvilli become polarized (e.g. restricted to the free surface of the blastomere), while the contact surfaces between neighbouring cells form small morphological blebs.[3] Fierro-Gonzalez et al.[4] recently reported that filopodia extend from some blastomeres to neighbouring cells, altering blastomere shape from round to elongated, cuboidal or crescent shape during early compaction. Before the next cell division, the filopodia retract, and cell shape reverts to a round morphology. Cycles of compaction proceed, and cell membranes flatten further, increasing cell-to-cell contact along the margins of these cells, until inter-cellular clefts are reduced to the point where individual blastomere boundaries are no longer visible. The fully compacted embryo resembles a single large cell with a smooth surface profile.

Compaction demonstrates consecutive morphogenic alterations associated with the fourth, fifth and possibly sixth mitotic divisions. Fully compacted morulae contain more cells than can be visualized; increased cell numbers, smaller blastomere sizes and positioning of cells (e.g. allocation of non-polarized cells to 'inside' and polarized cells to 'outside' positions) result in further differentiation of cells that becomes apparent at the blastocyst stage; inner non-polarized cells give rise to the inner cell mass, while outer crescent-shaped polarized cells give rise to trophectoderm. These alterations can now be studied in real time using time-lapse imaging.[5] The allocation of cells to inside or outside positions is believed to be random, not predetermined, but rather linked to the position of the daughter blastomeres after division.[2]

At the later stages of compaction, cell number may be the most important predictor of future blastocyst quality; having more cells translates to a higher probability of having a distinct inner cell mass and a well-formed trophectoderm with multiple cells. Impaired fourth and fifth mitotic divisions may still compact and form a blastocoel cavity, but the trophectoderm cells will be fewer and larger. The inner cell mass may be flat and difficult to visualize, with relatively few cells, or it may be absent altogether. It is not unusual for compaction to not occur at or around the eight-cell stage, or on day 4, and it may be delayed until day 5. With early compaction on day 3, if cell numbers are low (e.g. fewer than six cells), the developmental prognosis is usually poor; these embryos usually arrest at the early compaction stage or develop into late compaction morulae with low cell numbers that do not form a healthy inner cell mass and/or trophectoderm.[6]

Polarization and compaction are both spatial (cell number and/or position) and temporal events; delayed compaction may indicate that gene expression and mitotic events are not synchronized. The impact of delayed compaction is not clear, as these embryos may yet develop into high-quality late-compaction morulae, implant and give rise to normal gestations. There are data to suggest, however, that embryos that do not compact until day 5 may have higher rates of aneuploidy.[7]

Asynchronous compaction among blastomeres is also common, where some blastomeres anchor to neighbouring cells, and others remain separate and maintain a round shape and are loosely organized. Compaction can proceed to completion, where all cells participate in the process, and it appears that there is no adverse effect on quality and implantation.

Partial compaction is different from asynchronous compaction; some blastomeres are never incorporated into the embryo and are excluded (set aside from the embryo). These excluded cells may be of different sizes, and some may contain multiple nuclei or vacuoles. Excluded cells are observed primarily in the perivitelline space, but they may be found in the blastocoel cavity or engulfed by other blastomeres. The final size of the morula is correspondingly reduced according to the extent and number of excluded cells. Fragmentation plays a similar role, with similar effects on morula formation. A small percent fragmentation, less than 10%, seems not to affect morula quality, but as fragmentation increases, the size of the morula decreases, and quality is reduced due to only having a smaller portion or number of cells participate in the compaction process.

31.3 Morphological Considerations for Grading

For pre-implantation embryos, the definition of 'morula' has been generally accepted to mean a 'ball of cells'; it is best applied to observations where the number of cells is not as easily determined; 'morulae' is the plural form. The morula-stage embryo is unique – its development spans several days of in vitro culture, though the fully compacted embryo is typically observed on day 4. Early stages of compaction and advanced numbers of blastomeres beyond the eight-cell stage may be evident on day 3, and delayed compaction may be evident on day 5.[5,6] Time-lapse imaging data with respect to the compaction process are growing. The time frame from early compaction events to blastocoel formation with the inner cell mass visible may span 24 hours, but variable time frames are also documented, along with morphological events that occur between different sub-stages. Ideally, time-lapse imaging will also allow identification of abnormalities that arise during this time.

Morulae selected for transfer on day 4 have comparable implantation rates to blastocysts selected for transfer on day 5,[8–10] supporting the option for selection and transfer on day 4 as a reliable choice for practitioners. In a large retrospective study, Tao et al.[8] transferred fewer good-quality morulae on day 4 compared to numbers of cleaving embryos replaced on day 3 while demonstrating the same or higher implantation and pregnancy rates. Carving out the data for only good-quality embryos, morulae demonstrated significantly higher implantation and pregnancy rates than good-quality cleaving embryos, replacing a mean of 3.5 'good quality' embryos on day 3 yielded 21.4% implantation, 45.0% clinical pregnancy and 40.0% ongoing pregnancy rates, while replacing a mean of 2.1 'good quality' morulae on day 4 yielded an implantation rate of 46.4%, clinical pregnancy rate of 68.0% and ongoing pregnancy rate of 62.3%.

Morula-stage embryo transfer and/or cryopreservation are not prevalent in the human assisted reproductive technology (ART) field, and grading of these embryos is not considered feasible, or simple, by many embryologists. As such, many programmes do not routinely evaluate embryos on day 4 of culture. A non-scientific poll of embryologists by one author found that the uncertainty of grading morula-stage embryos appears to be based on the facts that (1) there is no widely acclaimed, clear and concise system for grading, and (2) embryologists are less experienced at grading morulae embryos than early cleavage- and blastocyst-stage embryos.

The morula-stage embryo is the product of mitotic cellular division that increases cell numbers while reducing blastomere size, but cell number evaluation is confounded or masked by morphological changes that include blastomere cell shape, cell-to-cell adhesion and arrangements of blastomeres and an overall appearance of compaction; these processes make it more difficult to develop a consistent and simple grading system for this stage. To facilitate grading, morulae can be divided into three sub-stages based on consecutive morphological alterations: early compaction, full compaction and late compaction. Consider also that morulae with early cavitation are still categorized as morula, not early blastocysts. Based on the pioneering work of Tao et al.,[8] an updated grading system has been proposed and is presented in Table 31.1; visual examples representing the different grades can be found in this same reference. Applying the grading table to photographs of morulae at different stages, for example, as found in Prado et al.,[11] can be a valuable tool for gaining proficiency in grading morulae.

31.3.1 The Grading System

There are three sub-stages of compaction: early, full and late. Each sub-stage can be scored as good, intermediate or poor, but not all grading criteria (descriptors) are applicable to all sub-stages (Table 31.1). To use this table, apply the descriptors under the column headers labelled 'All stages' to all morulae. Then identify the appropriate sub-stage for the degree of compaction (early, full and late), and evaluate the embryo according to the descriptors in the appropriate columns (two columns per sub-stage). For an embryo to be graded as 'good', all descriptors within the 'good' row must agree with the stage-specific row × column descriptors. An embryo may be graded as 'intermediate' if one descriptor falls within the 'intermediate' category and all remaining descriptors fall within the 'good' category.

31.3.2 Notes: Grading Examples

- **A good-quality late compact morula:** >75% cell-to-cell adhesion, <15% fragmentation, >30 cells, an identifiable inner cell mass
- **An intermediate early compact morula:** 60–75% cell-to-cell adhesion, 15%–45% fragmentation, six to eight cells, slight differences in blastomere uniformity
- **A poor-quality full compact morula:** <60% cell-to-cell adhesion, >40% fragmentation, irregular embryo shape, with large cells, multi-nuclei and/or engulfed cells

31.4 Cryopreservation

Selection of the ideal embryo for transfer has evolved, in many laboratories, to the period of time after embryonic genome activation, focused more so on the blastocyst-stage embryo. Selection of embryos for transfer at the morula stage is a viable option; in terms of cryopreservation and survival, Tao et al.[12,13] were the first to demonstrate that cryopreserved human morulae have similar high survival, after thawing, as other developmental stages, including the blastocyst stage. Well-established cell-to-cell connections and the concomitant formation of a large, fluid-filled cavity in the blastocyst-stage embryo can interfere with movement of water during exposure to cryoprotectants prior to and during cooling. Applying artificial collapse of the blastocoel may improve post-cryopreservation embryo survival, but for morula-stage embryos, collapse is not required.[14] Both

Table 31.1 Schematic for Morula Embryo Grading

Apply to	All stages	All stages	Early compact.	Early compact.	Full compact.	Full compact.	Late compact.	Late compact.
Embryo grading	% cell join compaction	Fragments, %	Cell no.	Cell size uniformity	Embryo shape	Large cells, multi-nuclei, engulfing	Cell no.	Identifiable potential ICM
A (good)	>75	<15	>8	Uniform	Sphere/smooth profile	No	>30	Yes
B (intermediate)	60–75	15–40	6–8	Slight differences	Close to sphere	Yes/no	15–30	Yes but low cell number
C (poor)	<60	>40	<6	Severe differences	Irregular	Yes	<15	Questionable or no ICM

Source: Modified from Tao et al.[8]

vitrification and slow-cooling methodologies are now represented in the literature with respect to cryopreservation of morulae.

31.4.1 Notes: Thawing Cryopreserved Morulae

Compared with early and fully compacted morulae, the late compaction stage may be optimal for cryopreservation. Early-compaction embryos may arrest, whereas embryos that have progressed to full and late compaction more readily proceed developmentally. At the late-compaction stage, cell boundaries are easily revealed again, so cell numbers can be readily evaluated, making it easier to predict the potential development of the inner cell mass and trophectoderm. It has been demonstrated that the majority of the late-compaction morulae are capable of developing to the blastocyst stage.

Morulae, specifically fully compacted morulae, do not have blastocoel cavities, there are no completely formed tight junctions restricting water or cryoprotectant movement across cells and between cell margins and penetration of cryoprotectants can be more efficient. Morulae also display unique morphological changes during freezing and thawing in relation to changes in the osmotic tension of the medium. As the relative concentrations of permeating cryoprotectant and non-permeating cryoprotectant increase immediately around the embryo, morulae demonstrate a reversal of compaction (e.g. early compaction reversed to cleavage stage, full compaction reversed to early compaction and late compaction reversed to full compaction). Corresponding changes during and after thawing are demonstrated with removal of cryoprotectants and decreasing osmotic tension (e.g. embryo compaction status reverts to pre-cryopreservation morphology). The significance of these osmotic-related morphological changes is that the change is instant, providing visible metrics for predicting or judging post-thaw recovery and competence. Decisions regarding the need to thaw additional embryos can be made sooner.

References

1. Van de Velde, H., Cauffman, G., Tournaye, H., Devroey, P. and Liebaers, I. The four blastomeres of a 4-cell stage embryo are able to develop individually into blastocysts with inner cell mass and trophectoderm. *Hum Reprod* 2008; 23:1742–7.

2. Sozen, B., Can, A. and Demir, N. Cell fate regulation during preimplantation development: a view of adhesion-linked molecular interactions. *Dev Biol* 2014; 395:73–83.

3. Nikas, G., Ao, A., Winston, R. M. L. and Handyside, A. H. Compaction and surface polarity in the human embryo. *Biol Reprod* 1996; 55:32–7.

4. Fierro-Gonzalez, J. C., White, M. D., Silva, J. C. and Plachta, N. Cadherin-dependent filopodia control preimplantation embryo compaction. *Nature Cell Biol* 2013; 15:1424–33.

5. Kovacs, P. Embryo selection: the role of time-lapse monitoring. *Reprod Biol Endocrinol* 2014; 12:124.

6. Iwata, K., Yumoto, K., Sugishima, M., Mizoguchi, C., Kai, Y. et al. Analysis of compaction initiation in human embryos by using time-lapse cinematography. *J Assist Reprod Genet* 2014; 31:421–6.

7. Kort, J. D., Lathi, R. B., Brookfield. K., Baker, V. L., Zhao, Q. et al. Aneuploidy rates and blastocyst formation after biopsy of morulae and early blastocysts on day 5. *J Assist Reprod Genet* 2015; 32:925–30.

8. Tao, J., Tamis, R., Fink, K., Williams, B., Nelson-White, T. and Craig, R. The neglected morula/compact stage embryo transfer. *Hum Reprod* 2002; 17:1513–18.

9. Kang, S. M., Lee, S. W., Jeong, H. J., Yoon, S. H., Koh, M. W. et al. Clinical outcomes of elective single morula embryo transfer

versus elective single blastocyst transfer in IVF-ET. *J Assist Reprod Genet* 2012; 29:423–8.

10. Lee, S. H., Lee, H. S., Lim, C. K., Park, Y. S., Yang, K. W. et al. Comparison of the clinical outcomes of day 4 and 5 embryo transfer cycles. *Clin Exp Reprod Med* 2013; 40:122–5.

11. Prado, F. J., Debrock, S., Lemmen, J. G. and Agerholm, I. The cleavage stage embryo. *Hum Reprod* 2012; 27(Suppl. 1):150–71.

12. Tao, J., Tamis, R. and Fink, K. Pregnancies achieved after transferring frozen morula/ compact stage embryos. *Fertil Steril* 2001; 75:629–31.

13. Tao, J., Craig, R. H., Johnson, M., Williams, B., Lewis, W. et al. Cryopreservation of human embryos at the morula stage and outcomes after transfer. *Fertil Steril* 2004; 82:108–18.

14. Vanderzwalmen, P., Bertin, G., Debauche, Ch., Standaert, V., van Roosendaal, E. et al. Births after vitrification at morula and blastocyst stages: effect of artificial reduction of the blastocoelic cavity before vitrification. *Hum Reprod* 2002; 17:744–51.

Embryo Assessment at the Blastocyst Stage in the IVF Laboratory

Tiencheng Arthur Chang, Shunping Wang and
Courtney Failor

Introduction

Embryo quality assessment and grading are major procedures in in vitro fertilization (IVF) laboratories and determining factors for clinical outcome success. Transferring in vitro–cultured embryos at the blastocyst stage (generally day 5 to 6 after insemination), including elective single-embryo transfer (eSET), allows better embryo selection and has been associated with higher implantation rates and better clinical outcomes, especially in good-prognosis patients having high numbers (six or more) of top-quality embryos on day 3.[1–7] Blastocyst transfer has become the preferred choice, replacing cleavage-stage (days 2 to 4) embryo transfer, among IVF laboratories worldwide. Recent advancements in embryo culture media, culture conditions and equipment, trophectoderm (TE) biopsy for pre-implantation genetic testing and the concept of selecting only a few high-implantation-potential embryos for cryopreservation have contributed to more clinics practicing extended embryo culture to the blastocyst stage. Therefore, blastocyst quality assessment has become an essential and important protocol. Developments in time-lapse imaging (TLI) in recent years provide a more dynamic assessment supplemental to traditional morphology grading. New, non-invasive embryo selection approaches using proteomics and metabolomics also hold promise. However, in most laboratories not using TLI and yet to apply emerging non-invasive embryo selection methods, blastocyst assessment using existing scoring systems remains crucial for decision making in embryo transfer, cryopreservation and discard. This chapter discusses essential steps for blastocyst assessment as a quick guideline and lists blastocyst grading criteria based on three commonly used scoring systems in the reference protocol.

32.1 Background

Embryo morphology evaluations at the cleavage stage (as discussed in Chapter 31) and the blastocyst stage are widely used by embryologists as the sole selecting criteria for choosing embryos for transfer and/or cryopreservation. Additional days of morula and blastocyst culture facilitate selection of high-implantation-potential embryos, which are more likely to result in viable offspring. A major issue in limiting the number of embryos transferred is the ability to accurately estimate the reproductive potential of individual embryos within a cohort of embryos. Important questions reproductive endocrinology and infertility (REI) clinicians and laboratory professionals today may have are what embryo selection technique will result in the greatest pregnancy rate, live birth rate and greatest cumulative pregnancy rate.

While no international consensus on blastocyst grading exists, several scoring systems have been developed by examining overall blastocyst formation, inner cell mass

(ICM) and trophectoderm (TE).[1,2,8–12] Many IVF laboratories use systems based on scoring protocols developed by Gardner and Schoolcraft,[8] the Society for Assisted Reproductive Technology (SART)[13] and the European Society of Human Reproduction and Embryology (ESHRE) and Alpha Executive.[12] Laboratories often adapt these guidelines with their own criteria to reflect inter-laboratory variances, different settings in embryo culture (e.g. oxygen concentration) and clinical outcome experiences. The key is to use an existing or modified system that is accurate, non-invasive, simple and robust; efficient for workload; and with minimal personnel variance. Detailed steps, including pre-assessment setup, embryo equilibration, scoring under inverted microscope and preparation for embryo transfer, cryopreservation and discard, should be listed in the laboratory protocols. Steps described in this chapter can serve as a reference and starting point for developing such a protocol.

32.2 Reagents, Supplies and Equipment

32.2.1 Reagents and Supplies

- Mixed gas (5–7% CO_2, 5% O_2, balance N_2)
- 0.2-μm syringe filter
- 10-ml serological pipette
- 5-ml³ syringe
- 5-ml serological pipette
- 5-ml snap-cap tube
- 35-mm/60-mm embryo culture dish
- Blastocyst culture medium, sequential or single-step/continuous
- Embryo handling medium (e.g. mHTF-HEPES)
- Embryo culture oil, mineral oil or light paraffin
- Embryo handling/'stripper' pipette tip (275–300 μm)
- 50/100/200-μl barrier tips for pipette

32.2.2 Equipment

- Stereo microscope
- 50- to 200-μl pipette
- Embryo manipulation/'stripper' pipette
- Inverted microscope with Hoffman modulation contrast (HMC) or equivalent optics, 10× oculars and 10×, 20×, 40× objectives
- Heated microscope stage
- Camera for inverted microscope
- Printer for embryo images
- Incubator, bench-top or upright
- Laminar flow hood/IVF workstation equipped with temperature-controlled work surface
- Nontoxic marking device (e.g. diamond marker pen)
- Laser for assisted hatching (optional)
- TLI system and software (optional)

32.3 Quality Control

1. All equipment should be maintained at optimal working condition and tested for proper function biannually. Backup items are recommended.
2. Reagents and consumables should be checked for expiration date. Each batch of supplies should be tested by mouse embryo assay (MEA) or human sperm survival assay before being use with human embryos.
3. Universal precautions should be applied when handling human embryos, preparing media and discarding biohazardous materials. Each laboratory should establish a safety practice policy that is in compliance with government regulations and accreditation agency requirements.
4. Laboratory personnel should participate in external proficiency testing programmes in embryo morphology grading (e.g. American Association of Bioanalysts Proficiency Testing Service (AAB-PTS) and College of American Pathologists (CAP)) to maintain consistency in quality control and minimize inter-personnel variance. Laboratory performance out of range of nationwide consensus should be corrected. Internal proficiency testing conducted monthly or between two external proficiency testings should be evaluated by the laboratory director to ensure consistency in embryo grading.

32.4 Procedure

32.4.1 Principle

Blastocyst-stage embryos on days 5, 6 and 7 after insemination are assessed to determine development progress and quality and estimate each embryo's developmental potential using criteria defined in this protocol.

32.4.2 Responsibility

• Embryologist

32.4.3 Specimen

• Human embryos on days 5 to 7 after insemination

32.4.4 Steps

1. All fertilized oocytes and embryos are monitored daily for developmental progress.
2. On days 5, 6 and 7 after insemination, embryos are cultured in equilibrated single-step/continuous or sequential blastocyst medium in an incubator with a balanced CO_2 or triple-gas/low-oxygen atmosphere.
3. Minimize temperature fluctuation throughout the grading process. Temperature-controlled workstation surface, heated stages and dishes should be used to maintain consistent temperature.
4. Grading may be performed with embryos staying in culture medium dish or placed in a handling medium (e.g. mHTF-HEPES) in ambient atmosphere. It is important to minimize the time embryos spend outside the incubator.
5. When using a handling medium dish to examine the embryo, label the dish with the patient's name and ID number using a nontoxic marking device (e.g. diamond marker

pen), and equilibrate the oil-covered handling medium dish at the designated controlled temperature (e.g. 37°C) prior to moving embryos into the dish. A second embryologist confirms the patient information. Embryo placement into a handling dish and back to a culture dish can be performed under a stereomicroscope.

6. Remove one dish of the patient's embryos from the incubator. Do not remove more than one dish of embryos at a time.

7. Quickly and cautiously place embryos under the inverted microscope for observation and scoring.

8. Assess blastocysts under the microscope at 200× to 400× with HMC or equivalent optics by applying the grading system of choice per laboratory policy.

9. Characteristics being assessed include overall blastocyst size, expansion and hatching, ICM quality, polar and mural TE quality, zona thickness and other abnormalities and cellular damage/necrosis, as well as cell number, if applicable.

10. Reference scoring systems are listed below. Downgrade one level if any abnormalities or significant morphological defects exist.

      Example: Blastocysts are given a number grade based on the level of blastocoel formation and letter grades for quality of both ICM and TE based on the Gardner and Schoolcraft system. This information is translated into a grade of good (G), fair (F) or poor (P) in compliance with the SART CORS standard.

11. Record the stage of blastocyst development and quality on the patient's embryo log sheet and/or in the electronic medical record system. Photographing all evaluated blastocysts is highly recommended. Names of the embryologist(s), date and time of assessment should be recorded as well.

12. Return embryos in the culture medium dish to the incubator. Confirm the location of embryos, or record new location of embryos in the incubator.

      WARNING: *When using an embryo handling medium dish for grading,* **do not** *return embryos in the handling medium dish to the incubator with an internal atmosphere designed for culture medium dishes.*

13. Repeat steps 6 to 10 with the next dish of embryos for grading.

14. After grading all embryos, check all applicable handling and embryo culture dishes outside the incubator on the microscope and workstation surface to ensure that no embryos are left behind.

15. If available, a second embryologist should confirm patient ID and clearance of all work surfaces.

16. Embryos with the highest scores are selected for embryo transfer. Others may be selected for cryopreservation, with the exception of freeze-all cycles due to ovarian hyperstimulation syndrome (OHSS) in the patient or elective embryo banking.

32.5 Notes

A. **Timing of blastocyst assessment.** The blastocyst should reach full size with a defined blastocoel cavity, tightly packed ICM cluster and an abundant number of cohesive and evenly spaced TE cells. Discrepancies in any characteristic could lead to developmental problems.

   a. Day 5: 154 hours after human chorionic gonadotrophin (hCG) or 112 to 120 hours after insemination

b. Day 6: 136 to 140 hours

c. Day 7: 160 to 164 hours (time frame less well defined because many laboratories use day 6 as cut-off for embryo culture)

d. Alternative timing for early or delayed embryo development outside the normal day 5 to 7 range: 24 hours after morula formation

B. **Morphology or normal ICM and TE.** A normal ICM should be oval or round, and its cells should be compacted and without apoptotic cells. The TE structure should be a homogeneous layer of differentiated cells without any irregular or apoptotic cells. Several studies indicate that both ICM and TE quality are important predictors of implantation. While some laboratories emphasize ICM quality more, others focus on the TE because a viable TE is essential for implantation initiation, interaction with the uterus and subsequent placenta formation.

C. **Embryo morphology: Gardner and Schoolcraft scoring system.** Blastocysts are assigned with a numerical score (1–6) based on expansion and hatching. For blastocysts graded 3 to 6, ICM and TE are assessed and assigned with an alphabetical score (A–C) in most cases.[8] A modified system developed by the Cornell programme has been commonly used in the United States as well.[9]

D. **Embryo morphology: SART grading and reporting in Clinical Outcomes Reporting System (SART CORS).** Early blastocyst, blastocyst or hatching blastocyst stage.

E. **Embryo morphology: ESHRE and Alpha Executive Istanbul Consensus.**[12]

F. Besides overall blastocyst formation and ICM and TE qualities, other nonstandard morphological patterns and abnormal development may include inclusion/cell debris in the blastocoel, split ICM, very small ICM, pre-compaction blastomeres, blastomere(s) inside or outside the blastocoel, vacuoles, fragmentation, dark mass or damaged cells and thick zona.

G. **Cell number and ICM size.** Newly expanded blastocysts on day 5 have a total of 50 to 66 cells and increase to 79 to 90 cells on day 6 and 107 to 145 on day 7. Number of ICM cell numbers range from 16 to 24 on day 5, doubles on day 6 and remains unchanged on day 7. TE cells are 32 to 45 cells on days 5 to 6 and 65 to 96 cells on day 7.[14] ICM size of 4,500 μm^2 on day 5 and 3,800 μm^2 on day 6 may be used as cut-off values to differentiate ICM quality.[10]

H. **Illustration of blastocyst development** (Figure 32.1). We recommend *An Atlas of Human Blastocysts*, by Veeck and Zaninović,[9] an embryo atlas developed by SART and the Society of Reproductive Biologists and Technologists (SRBT) (www.SART.org, updated in 2015) and the *ESHRE Atlas of Human Embryology* [15] for further reading.

I. The blastocyst grows dynamically and rapidly. Assessment should be performed through multiple focal planes under the inverted microscope to examine the TE layer and cell distribution. Gently rolling/turning the embryo by using a handling pipette is often beneficial to locate and examine the ICM. Pay attention to the ICM, which is a cluster of cells, and distinguish it from a single blastomere inclusion that often has a more uniformed monotonic appearance. Handle the blastocyst carefully, as the blastocyst is sensitive to external environmental conditions (e.g., physical stress, chemical and osmotic changes and temperature fluctuation).

J. Multiple sequential observations, while minimizing the exposure of embryos to ambient atmosphere, may be necessary to obtain a more accurate assessment, especially when blastocoel collapse was found during the initial assessment.

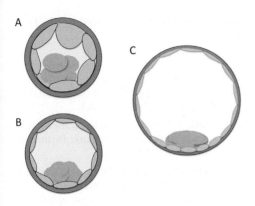

Figure 32.1 Example stages of blastocyst development: (A) early blastocyst; (B) blastocyst, unexpanded; (C) expanded blastocyst. Characteristics to note include compaction of ICM, more epithelial structure of TE and thinning of the zona pellucida.

K. **Expansion, collapse and re-expansion of the blastocoels.** Cavitation and expansion of the blastocoel, caused by ionic gradient changes, osmotic pressure changes and effective tight junctions of TE cells, is time dependent, and progress may vary by laboratory. Collapse and re-expansion of the blastocoel are not unusual phenomena for blastocysts cultured in vitro before the blastocysts start hatching. External environment conditions including temperature fluctuation, mechanical stress and chemical and osmotic changes may also induce blastocyst collapse.[9] While collapse often occurs rapidly, re-expansion takes a much longer time. When examining collapsed blastocysts, it is recommended to check morphology again a few hours later. If the embryo transfer (ET or FET) procedure does not allow enough time for the blastocyst to re-expand (e.g. due to clinical scheduling), record the quality of the collapsed blastocyst as is, with overall survival and any identifiable ICM and TE morphology.

L. **Sequential grading and cumulative scores.** Blastocyst grading is independent of cleavage-stage embryo grading. Embryos assigned with same score at the blastocyst stage may have different scores from previous stages. Many laboratories perform a sequence of multiple grading events throughout fertilization to day of transfer/cryopreservation and may elect to use cumulative scores to determine the best embryo for transfer/cryopreservation, especially when multiple top-quality blastocysts become available at the time of transfer.

M. **Frozen-thawed blastocyst grading.** After applying the thaw protocol (see Chapters 34 and 35), allow the blastocyst to re-expand. Grade the blastocyst using the same criteria as for fresh cycles. Record observations of post-thaw embryo survival based on morphology: overall, ICM and TE. Dark and degenerated cells often indicate signs of non-survival. Degenerated ICM cells usually indicate a more severe problem than apoptotic mural TE cells.

N. **Assessing post–assisted hatching (AH) blastocysts.** For embryos undergone assisted hatching on days 3 to 4, the embryologist should note any hatching event observed during days 5 to 7 and the correlated size of the blastocyst and zona thickness. Unexpanded blastocysts with herniated TE caused by assisted hatching should be recorded.

O. **Non-viable embryos.** If an embryo has not progressed for at least 24 hours or all of its cells have degenerated, the embryo is considered arrested and non-viable. Some suboptimal quality blastocysts assessed on day 5 that do not undergo transfer or cryopreservation may appear degenerated on days 6 to 7 and be deemed non-viable.

P. **Assessing blastocyst quality with TLI and pre-implantation genetic testing (PGT: PGD/PGS).** See relevant chapters in this book.

References

1. Dokras, A., Sargent, I. L. and Barlow, D. H. Human blastocyst grading: an indicator of developmental potential? *Hum Reprod* 1993; **8**:2119–27.

2. Balaban, B., Urman, B., Sertac, A., Alatas, C., Aksoy, S. et al. Blastocyst quality affects the success of blastocyst-stage embryo transfer. *Fertil Steril* 2000; **74**:282–7.

3. Gardner, D. K., Lane, M., Stevens, J., Schlenker, T. and Schoolcraft, W. B. Blastocyst score affects implantation and pregnancy outcome: towards a single blastocyst transfer. *Fertil Steril* 2000; **73**:1155–8.

4. Racowsky, C., Combelles, C. M., Nureddin, A., Pan, Y., Finn, A. et al. Day 3 and day 5 morphological predictors of embryo viability. *Reprod Biomed Online* 2003; **6**:323–31.

5. Gardner, D. K. and Balaban, B. Choosing between day 3 and day 5 embryo transfers. *Clin Obstet Gynecol* 2006; **49**:85–92.

6. Blake, D. A., Farquhar, C. M., Johnson, N. and Proctor, M. Cleavage stage versus blastocyst stage embryo transfer in assisted conception. *Cochrane Database Syst Rev* 2007; CD002118.

7. Glujovsky, D., Blake, D., Farquhar, C. and Bardach, A. Cleavage stage versus blastocyst stage embryo transfer in assisted reproductive technology. *Cochrane Database Syst Rev* 2012; 7:CD002118.

8. Gardner, D. and Schoolcraft, W. In vitro culture of the human blastocyst. In *Towards Reproductive Certainty: Infertility and Genetics Beyond*, ed. R. Jansen and D. Mortimer (pp. 378–88) (Carnforth, UK: Parthenon Publishing, 1999).

9. Veeck, L. L. and Zaninović, N. *An Atlas of Human Blastocysts* (New York: Parthenon Publishing, 2003).

10. Richter, K. S., Harris, D. C., Daneshmand, S. T. and Shapiro, B. S. Quantitative grading of a human blastocyst: optimal inner cell mass size and shape. *Fertil Steril* 2001; **76**:1157–67.

11. Kovacic, B., Vlaisavljevic, V., Reljic, M. and Cizek-Sajko, M. Developmental capacity of different morphological types of day 5 human morulae and blastocysts. *Reprod Biomed Online* 2004; **8**:687–94.

12. Alpha Scientists in Reproductive Medicine, ESHRE Special Interest Group of Embryology. The Istanbul consensus workshop on embryo assessment: proceedings of an expert meeting. *Hum Reprod* 2011; **26**:1270–83.

13. Racowsky, C., Vernon. M., Mayer, J., Ball, G. D., Behr, B. et al. Standardization of grading embryo morphology. *Fertil Steril* 2010; **94**:1152–3.

14. Hardy, K., Handyside, A. H. and Winston, R. M. The human blastocyst: cell number, death and allocation during late preimplantation development in vitro. *Development* 1989; **107**:597–604.

15. Magli, M. C., Jones, G. M., Lundin, K. and van den Abbeel, E. Atlas of human embryology: from oocytes to preimplantation embryos. *Hum Reprod* 2012; **27**(Suppl. 1):i1.

Markus H. M. Montag

Chapter 33

Embryo Culture and Assessment via Time-Lapse Microscopy in the IVF laboratory

Introduction

Time-lapse imaging (TLI) allows the culture of embryos in an undisturbed environment over the entire culture period. Continuous monitoring of the growing embryos enables a new way of assessing and documenting their development. Any morphological event can be mapped to the specific time point at which it occurred. The exact definition of these so-called morphokinetic variables and how and when to annotate them results in an objective and standardized method of embryo assessment. In combination with a proper annotation strategy, one can create a workflow that allows for a minimal workload and a maximum of information for an objective and transparent decision on which embryo to transfer.

33.1 Background

Following the development of an embryo at any time during in vitro culture has become real with dedicated TLI systems.[1] Continuous imaging provides more information about the embryo, in particular, the correlation with the exact time point at which an event occurred or became visible. This morphokinetic information can be used to better characterize and assess the potential of an embryo to implant. The availability of this information at any time enables standardized embryo classification via proper training of fellow embryologists as well as knowledge sharing with others.

A proper implementation of this new technology is needed to use it to its full capacity. This applies to all TLI systems and includes on how to get started and how to expand gradually towards more advanced features such as modelling and the use of morphokinetic deviations as an early warning system for potential laboratory problems. Embedded in the clinical network, TLI systems can be used for a transparent information flow from the embryologist to the clinicians and further on to the patients.

33.2 Supplies and Equipment

Time-lapse imaging equipment is available either as stand-alone units that incorporate a camera in a bench-top-like incubator or as separate camera inserts for big-box incubators. Embryos are cultured in dishes that are designed to fit to a specific TLI system and hold the embryo in the proper position for the imaging process and during the entire culture period.

Image acquisition occurs at time intervals of 5 to 15 minutes at different focal planes. Interactive software solutions allow for translating morphokinetic time-lapse information into databases for documentation and further evaluation.

Other items required include
- Stripper with tips (170 μm)
- Multi-dispenser pipette (200 μl maximum volume, adjustable to 25 μl)
- Culture medium and oil for overlay

33.3 Quality Control

Standard quality control applies in regards to temperature and gas control using external calibrated measuring devices. Additional quality control should be implemented for standardizing annotation of morphokinetic events by embryologists, as outlined in Section 33.4.

33.4 Procedures

33.4.1 Getting Started with TLI

1. As TLI the attention of every embryologist in the laboratory, a TLI coordinator should be nominated, who will coordinate the implementation of TLI in clinical routine and training of staff.
2. First steps include preparation of the TLI culture dishes, where special attention has to be paid to air bubbles (avoidance/removal). For dishes with micro-wells, it is advisable to fill first all micro-wells with a minimal amount of medium and then top up culture medium with multi-dispenser pipettes followed by oil overlay. Care has to be taken to work fast and to avoid evaporation. TLI culture dishes should be prepared on the day before and incubated over night at appropriate CO_2 and O_2 settings in an incubator. If air bubbles are present at the time of dish preparation, these can be removed much better following one to two hours of incubation as the bubbles round up. Loading and unloading of embryos can be trained by using immature or unfertilized oocytes.
3. Some companies provide a training database that allows annotation of embryos by several users for annotation comparison. This helps to align embryo characterization among all embryologists within one laboratory and to train specific aspects according to personal needs. The accessibility of images and videos for the entire embryo development helps to address difficult-to-classify or uncommon embryo behaviours and enhances knowledge sharing in front of the screen.

33.4.2 Clinical Implementation of TLI Cultures

1. Prior to starting with embryos from a clinical treatment cycle, some laboratories may prefer a mouse embryo assay (MEA) to ensure the safety of the system, while others may start directly with culturing human embryos.
2. It is essential to calibrate any (TLI) incubator to achieve the same CO_2/pH correlation as in standard incubators. The use of reduced oxygen is recommended, and the target value of O_2 concentration must be confirmed by calibration, too.
3. In order to assess the potential of undisturbed TLI culture, a sibling oocyte approach should be used, where immediately after intracytoplasmic sperm injection (ICSI), half the oocytes from a patient are cultured by the established traditional culture method, and the other half are cultured in the TLI system. The endpoint is overall embryo development and the rate of top-quality embryos on days 3 and 5, as well as the total rate

of useable embryos for cryopreservation and transfer at the time of transfer. A first evaluation should be performed after culture of 10 to 20 patients, or approximately after 50 to 100 embryos in each arm. The number of useable embryos should be assessed in both arms by the same morphological criteria in order to allow for a direct comparison. This kind of evaluation is independent of using further information that can be gained by annotation using TLI.

33.4.3 Starting with a Proper Workflow

Not all embryos will develop to the desired cell stage at the day of transfer. Therefore, one can adapt an easy strategy that minimizes the number of embryos that have to be annotated.

1. In an ICSI case, one should check the number of pronuclei (PNs) at 16 to 18 hours after ICSI, and all oocytes that have two PNs should be marked as such in the software. All unfertilized oocytes or those with one PN and three or more PNs should be marked as being potentially discarded.
2. There is no need to characterize embryos on day 2 unless embryo transfer is scheduled for day 2.
3. One should look on the embryos on day 3 and mark in the software all embryos that are not at the appropriate cell stage (e.g. having at least six blastomeres) as being 'discard' (although the embryos will still be kept in TLI culture). All remaining and eligible embryos can be annotated up to day 3.
4. The next check would be required on day 5, where one will again 'discard' all embryos that are not at the appropriate cell stage. Next, one will annotate the embryos that have reached the blastocyst stage and select among them for embryo(s) for transfer.
5. This workflow is optimized for a minimal workload. As the pictures of the non-annotated embryos become available even after the cycle has finished, one can always go back and re-annotate these embryos.

33.4.4 Which Morphokinetic Variables Should Be Annotated?

An overview of annotation definitions and the nomenclature used can be found in a recent publication from a TLI user group.[2] The use of TLI for morphokinetic annotation enables one to acquire a lot of information from all embryos of a patient.

1. In the beginning, it is important that the laboratory establish a list of the most relevant morphokinetic variables that have to be annotated with every embryo that is considered to be eligible for embryo transfer. This list should contain variables that are linked to cell division, as well as morphological variables.
2. The most versatile cell division variables are the number of PNs at 16 to 18 hours (two PNs), the time when the pronuclei are faded (tPNf) and the time to the division to two (t_2), three (t_3), four (t_4), five (t_5) and eight cells (t_8) and blastocysts (t_B). Some may add the time of formation of the morula (t_M) and the start of blastocoel formation (t_{SB}). The exact annotation of a t-value is the time point when the blastomeres are completely separated after division.
3. Morphologically relevant variables are symmetry (even/uneven), multi-nucleation (MN) and fragmentation (Frag) at the two- and four-cell stages. Using appropriate software, recording of the division events allows visualization and assessment of the length of the cell cycle of any particular stage of development. This enables one to look for

morphological events at the correct time point, which is in the middle of the cell cycle of the two- and four-cell stages. Nuclei are not visible immediately after cell division, and thus, multi-nucleation assessment in traditional incubation will not give the real picture.[3,4] Symmetry and fragmentation may vary from the time when an embryo has just divided until the embryo reaches the middle of the cell cycle.[5]

4. Further variables can be added based on the needs or interests of the laboratory.

33.4.5 Using Morphokinetic Variables in the Decision Process

Annotation of morphokinetic variables allows the use of this information in deciding which embryo to transfer. Since the introduction of TLI, the relevance of different variables has been discussed in numerous publications.[6–8]

1. Criteria for de-selection of embryos are much easier to obtain and to implement. For example, direct cleavage of an embryo from the one-cell to the three-cell stage has been shown to be associated with very low implantation rates.[9] The same holds true for reverse cleavage, which characterizes an embryo where one blastomere (mostly at the two-, three- or four-cell stage) divides into two daughter cells, which then fuse back to one cell.[10] Other criteria with low prognosis are uneven blastomere size at the two-cell stage and multi-nucleation at the two- or four-cell stage.[3,4]

2. The use of fixed time values for certain division events such as t_2, t_3, t_5 or t_8 has been shown to be of good prognostic value in some laboratories, but the same time values cannot be applied in another laboratory.[11] This is due to external factors that influence the development of embryos. A very prominent example is the concentration of oxygen during embryo culture. Incubation in 5% O_2 will lead to faster development and lower t-values than incubation at 20% O_2.[12] Thus, a model developed on fixed time points in ambient air cannot be copied from a laboratory that uses reduced oxygen.

33.4.6 Starting with Algorithms for Embryo Implantation Assessment

Starting with algorithms for embryo implantation assessment can be done by two different options:

1. The first option is based on using an algorithm that has been developed on known implantation data (KID) of embryos from a large database that hosts data from multiple centres that work under different culture conditions. Such a versatile algorithm will help to rank embryos and support the decision process for embryo transfer. Furthermore, such an algorithm can be used from the first cycle onwards, provided that the relevant variables that are the basis for the algorithm are properly annotated. Usually such algorithms are based on mathematical models that are independent of or not influenced by fixed time points.

2. The second option requires that a centre assemble sufficient data from its own TLI system and incubation conditions for statistic analysis of the morphokinetic variables present in KID embryos. Comparing confidence intervals for time values from KID-negative with KID-positive embryos may allow finding variables that are suitable to get a good differentiation between implanting and non-implanting embryos. Mostly the confidence intervals will be overlapping, but this information can be used in algorithm construction. Centres that perform predominantly single-embryo transfer will acquire the necessary amount of data much faster than others.

33.4.7 TLI to Assess Laboratory Conditions

1. In a centre with a sufficiently large number of cycles incubated in time lapse, the data on all embryos within a given time period can be used to calculate the mean value and standard deviation for each morphokinetic variable. Using the principle of rolling averages, one can use the mean value of morphokinetic variables from overlapping time periods to detect eventual changes. Such changes can be due to the patient cohort, but in a worst-case scenario, they can be the first sign of something that negatively influences the growth of the embryos.[13] Detecting that at such an early stage may allow investigation of the underlying reason and the finding of a solution at an early stage instead of being confronted with negative pregnancy outcome two to three weeks later. The time period for rolling averages depends on the actual cycle number and the number of embryos available for analysis.

33.5 Notes

A. Different TLI companies present excellent teaching materials on their respective webpages.

B. Different types of TLI systems are available that are designed either as stand-alone incubators with an integrated TLI system or that are designed as camera inserts that fit into a larger incubator. Stand-alone systems are available that work with an integrated gas mixer, and one system requires pre-mixed gas. Camera inserts can be fitted into any suitable incubator that is large enough and enables cable connections from outside into the incubation chamber.

C. Currently, two algorithms are available. One is designed as a blastocyst prediction model based on automatic detection of the first cell divisions up to day 2 and the correlated time points. Another algorithm is designed on morphokinetic variables derived from embryos with known implantation data that were transferred on day 3. Suppliers may present further algorithms.

References

1. Herrero, J. and Meseguer, M. Selection of high potential embryos using time-lapse imaging: the era of morphokinetics. *Fertil Steril* 2013; 99:1030–4.

2. Ciray, H. N., Campbell, A., Agerholm, I. E., Aguilar, J., Chamayou, S. et al. Proposed guidelines on the nomenclature and annotation of dynamic human embryo monitoring by a time-lapse user group. *Hum Reprod* 2014; 29:2650–60.

3. Ergin, E., Caliskan, E., Yalcinkaya, E., Öztel, Z., Cökelez, K. et al. Frequency of embryo multinucleation detected by time-lapse system and its impact on pregnancy outcome. *Fertil Steril* 2014; 102:1029–33.

4. Goodmann, L. R., Goldberg, J., Falcone, T., Austin, C. and Desai, N. Does the addition of time-lapse morphokinetics in the selection of embryos for transfer improve pregnancy rates? A randomized, controlled trial. *Fertil Steril* (in press).

5. Montag, M., Liebenthron, J. and Köster, M. Which morphological scoring system is relevant in human embryo development? *Plazenta* 2011; 32(Suppl. 3):S252–6.

6. Liu, Y., Chapple, V., Roberts, P. and Matson, P. The prevalence, consequence, and significance of reverse cleavage by human embryos viewed with the use of the EmbryoScope time-lapse video system. *Fertil Steril* 2014; 2:1295–1302.

7. Meseguer, M., Herrero, J., Tejera, A., Hilligsoe, K. M., Ramsing, N. B. et al. The

use of morphokinetics as a predictor of embryo implantation. *Hum Reprod* 2011; 26:2658–71.

8. Rubio, I., Galán, A., Larreategui, Z., Ayerdi, F., Bellver, J. et al. Clinical validation of embryo culture and selection by morphokinetic analysis: a randomized, controlled trial of the EmbryoScope. *Fertil Steril* 2014; 102:1287–94.

9. Cetinkaya, M., Pirkevi, C., Yelke, H., Colakoglu, Y. K., Atayurt, Z. et al. Relative kinetic expressions defining cleavage synchronicity are better predictors of blastocyst formation and quality than absolute time points. *J Assist Reprod Genet* 2015; 32:27–35.

10. Rubio, I. R., Kuhlmann, R., Agerholm, I., Kirk, J., Herrero, J. et al. Limited implantation success of direct-cleaved human zygotes: a time-lapse study. *Fertil Steril* 2012; 98:1458–63.

11. Freour, T., Le Fleuter, N., Lammers, J., Splingart, C., Reignier, A. et al. External validation of a time-lapse prediction model. *Fertil Steril* 2015; 103:917–22.

12. Kirkegaard, K., Hindkjaer, J. J. and Ingerslev, H. J. Effect of oxygen concentration on human embryo development evaluated by time-lapse monitoring. *Fertil Steril* 2013; 99:738–44.

13. Wolff, H. S., Fredrickson, J. R., Walker, D.L. and Morbeck, D. E. Advances in quality control: mouse embryo morphokinetics are sensitive markers of in vitro stress. *Hum Reprod* 2013; 28:1776–82.

Chapter 34

Cryopreservation of Pre-Compaction Embryos for IVF

Cecilia Sjöblom

Introduction

Improvement in the success of cryopreservation has increased the use of human embryos produced from ovarian hyper-stimulation and in vitro fertilization (IVF)/intracytoplasmic sperm injection (ICSI). High survival and implantation rates of frozen-thawed embryos have allowed for a decrease in the number of embryos transferred and even made way for a modern 'freeze all' approach, where all embryos derived from a fresh cycle are frozen and transferred in a subsequent frozen embryo transfer cycle.[1,2]

In recent years, cryopreservation has evolved to include vitrification, with many laboratories preferring this sometimes faster method, which also requires less complex equipment. However, slow freezing can often be more successful, cost-effective and faster than vitrification, particularly in zygotes and cleavage-stage embryos.

For most vitrification approaches, the process is the same, independent of the embryo's stage of development. Blastocyst vitrification, described in Chapter 20, can be applied for cleavage-stage embryos, and this chapter will focus on slow freezing of pre-compaction embryos.

34.1 Background

The first successful pregnancy after freezing and thawing of human embryos was reported by Trounson and Mohr[3] in 1983 using dimethyl sulfoxide (DMSO) and high levels of serum in a slow-cooling, slow-warming approach. The first live birth was reported the year after [4]. Modern-day slow-freezing protocols are mostly variants of the protocol developed by Lassalle and Testart,[5,6] as this approach was found to be more successful and faster than the DMSO protocol developed by Trounson and Mohr. Embryos are dehydrated using 1,2-propanediol (PROH) and sucrose, followed by a controlled rate cooling from room temperature to $-7°C$ at a rate of -1 to $-2°C$ per minute, when induction of ice crystals (seeding) is performed. The cooling is then continued at $-0.3°C$/minute to $-30°C$, when the vessel holding the embryos is plunged into liquid nitrogen and stored. Subsequent thawing is done by stepwise removal of cryoprotectants.

The first pregnancy by the vitrification technique was reported in 1999 using vitrified oocytes,[7] followed the year after by reports of pregnancies from vitrified embryos.[8] Today, most laboratories use vitrification for cryopreservation of embryos at all developmental stages from zygote to blastocyst, with the perception that this approach is faster and more successful than the slow-freezing protocol.[9]

The conclusion that vitrification is more successful can surely be questioned and could depend on the vitrification approach having fewer variables.[10] The success of slow freezing is highly dependent on a number of factors – such as the quality and stage of the embryo together with the performance, accuracy and maintenance of the controlled-rate freezer.

Studies have shown that the implantation potential of slow-frozen pre-compaction embryos depends on the number of cells and degree of fragmentation at the time of freezing and the number of blastomeres that survive after thawing.[11] Moreover, the ability of the thawed embryo to cleave after on culture has been suggested as a strong indicator for live birth.

At Westmead Fertility Centre we have successfully continued to use slow-freezing as the preferred method for pre-compaction embryos. A combination of using the improved cryoprotection protocol developed by Edgar et al.[12] and close attention to quality control (QC) and performance of the controlled freezer has resulted in survival rates of greater than 80% in cleavage-stage embryos (>90% for good-quality embryos). We have found that slow freezing is faster, as we cryopreserve a high number of embryos every day, and use of the Edgar and Geek one-step approach, where the 10-minute incubation is done in the straw, allows us to efficiently finish all cleavage-stage freezing in five to ten minutes.

Careful attention to the selection of embryos suitable for freezing can improve the cryo-survival, but poorer-quality embryos can be frozen in groups and subsequently thawed and cultured over night or to day 5 for blastocyst single-embryo transfer.

Embryos with two to four cells on day 2 or six to eight cells on day 3 with less than 30% fragmentation are frozen singly, and all embryos with poorer quality are frozen in groups for an 'on-culture' approach. The timing of the freezing is also crucial for the outcome and if embryos are found to be cleaving or having an uneven number of cells, the freezing is postponed for an hour or two until the embryo is in a steady state.

34.2 Reagents, Supplies and Equipment

34.2.1 Reagents

- Cleavage-stage embryo cryopreservation is done using PROH and sucrose as cryoprotectants according to Lassalle et al.[1] modified by Edgar et al.[2]
- All solutions are made up from handling medium such as HTF-HEPES with human serum albumin (HSA) or similar.
- 1,2-Propanediol (Sigma 398039).
- Sucrose (Sigma S1888).
- Embryo freezing solution (EFS) 1.5 mol/l PROH + 0.2 mol/l sucrose in HTF-HEPES.
- Embryo thawing solution (ETS).
- ETS1: 0.5 mol/l sucrose.
- ETS2: 0.2 mol/l sucrose.
- ETS3: 0 mol/litre of sucrose (handling medium).

Cryosolutions are available from different suppliers, and procedure protocols may vary slightly.

34.2.2 Disposables

- 4/5 well dishes
- Organ culture dishes
- Embryo cryopreservation straws

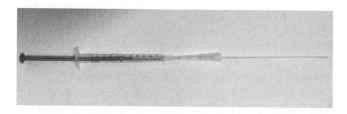

Figure 34.1 Syringe attached to pipette tip and straw for loading/expelling of straw. (A black and white version of this figure will appear in some formats. For the color version, please refer to the plate section.)

- 1-ml syringe
- 100-µl sterile pipette tips
- Attach pipette tip as per Figure 34.1
- Sterile single-use scissors

34.2.3 Equipment

- Controlled-rate freezer
- Thermocouple with PT100 probe (Note A)
- Timer

All measuring devices need to be calibrated annually against international standards and have a calibration certificate.

34.3 Quality Management

Quality control during controlled freezing is paramount and is required each time embryos are cryopreserved. Quality control should be done using a secondary temperature measuring device and timer parallel with the controlled freezer display reading for temperature and time. The secondary thermocouple probe should be designed to fit inside the chamber of the controlled freezer (Note A).

The quality control log should contain a standard graph with the cooling slope (temperature on the x-axis and time on the y-axis). Alternatively, a table can be made up with time points for the cooling run and corresponding temperatures. The quality control log should clearly state acceptance limits and clear action to take when the readings fall outside the accepted limits.

Record time/display temperature/actual temperature at time points:

1. t_0
2. Seeding
3. Random time during freeze run (30–40 minutes after seeding)

Plot each reading on the standard graph or table, and sign if found to be in agreement with the graph/table. Take immediate action if a reading is not in agreement with graph/table (Note B).

The controlled-freezer cooling programme should be verified biannually. Three repeated mock runs are undertaken with continuous measurement of time versus chamber temperature (using the secondary measuring device). The results should be summarized in a graph comparing the actual cooling curve to the programme and documented in a verification report including the standard error of each measurement. If the verification results lie outside the acceptance limits, the equipment must be serviced and calibrated by the manufacturer/service provider. In addition, the controlled freezer should be serviced by the manufacturer / service provider annually.

The key performance indicators (KPIs) for cryopreservation need to be monitored monthly, with the KPI report including embryo survival rate, ability to form blastocysts after culture (for cycles in which a group of embryos are thawed and cultured from cleavage stage to blastocyst) and clinical pregnancy rate. Every laboratory needs to set lower acceptable limits and actions that will be taken if the KPIs fall below the agreed limit.

It is recommended that the cleavage-stage embryo cryopreservation process be validated yearly using cleavage-stage mouse embryos. The mouse embryos are taken through the normal process of freezing and thawing, and the report should contain both the survival rate of embryos and their ability to grow to the blastocyst stage. Each laboratory needs to determine limits for acceptance of the process (Note C).

34.4 Procedures

34.4.1 Cryopreservation Setup

1. Assess the embryos, and record their scores in the patient's laboratory notes.
2. Complete the records and database for numbers of embryos to freeze, select storage cassette colour and organize tank location (Notes D and E).
3. Turn off heated stage.
4. Clean the IVF workstation area.
5. Label dishes, straws and storage cassette with the patient's couple number (Note F), initial and surname, date of birth, freeze date (e.g. 'C. Sjoblom 12345 1/2/87 FZ 12/12/ 2016'). Remember to label the top strip of the storage cassette with the couple number for easy identification once stored in the tank.
6. Prepare freezing dish(es), and allow the medium to reach room temperature (Note G).
7. Perform double witnessing when embryos are introduced to the work area. Confirm identifiers on all dishes and straws, and sign witnessing section on patient laboratory sheet (Note H).

34.4.2 Cryoprotection

1. Wash embryos carefully in handling medium (solution 1) in order to remove residues of culture medium (mostly carbonate, which can cause gas bubbles during cooling and warming).
2. Place the embryos in EFS (solution 2), and start the timer for 10 minutes. Begin loading straws as soon as embryos are placed in EFS according to Figures 34.1 and 34.2, and seal the straw using a heat sealer (Note I). The 10-minute incubation is primarily done inside the straw, and when the straw has been sealed, it can be placed in the controlled freezer.

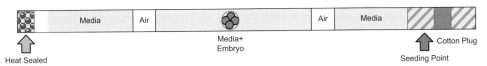

Figure 34.2 Schematic diagram of embryo loading and seeding. (A black and white version of this figure will appear in some formats. For the color version, please refer to the plate section.)

34.4.3 Controlled-Rate Freezing Programme

1. 18°C to −7°C at a rate of −2°C per minute
2. Seeding
3. Hold at −7°C for 10 minutes
4. −7°C to −30°C at a rate of −0.3°C per minute
5. Plunge/free fall to −196°C

34.4.4 Freezing Process

1. Witness that the controlled freezer is set to the correct programme.
2. Take note of the t_0 time and temperature as per quality control protocol, and note in logbook.
3. Start the controlled freezer 10 minutes after the embryos are loaded into EFS.
4. Set timer for 13 minutes.
5. After 13 minutes, the chamber should have reached −7°C.
6. Seed at the cotton plug using forceps chilled in liquid nitrogen (Note J).
7. Take note of the seeding time and temperature as per quality control protocol, and note in logbook.
8. Approximately 30 to 40 minutes after seeding, take note of the time and temperature as per quality control protocol, and note in logbook.
9. Remove the embryo straws from the chamber, and place them inside the storage cassette at the end of the freezing programme or when the chamber reaches −30°C (Note K).
10. Place the embryos in the allocated storage location (liquid or vapour) with two embryologists witnessing the location and signing the laboratory notes.

34.4.5 Embryo Thawing Setup

1. Confirm that the patient(s) have signed the thaw consent forms (Note L).
2. Make up a culture dish in accordance with the laboratory culture protocol.
3. Prepare a 15-ml tube with sterile water in a 30°C warming block.
4. Turn off the heated stage.
5. Clean the IVF workstation area.
6. Connect the syringe to the pipette tip and aspirate air into the syringe.
7. Print patient's laboratory thaw sheet.
8. Label dishes with patient name and identifier.
9. Prepare thaw dish(es), and allow the medium to reach room temperature (Note G).
10. Perform double witnessing when embryos are introduced to the work area. Confirm identifiers on all dishes, and sign the witnessing section on the patient's laboratory thaw sheet (Note H).

34.4.6 Embryo Thawing

1. Take the embryos out of the liquid nitrogen.
2. Quickly double witness the name and identifiers on the straw and dishes while holding the straw in the air for 30 seconds (sign the laboratory thaw sheet).

3. Immerse the straw in the tube containing 30°C water, and allow the straw to fully thaw.
4. Cut off the straw at the cotton end.
5. Attach the straw to the syringe/tip device.
6. Cut off the heat-sealed end.
7. Expel the embryo(s) into ETS1, and incubate at room temperature for five minutes (Note M).
8. Carefully move the embryo(s) to ETS2 and incubate at room temperature for five minutes.
9. Carefully move the embryo(s) to ETS3 and incubate at room temperature for five minutes.
10. Move the embryo(s) to the culture dish (double witnessed), observe quality/survival, note in the laboratory thaw sheet and place the dish in the incubator awaiting embryo transfer.
11. Finalize the patient's laboratory notes and database.

34.5 Notes

A. Probe and thermocouple need to be calibrated for measurements of −7°C, −15°C and −30°C.
B. If there is a problem with the cooling rate as confirmed by the external probe, the best immediate action is to immediately abort the run; thaw the embryos as per thawing instructions. Place the embryos in culture, and verify the controlled freezer (call for service/repair, etc.). Allow the embryos to remain in culture for at least 24 hours before re-freezing using slow freezing or vitrification as suitable.
C. Process validation using mouse embryos is not possible in some laboratories due to local/national/regional legislation and guidelines.
D. Confirm that patient(s) have signed consent forms for cryopreservation.
E. Confirm patient blood screening status, and allocate embryo storage accordingly.
F. In order to ensure patient safety, it is recommended that samples be labelled with unique identifiers. As name and date of birth cannot be considered unique, a patient-specific number such as a clinic-generated couple number or medical records number is required together with the name and date of birth.
G. The two solutions used for freezing can be placed in one four- or five-well dish where the handling medium for the wash step is placed in one well and the EFS is placed in two wells. Alternatively, use two organ culture dishes with handling medium in one dish and EFS in both the centre well and moat of this dish. The EFS in the spare well or moat is to be used for filling the straw and minimizing the risk of accidentally loading embryos. Similarly for ETS1 to ETS3, these can be placed in a four- or five-well dish or in individual organ culture dishes.
H. If a designated area is used for freezing/thawing, the area and all dishes/straws can be witnessed at one time with no need of further witnessing of material inside the area. However bringing embryos into/out of the area has to be double witnessed.
I. When you load straws, it is important to seal the cotton plug. This is done by carefully aspirating the medium in the straw to a point where it is soaked up by the first part of the cotton plug.
J. Timing and technique of seeding are crucial for success of slow freezing. The seeding should always be done exactly when the chamber and straw reach −7°C. Pinch the cotton or top end of the straw with super-cooled forceps, and observe the formation of

ice crystals at the top of the straw. Place the cover back on the chamber. The seeding is followed by a 10-minute holding time at −7°C to allow time for the ice crystals to migrate down through the straw. Many times the 10-minute holding is perceived as being a grace time for seeding, but this is incorrect. Never, ever seed mid-straw near the embryos, as this will risk super-cooling of the embryos.

K. It is safe to plunge the straws into liquid nitrogen at −30°C as all water has reached crystallized form at this point. However, this can only be done with certain makes of controlled-rate freezers.

L. Clinics should ensure that the signature of partner two (usually the male partner) is witnessed by an official such as the patient's referring clinician, a general practitioner or justice of the peace with a copy of identification. This is to ensure that the second partner is aware and consenting to the frozen embryo being thawed.

M. Always expel the embryos into ETS1. Never expel the embryos onto a naked dish and then move them to ETS1. Remember that the embryo is dehydrated and susceptible to mechanic stress and should not be moved at this stage.

References

1. McLernon, D. J., Harrild, K., Bergh, C., Davies, M. J., de Neubourg, D. et al. Clinical effectiveness of elective single versus double embryo transfer: meta-analysis of individual patient data from randomised trials. *British Med J* 2010; 341: c6945.

2. Blockeel, C., Drakopoulos, P., Santos-Ribeiro, S., Polyzos, N. P. and Tournaye, H. A fresh look at the freeze-all protocol: a SWOT analysis. *Hum Reprod* 2016; 31(3):491–7.

3. Trounson, A. and Mohr, L. Human-pregnancy following cryopreservation, thawing and transfer of an 8-cell embryo. *Nature* 1983; 305(5936):707–9.

4. Zeilmaker, G. H., Alberda, A. T., Vangent, I., Rijkmans, C. and Drogendijk, A. C. Pregnancies following transfer of intact frozen-thawed embryos. *Fertil Steril* 1984; 42(2):293–6.

5. Lassalle, B., Testart, J. and Renard, J.P. Human-embryo features that influence the success of cryopreservation with use of 1,2-propanediol. *Fertil Steril* 1985; 44(5):645–51.

6. Testart, J., Lassalle, B., Belaisch-Allart, J., Hazout, A., Forman, R. et al. High pregnancy rate after early human embryo freezing. *Fertil Steril* 1986; 46:268–72.

7. Kuleshova, L., Gianaroli, L., Magli, C., Ferraretti, A. and Trounson, A. Birth following vitrification of a small number of human oocytes: case report *Hum Reprod* 1999; 14(12):3077–9.

8. Yokota, Y., Sato, S., Yokota, M., Ishikawa, Y., Makita, M. et al. Successful pregnancy following blastocyst vitrification: case report. *Hum Reprod* 2000; 15(8):1802–3.

9. Balaban, B., Urman, B., Ata, B., Isiklar, A., Larman, M. G. et al. A randomized controlled study of human day 3 embryo cryopreservation by slow freezing or vitrification: vitrification is associated with higher survival, metabolism and blastocyst formation. *Hum Reprod* 2008; 23(9):1976–82.

10. Edgar, D. H. and Gook, D. A. A critical appraisal of cryopreservation (slow cooling versus vitrification) of human oocytes and embryos. *Hum Reprod Update* 2012; 18(5):536–54.

11. Edgar, D. H., Archer, J., McBain, J. and Borne, H. Embryonic factors affecting outcome from single cryopreserved embryo transfer. *Reprod Biomed Online.* 2007; 14(6):718–23.

12. Edgar, D. H., Karani, J. and Gook, D. A. Increasing dehydration of human cleavage-stage embryos prior to slow cooling significantly increases cryosurvival. *Reprod Biomed Online* 2009; 19:521–5.

Chapter

35

Cryopreservation of Post-Compaction Embryos for IVF

Mitchel C. Schiewe

35.1 Cryopreservation: General

35.1.1 Background

At the beginning of this century, the application of vitrification technology was gaining momentum in clinical medicine with the use of various 'open vitrification systems' (i.e. direct embryo–solution contact with liquid nitrogen), which offered high cooling rate potential and high levels of completely intact embryo survival using mixed dimethyl sulfoxide (DMSO)/ethylene glycol (EG) solutions. Not surprisingly, the combined use of blastocoele collapsing proved effective at ensuring high rates of complete survival (>90%).[1,2] By the mid-2000s, 'closed vitrification systems' (i.e. embryo–solution sealed in a container/device) began to be used efficiently and, to date, have achieved success rates comparable with and higher than those of other open-system devices.[3,4] The latter aseptic closed systems completely eliminate risks and concerns associated with potential contaminants found in liquid nitrogen during storage. It has been shown that pre-vitrification blastocoele collapsing is not an essential prerequisite for vitrification solutions devoid of DMSO,[4,5] as less permeable cryoprotectants (e.g. glycerol) and a more concentrated solution can induce and sustain blastocoele shrinkage during vitrification.

Today we know that the efficacy of vitrification success is more highly dependent on warming rates than cooling rates.[6,7] Independent of the vitrification device or open/closed system used, the warming rate must exceed the cooling rate to ensure high survival rates. High warming rates minimize the opportunity for any ice growth (i.e. re-crystallization of nucleated impurities in cryosolutions) during the devitrification phase of warming. Therefore, it is not surprising that device familiarity is an important factor regarding technical variation and successful outcomes. It is this concept of 'technical signature'[5] that explains why repeatability between programmes may be problematic.

When assessing the completeness of vitrification devices for your potential use, there are several quality control factors that should be taken into account, including

1. **Recovery potential/survivability**. Is the device design prone to potential problems in the guaranteed recovery of embryos, and will they reliably vitrify and maintain complete cellular integrity after warming?
2. **Liquid nitrogen storage capacity**. Does the device offer security and safety from possible contaminants as an aseptic closed system? Can the device be simply and safely handled and identified? Is its storage potential space efficient?

3. **Labelling potential**. Can labels be securely adhered? Are they tamperproof? Do they offer dual colour identification potential? Does it require a secondary label, and can the label be easily removed for record-keeping purposes (i.e. patient verification) after warming?

4. **Technical ease**. Can embryos be easily loaded into/onto the device in a timely manner, and can they be easily identified and tracked after warming?

5. **Procedural simplicity/repeatability**. Does the vitrification method offer simplicity and reliability that easily allows for repeatability, which minimizes variation between technicians (internal) and programmes (external)?

Today's vitrification technology gives us a powerful and highly effective tool to reliably maintain the complete integrity of a cryopreserved embryo. Unlike conventional slow freezing using one of two containers (straw or vial) or cryoprotectants (propanediol or glycerol), clinical vitrification employs numerous methods, device systems and a combination of cryoprotectants. This chapter will briefly describe an aseptic, closed microSecure vitrification (µS-VTF) technique we developed and validated[4,8] and have applied successfully to post-compaction human embryos using a DMSO-free vitrification solution.[4,9] In addition, the chapter will highlight quality control tips and procedural differences pertaining to vitrification systems.

35.1.2 Materials

A. Media/reagents (type, storage requirements, recommended shelf life, comments):

1. Constituted vitrification medium, 4°C, one month from the date of opening, commercial source variation exists.

   a. Generally, this includes an equilibration solution (ES, or V1), possibly an intermediate solution (IS, or V2) and a vitrification solution (VS, or V3).

   b. We use a glycerol-glycol permeating cryoprotectant-based solution (BL-VTF solution: ≥ 7.9 M), whereas other commercial preparations are typically ethylene glycol (EG)/dimethyl sulfoxide (DMSO) (30%–40% v/v) but could be EG/propylene glycol (32% v/v; PPG). (Mixed solutions are typically used to reduce cryo-toxicity concerns.)

   c. Non-permeating additives such as sucrose, ficoll, albumin and/or sodium hyaluronate may be present to add viscosity and cellular support.

2. HEPES-buffered medium (e.g. H-HTF, LG-H) with non-essential AA, 4°C, manufacturer specified.

3. Protein supplement, 4°C, manufacturer specified, purchase low-endotoxin lots.

4. Sucrose, room temperature, up to one year after opening (see Appendix 35A).

B. Supplies:

1. Acrodisc syringe filters (0.2 µm)

2. Aluminum cane

3. CBS embryo straw (hydrophobic plug) or embryo/semen straw (cotton-PVP plug), 0.3 ml, individual sterile

4. Colour, weighted ID rods, 40 mm

5. Conical tubes, 15 ml; snap-cap tubes, 10 ml
6. Coloured cane tabs
7. Cryosleeves
8. Flexipettes, sterile (300-μm ID)
9. Goblet
10. Large forceps
11. Multi-well dishes (e.g., six-well, four-well)
12. Powder-free gloves
13. Petri dishes (35, 60, 100 mm)
14. Pipette tips
15. Serological pipettes (1, 5, 10 ml)
16. Sterile scissors (dissection)
17. Sterile 4 × 4 gauze pads
18. Straw labels (Thermal Brady labels or coloured cryogenic labels)
19. Syringes (10, 20, 60 ml)
20. Sucrose, granular
21. Tissue culture flasks, 50 ml
22. Vitrification device (e.g. HSV, Rapid-i, Cryotop, Cryolock, Vitrisafe)

C. Equipment:
1. Brady thermal straw labeller (if not hand writing labels)
2. Cryobiological storage tank(s)
3. Dewar flask, stainless steel (0.5 litre) or Cryo-bath
4. Heat-sealing device (e.g. Syms sealer, impulse sealer, etc.)
5. Pipette aid
6. Pipetting devices
7. Stereomicroscope
8. Timer

35.1.3 Quality Control Considerations

1. Use different colours (e.g. pens, labels, ID plugs/rods) to distinguish patients if cryopreserving more than one group of embryos at a time.
2. Use different dishes and pipettes for each patient.
3. Minimize the volume of medium transferred when moving blastocysts from one solution to another.
4. Typically, one blastocyst should be cryopreserved per straw/device.
5. Maintain sterile technique, and adhere to all safety precautions.
6. Confirm physician's order and confirm signed patient consent before initiating procedures. Check the disposition of the patient's embryo(s) in inventory.
7. If blastocysts are transferred to another facility, a 'Release of Liability and Consent for Transport' must be signed by all autologous gamete source providers and a witness (e.g. notary, onsite staff).
8. Procedural considerations:
    a. Media and protein quality control, as appropriate, to include bioassays, endotoxin determinations and expiration/lot number verification and tracking.

b. Clinical cryopreservation outcome monitoring and evaluation, as described in your quality management practices, should include panic values, including

    i. Recovery rates < 95%
    ii. Survival rates < 80%
    iii. Clinical pregnancy rates using single euploid blastocysts < 50%

35.2 Blastocyst Vitrification (VTF)

35.2.1 Cryopreservation Procedure

1. Preparation:

    a. Complete the appropriate paperwork to include entering data into the worksheets and the cryopreservation database and inventory log(s).

    b. Prepare fresh cryopreservation solutions or use a commercial source (recommended one-week to one-month shelf life once in use, 4°C storage).

    c. Label each straw/device and Cryo-goblet with the patient's name and unique ID number (e.g., Social Security Number, date of birth, patient ID number) using the cryo-marker, and the date of VTF, as well include each a unique number on each straw/device (e.g. 1, 2, 3, 4).

Tip 1:

For μS-VTF, the label is secured onto a 30- to 40-mm colour-weighted ID rod, inserted and sealed into a 0.3-ml CBS embryo straw and then returned to its individual sterile package until use (see Appendix 35B).

    d. Identify each cane with a unique inscribed ID number or with an ID tag using the patient's first and last name and date of VTF. In addition, full ID information, including unique secondary ID (e.g., date of birth) and embryo description (stage, quality grade) can be written onto the upper cane surface using a Sharpie marker.

    e. Prepare fresh dishes (100 mm), labelling the under-surface with the patient's name and solution ID and embryo/holding droplet ID (Figure 35.1A). In our case, set up four rows of droplets – isotonic HEPES-buffered media: V1 (ES), V2 (IS), V3 (VS) – and the embryo ID by labelled columns.

Tip 2:

We use a series of 25- to 50-μl wash droplets ($n = 3$) to ensure that each individual final 10- to 15-μl equilibration droplet is pure and undiluted. Using this approach, up to 500 individual embryos can by vitrified using a single dish. Keep dish covered when not in use to avoid any room-temperature evaporation/dehydration of the droplets.

Tip 3:

Each commercial supplier has specific instructions for droplet setups, of which some involve the eventual merging of ES-VS solution droplets in close proximity to each other.

(A)

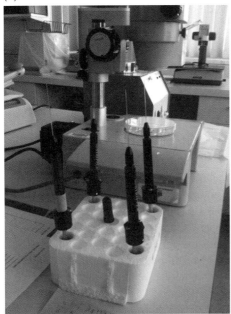

(B)

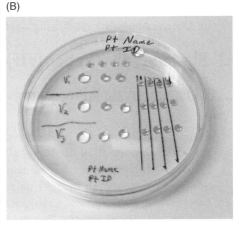

Figure 35.1 Micro-secure VTF setup includes a VTF dish (A) with distinct rows of solutions, which use three wash droplets before placement in distinct, numbered equilibration droplets. Additionally, individual pipetters with shortened VTF tips (i.e. 300-μm ID flexipettes) are secured and organized in a Styrofoam tube rack (B), which can be rotated for orderly use. A black and white version of this figure will appear in some formats. For the color version, please refer to the plate section.

    f. For μS-VTF, prepare sterile flexipettes by cutting 3 cm from the base end, insert onto individual pipetters (set at 3 μl) and secure the VTF tips upright in a Styrofoam tube rack (Figure 35.1B).

2. Embryo selection:

    a. Confirm patient/specimen identification.

    b. Blastocysts are graded and classified according to the Gardner method[10] with a numeric classification of 1 to 6 used for early to hatched blastocysts, respectively, and an A, B or C grade assigned to the inner cell mass (ICM) and trophectoderm (TE). For blastocyst biopsying, we pre-hatched the zona pellucida by laser ablation on day 3 to promote the early herniation of the TE.[9]

    c. Our preference is to cryopreserve grade 3 or higher blastocysts of BB quality or greater on day 5 or 6. However, vitrified blastocysts of lower quality (C) and post-compaction embryos at earlier stages (including late morula to grade 1 or 2 blastocysts) can certainly survive warming completely intact and yield viable embryos capable of achieving live births.

    d. The blastocoele of each blastocyst should be collapsed directly prior to the onset of the cryodilution process by means of micro-puncturing a TE junction or laser pulse ablation of a TE cell.

3. Cryodilution and blastocyst loading:

    a. Confirm patient/specimen identification (quality control by secondary source).

b. Confirm blastocyst development, update the cryo data sheet and pipette blastocyst(s) into an isotonic holding droplet.

c. Using a VTF flexipette (i.e. VTF tip), isolate blastocyst(s) into individual isotonic holding droplets.

d. Blastocyst(s) are individually moved to V1 (ES) solution by pre-filling the flexipette with V1 solution. Mix half the content onto the embryo, pipette the embryo and move it to the first V1 wash droplet. Pipette the embryo two to three times around the perimeter, and clear the pipette contents into the droplet (avoiding bubble formation). Fill the VTF tip with the next V1 wash drop, and repeat pipetting of embryo(s). Repeat a third time, and move the blastocyst(s) to an individual V1 holding drop. The dilution/washing steps should take 30 to 45 seconds. Pre-load each VTF tip with the next solution (e.g. V2), insert pipetter into rack and use the next pipetter.

Tip 4:

Since the total exposure time in our DMSO-free V1 and V2 solutions is five minutes each, the pipetting of individual blastocysts should be evenly staggered within that interval, considering that the final V3 step will require at least one minute per blastocyst to perform. For example, if you have four BLs in a VTF grouping, pipette blastocysts 1, 2, 3 and 4 at intervals of 1 minute and 15 seconds.

e. Repeat step d using V2 (IS) solutions.

f. Repeat step d using V3 (VS) solutions.

g. Upon placing each blastocyst in the V3 holding droplet, clear residual solution and bubbles from the VTF tip (outside the droplet). To initiate loading of the VTF tip, fill tip completely with clean V3 solution around the embryo. Next, expel approximately one-third of the volume, and pipette the blastocyst(s) and remaining V3 solution completely into the VTF tip.

h. Remove the VTF tip from the pipetter, wipe the tip dry of residual V3 on its outer tip surface on a sterile gauze pad and then insert the tip end first into the open end of the pre-labelled CBS straw. A dry tip is critical to preventing possible inner straw adherence.[8]

Tip 5:

For most open blade (e.g. Cryotop, Cryolock, Cryotech or Rapid-i), gutter (e.g. HSV or VitriSafe) or microdrop/straw (e.g. CSS or ICE) methods, step g is modified by pipetting the blastocyst(s) into ≤1 μl of VS and then transferring it onto the device surface, at which point residual VS can be extracted down to a final volume of 0.l μl depending on the method/preference (see Appendix 35C).

i. Invert the straw label end down, observe the tip at the inner plug and safely seal the open end with a 1-cm airspace, preferably with an automatic sealing device (e.g., Syms I or II sealer) to eliminate technical variation.

Tip 7:

The advantage of using CBS straws (e.g. HSV, μS-VTF) is that their ionomeric resin plastic creates a reliable 'weld' seal using any properly operated sealing device.

j. Once sealed, the closed straw is plunged directly into liquid nitrogen in a stainless steel Dewar flask, and the straw(s) are placed into the open goblet attached to the patient's cane for storage. Because μS-VTF straws use 40-mm weighted ID rods to offset the buoyancy of the air-filled straw, the use of inverted goblets or empty cryovials to cover the specimen(s) is not required unless transportation is involved.

Tip 8:
Other aspetic closed VTF systems (e.g. HSV, CSS, VitriSafe) involve the insertion of their device into a straw at room temperature, sealed and then plunged into liquid nitrogen for rapid cooling (1,000–2,000°C/minute).

Tip 9:
Many other devices (i.e. especially open systems) will complete step h, directly place their device in liquid nitrogen (10,000–20,000°C/minute) and then place a protective cover over the device tip. Frequently, this involves the placement of a weighted partial straw cover held in liquid nitrogen, pushed over the device and secured to the wand handle (e.g. Cryotop, Cryotech). Obviously, care must be taken here not to accidentally touch the straw opening upon insertion, which could result in 'flicking or scrapping' the device tip, thus creating a potential for specimen loss.

Tip 10:
Other attempts may include the placement of the device into a super-cooled straw resting in liquid nitrogen either before ultra-rapid cooling (e.g. Rapid-i) or after (e.g. Closed Cryotop), each warranting concern over the possible presence of liquid nitrogen vapours or even liquid in the straw. The introduction of a warm device into a super-cooled straw will generally trigger a 'kinetic reaction', thus requiring the straw's opening to be covered (i.e. with fingertip or hand) to prevent expulsion of the device out of the straw. Alternatively, ultra-rapid cooling devices (see Tip 9) placed into a straw container to be sealed while in the liquid nitrogen bath must heed concern over trapped liquid nitrogen vapours in the straw, which could become explosive upon rapid warming in a water bath. In either scenario, the device could be compromised and potentially result in the contamination or loss of the embryo(s).

4. Warming and cryo-solution elution/dilution:
   a. Confirm physician's order regarding VFET date, scheduled time and embryo details (number to thaw/transfer, specific embryo number if PGS tested, etc.).
   b. Prepare fresh warming solutions (1.0 M sucrose stock solution; Appendix 35B) and/ or use a commercial source (recommended one-week to one-month shelf life once in use, 4°C storage).
   c. Warm (37°C) 1 × 10-ml tube each of 1.0 M sucrose solution and H-HTF medium/ patient for μS-VTF warming bath use.
   d. Prepare fresh thawing dishes (six-well plate), label the cover surface with the patient's name and solution IDs. In our case, we use (1) T1 wash (200 μl without oil overlay), (2) T1 (100 μl) with 1 ml oil, (3) T2 (100 μl) with oil, (4) T3 (100 μl) with oil, (5) T4 (100 μl)

with oil and (6) T5 (200 μl isotonic HEPES-buffered medium with 10% human serum albumin (HSA) without oil overlay).

Tip 11:

If a commercial source is not available, a universal sucrose solution step-down protocol can be applied: T1 = 1.0 M; T2 = 0.5 M; T3 = 0.25 M and T4 = 0.125 M. These same solutions, and the preceding protocol, can be effectively used for old slow-frozen blastocysts.

    e. Thaw one patient's materials at a time/workstation

Tip 12:

The embryologist should (1) confirm the cycle before warming the indicated number (i.e. one or two blastocysts), and (2) assess survival/probable viability and, if questionable, contact the physician and/or patient before warming another blastocyst.

    f. Confirm patient/specimen identification (with secondary quality control check).
    g. Place patient cane in a Dewar flask filled with liquid nitrogen, and isolate/ID the straw to be warmed.
    h. Bring the six-well dilution dish to the stereomicroscope stage, and using a 60-mm Petri dish, add the warmed sucrose and H-HTF solutions to create a 0.5 M sucrose warming bath (uncovered).
    i. Hold the upper straw seal to confirm ID above the liquid level, and then grasp and secure the straw below the internal plug using a Mayo scissors (VTF tip still submerged in liquid nitrogen).
       (Details can be visualized in an YouTube videos, *MicroSecure Vitrification*)

Tip 13:

Firmly tap scissors on the Dewar flask a couple times to jar the VTF tip from the inner straw sidewall as a quality control precaution, if adherent, ensuring the base drops to the sealed end opposite the labelled end, thus providing an airspace near the plug end.

    j. Lift the straw with the scissors into ambient air in a horizontal position (next to or below the stereoscope surface), grasp the non-labelled end (label to the right side), cut straw at the inner plug, lift above warming bath dish and pour the VTF tip into the warm sucrose bath at a 60-degree angle until completely extruded and rapidly warmed (>6,000°C/minute). The base of the flexipette will rest up above the dish sidewall.[8]

Tip 14:

The VTF tip should free fall into the bath. Gently tap the upper straw surface if the tip does not immediate come out. If it only appears partway, you can assist extrusion by grasping the shaft of the flexipette with the scissors or a fine forceps.

    k. After five to ten seconds, grasp to pipette base, insert into a micro-cap pipetting device (i.e. a hole in the bulb acts to release pressure upon insertion) and then cover bulb hole with an index finger and gently squeeze the bulb to release the vitrified blastocyst into the T1 wash (number 1), while viewing by stereomicroscopy. Once confirmed, clear the residual V3 (VS) solution and bubbles into the centre discard well. Start the five-minute timer.

l. Remove the VTF tip and replace it onto a stripper pipetter. Proceed by moving the embryo into T1 number 2 under oil for the remaining time.

Tip 15:

If more than one straw needs to be warmed, immediately warm the second straw and VTF tip (repeating steps i–k) before initiating step l, and move both blastocysts together for a minimum elution in T1 (1.0 M sucrose) of >3 minutes.

m. Pre-fill the flexipette with the next solution; then move and dilute the blastocyst(s) in T2, T3 and T4 at three-minute intervals. If the zona pellucida has not been previously laser ablated (i.e. hatched), do so in T4.

n. Equilibrate blastocysts in T5 for five minutes on a warm surface (37°C).

o. Assess the survival and then place into embryo culture for 30 minutes to six hours before ET, at which time the embryo(s) is re-examined and documented before transfer (*Note:* BL re-expansion is not necessary to transfer a viable embryo.) If more than one viable blastocyst exists at the time of ET and the patient opts to ET only one blastocyst, the supplemental blastocyst can then be successfully re-vitrified (rVTF) by repeating steps d–j described earlier. We have experimentally performed rVTF up to six times without any apparent effect on survival/viability and have numerous live births following single rVTF events.

Appendices: Procedural Notes

Appendix 35A: Sucrose Solution Preparation

Due to risks of endotoxin accumulation in sucrose granules upon repeated openings, 17.1 g of sucrose should be aliquoted into 50-ml sterile flasks upon the initial opening (e.g. weekly supply source). Subsequently, when mixing pre-weighed granular sucrose into solution (1.0 M stock = 3.42 g/10 ml H-HTF), warming to 37°C increases its solubility in conjunction with repeated inversions to final mixing. Filtration (0.22-μm filter) through positive-pressure filtration units is recommended for viscous solutions (>0.5 M sucrose) or high volumes. Hand-pressure pumps are sufficient and inexpensive, whereas an electrical pump is noisy, causes vibrations and is simply not required.

Appendix 35B: Labelling

Depending on the straw/device system used, Brady labels or handwritten labels maybe affixed to an ID handle (straw connector), directly onto the straw/device or onto a CBS ID rod before internal insertion and weld sealing (i.e., tamperproof labelling) For non-labelling, a secondary label is highly recommended.

Appendix 35C: Embryo Loading and Manipulation

Care must be taken not to extract too much VS, which could make the BL(s) susceptible to excessive dehydration and potentially deleterious osmotic damage. Nor should the droplet be too large, making it unstable (i.e. reduced surface tension) and susceptible to possible displacement before vitrification or in storage, which in an open system could result in loss of the embryo(s) before warming. This is a distinct quality control advantage of the μS-VTF method, where the same volume is repeatedly pipetted and retained safely in an unsealed tube by capillary reaction before, during and after VTF/warming.

References

1. Mukaida, T., Oka, C., Goto, T. and Takahashi, K. Artificial shrinkage of blastocoeles using either a micro-needle or a laser pulse prior to the cooling steps of vitrification improves survival rate and pregnancy outcome of vitrified human blastocysts. *Hum Reprod* 2006; 21:3246–52.

2. Liebermann, J. and Conaghan, J. Artificial collapse prior blastocyst vitrification: improvement of clinical outcomes. *J Clin Embryol* 2014; 16:107–18.

3. Panagiotidis, Y., Vanderzwalmen, P., Prapas, Y., Kasapi, E., Goudakou, M. et al. Open versus closed vitrification of blastocysts from an oocyte-donation programme: a prospective randomized study. *Reprod Biomed Online* 2013; 26:470–6.

4. Schiewe, M. C., Zozula, S., Anderson, R. E. and Fahy, G. M. Validation of microSecure

vitrification (mS-VTF) for the effective cryopreservation of human embryos and oocytes. *Cryobiol* 2015; 71:264–72.

5. Stachecki, J. J., Garrisi, J., Sabino, S., Caetano, J. P. J., Wiemer, K. et al. A new safe, simple, and successful vitrification method for bovine and human blastocysts. *Reprod Biomed Online* 2008; 17:360–7.

6. Seki, S. and Mazur, P. Effect of warming rate on the survival of vitrified mouse oocytes and on the recrystallization of intracellular ice. *Biol Reprod* 2008; 79:727–37.

7. Mazur, P. and Seki, S. Survival of mouse oocytes after being cooled in a vitrification solution to −196°C at 95°C to 70,000°C/min and warmed at 610°C to 118,000°C/min: a new paradigm for cryopreservation by vitrification. *Cryobiol* 2011; 62:1–7.

8. Schiewe, M. C., Zozula, S., Nugent, N., Waggoner, K., Borba, J. and Whitney, J.B., Modified microSecure vitrification: A safe, simple and highly effective cryopreservation procedure for human blastocysts. J Vis Exp 2017; 121: (in video release).

9. Whitney, J. B., Anderson, R. E., Nugent, N.L. and Schiewe, M. C. Euploidy predictability of human blastocyst inner cell mass and trophectoderm grading. *Ann Clin Lab Res* 2015; 3:4–7.

10. Gardner, D. K. and Lane, M. Culture and selection of viable blastocysts: a feasible proposition for human IVF? *Hum Reprod Update* 1997; 3:377–85.

Chapter 36

Embryo Biopsy by Laser on Day 5 in the IVF Laboratory

Anick De Vos

Introduction

At present, the blastocyst stage is considered to be the optimal time to perform biopsies for pre-implantation genetic diagnosis (PGD) or screening (PGS). Trophectoderm biopsy does not adversely affect the embryos in contrast to cleavage-stage biopsy. Vitrification with transfer in a subsequent cycle might be necessary to allow time for the genetic analysis. However, clinical outcomes have been proven equivalent after transfer of euploid bastocysts during fresh in vitro fertilization (IVF) and cryopreserved blastocyst transfer cycles. Laser energy is used to open the zona pellucida either on day 3 to 4 or on day 5. Trophectoderm cells can be aspirated from herniating blastocysts, and with laser energy, these are dissected from the blastocyst. Trophectoderm biopsies contain multiple cells, typically five to seven.

36.1 Background

Trophectoderm biopsy in human blastocysts was first described by Dokras et al. in 1990,[1] showing the feasibility of the procedure and that sufficient extra-embryonic material can be obtained for PGD without impairing further development of the blastocyst. Compatibility of trophectoderm biopsy with implantation and development to term was first reported by Kokkali et al. in 2005.[2] In view of PGD, blastocyst biopsy has been associated with an implantation rate as high as 41%[3] and even significantly higher than when the biopsy is taken on day 3 (43% compared with 26%).[4] Many, if not most, centres performing PGS have now shifted towards trophectoderm biopsy for two main reasons. First, the high frequency of mosaicism at the cleavage stage makes this earlier stage less appropriate for screening. Additionally, biopsy at the blastocyst stage is less invasive to the embryo[5] because only a few trophectoderm cells are removed, whereas the inner cell mass (ICM) is left intact.

So far, trophectoderm biopsy in combination with comprehensive chromosome screening (CCS) has given an interesting insight into the euploidy rates in human blastocysts not only according to female age[6] but also according to blastocyst morphology.[7] Euploid blastocysts definitely have a high implantation potential. However, the benefit and cost-effectiveness of second-generation PGS in different IVF populations needs more evidence-based comparisons on an 'intention-to-treat basis', including cumulative live birth rates using all remaining cryopreserved embryos.[8,9]

Reporting trophectoderm biopsy for the first time in Data Collection VI (i.e. cycles from 2003),[10] the European Society of Human Reproduction and Embryology (ESHRE) PGD Consortium still only reports a small minority of cycles with blastocyst biopsy.[11] However,

111 cycles over seven years (2003–9) compared with 86 cycles in 2010 might indicate a future increase. So far, trophectoderm biopsy is performed more frequently for PGD (142 cycles) than for PGS (55 cycles), at least in the reporting countries.

Trophectoderm biopsy requires an appropriate blastocyst culture system as well as a good vitrification programme if the genetic result is not obtained fast enough to allow a fresh transfer.

36.2 Reagents, Supplies and Equipment (Note A)

36.2.1 Equipment
- Laminar airflow
- Mini table incubator
- Inverted microscope
- Intracytoplasmic sperm injection (ICSI) workstation
- Oil-filled injectors
- Laser system

36.2.2 Supplies
- Biopsy dishes (type injection dish)
- Pipetting capillaries
- Holding pipettes
- Aspiration pipettes
- Micro-droplet culture dishes

36.2.3 Reagents
- Sequential culture media
- HTF-HEPES
- Polyvinylpyrrolidone (PVP)
- Oil for embryo culture

36.3 Quality Control

1. Annual maintenance for the laser system is scheduled to guarantee proper function.
2. Extended culture performance is monitored on a monthly basis in order to have an idea of blastocyst formation and quality (Note B).
3. Trophectoderm biopsy is performed by skilled technicians with experience in cleavage-stage biopsy using a laser. These technicians underwent a specific training on a limited number of vitrified, warmed blastocysts that were donated for research.
4. At the start of the biopsy procedure, the patient's identity is verified by two witnesses. Blastocyst identity is double-witnessed both before and after the procedure, taking the blastocyst from and putting it back into the patient's micro-well dish.
5. For every blastocyst, we use a new aspiration pipette in order to fully exclude any DNA carry-over from one blastocyst to the next (Note C).

36.4 Procedures

36.4.1 Zona Opening

There are two options for zona opening in view of trophectoderm biopsy. The opening can be postponed until day 5 at the blastocyst stage.[2] The ICM is then visible and can be held on the opposite side. In this case, time is needed for herniation (one to four hours). If the opening is created on day 3 or day 4 of development,[3] as the blastocyst and trophectoderm grow, herniating blastocyts can be biopsied more rapidly on day 5 (Note D). The size of day 5 openings is not well specified,[2] except that the lowest energy setting of the laser is used, most probably as a precaution against harming the trophectoderm or avoiding blastocyst collapse as the zona is very thin and close to the trophectoderm at that point (especially in fully expanded blastocysts). Day 3 openings may vary from 5 μm,[12] 6 to 9 μm,[13] up to 25 to 30 μm (comparable to cleavage-stage biopsy).[3]

1. On day 3 of development, the medium is switched from cleavage medium to blastocyst medium. Embryos are then placed in a micro-well dish (avoidance of mixup).
2. On day 4 of development, zona opening can be performed in the micro-well dish itself (no micro-tools are involved to hold the embryo).
3. On the inverted microscope, the embryo is placed with the zona pellucida under the laser target. No specific location is chosen because the ICM is not yet formed. In cases of early cavitation on day 4, where an eventual start of the ICM can be seen, obviously the opposite side is chosen for opening. Laser settings should allow creation of an opening of around 30 μm with two or three pulses (Saturn 5, 0.594 ms; Octax Laser Shot, 2–3 ms; Fertilase, 7 ms).
4. If all available embryos are zona opened, the micro-well dish is returned to the incubator for further culture until day 5 or 6.

36.4.2 Inclusion Criteria for Trophectoderm Biopsy

As the blastocysts grow, they will start to herniate overnight (i.e. trophectoderm cells begin to come out of the zona pellucida) (Figure 36.1, herniating blastocyst). On day 5, blastocyst development is assessed based on the Gardner score.[14] Expanding and expanded blastocysts with an ICM of grade A or B and a trophectoderm of grade A or B are included for biopsy of herniating trophectoderm cells. Cavitating morulas and early blastocysts remain in culture, and biopsy is attempted 24 hours later on day 6 of development based on the same inclusion criteria used on day 5 (Notes E and F).

36.4.3 Preparation of Biopsy Dishes

Biopsy dishes contain four droplets of 10 μl human tubal fluid (HTF)–HEPES to contain blastocysts and an additional two 10-μl droplets to be used for rinsing. One additional 5-μl droplet of HTF-HEPES is placed to be replaced by PVP at the time of biopsy. The droplets are covered with oil.

36.4.4 Trophectoderm Aspiration and Laser Ablation

1. Micropipettes (holding and aspiration pipettes) are mounted on the inverted microscope.

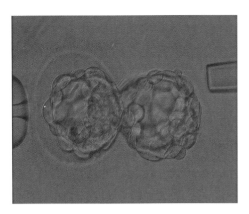

Figure 36.1 Herniating blastocyst. When opening the zona pellucida on day 3 or 4, as the blastocyst grows, it will start to herniate; that is, trophectoderm cells will begin to come out of the zona pellucida. (A black and white version of this figure will appear in some formats. For the color version, please refer to the plate section.)

2. Then 5 µl of PVP is placed in the biopsy dish (replacement of the 5-µl medium droplet), and a blastocyst is transferred from the culture dish to the biopsy dish (double-witnessed for patient identity and blastocyst identity). The dish then is placed on the heated stage of the inverted microscope.

3. The micro-tools are visualized, and proper functioning of both injectors is checked by aspiration and expulsion of medium. The inner wall of the aspiration pipette is covered with a thin film of PVP (by aspiration and removal again) in order to avoid sticking of trophectoderm cells to the pipette.

4. Herniating trophectoderm cells are aspirated. Tension is applied to the blastocyst by both holding and aspiration pipettes in order to stretch the blastocyst, showing a narrow bridge of trophectoderm cells between the aspirated cells and the cells still inside the zona pellucida (Figure 36.2).

5. Ablation of the aspirated trophectoderm cells is done by firing the laser onto the narrow bridge of cells (Notes G and H).

6. When the biopsy piece is fully detached, it is left in the biopsy dish next to the blastocyst (Figure 36.3). The blastocyst is then removed from the biopsy dish and returned to the culture dish (double-witnessed). Capillaries are well rinsed in between blastocysts using an extra tube of HTF-HEPES medium as a measure to avoid DNA carry-over.

7. The aspiration pipette is renewed before starting with the next blastocyst. All these steps are repeated for each blastocyst available.

8. Biopsy dishes with trophectoderm biopsy pieces are given to the diagnostic laboratory. Culture dishes with blastocysts are returned to the incubator. Subsequently, when the biopsy pieces are tubed, the blastocysts can be frozen individually by vitrification.[15] The genetic diagnosis will come later.

36.5 Notes

A. Several options exist for equipment, supplies and reagents. Three types of lasers are currently and mainly used: Octax Laser Shot, MTG GmbH, Germany (similar to the older version named Fertilase); Zilos-tk, Hamilton Thorne, USA and Saturn 5, Research Instruments, UK. All represent 1.48-µm infrared diode lasers, with laser power, respectively, of 100 to 150, 300 and 400 mW. The use of micro-well dishes allows us to keep embryos/blastocysts separated in one dish, avoiding any risk of mix-up due to

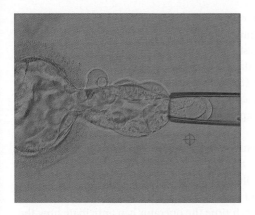

Figure 36.2 Aspiration of herniating trophectoderm cells. Tension is applied to the blastocyst by both holding and aspiration pipettes in order to stretch the blastocyst, showing a narrow bridge of trophectoderm cells between the aspirated cells and the cells still inside the zona pellucida. (A black and white version of this figure will appear in some formats. For the color version, please refer to the plate section.)

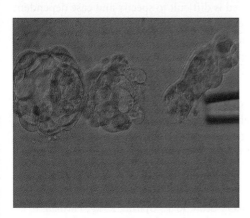

Figure 36.3 Fully detached biopsy piece. The trophectoderm biopsy piece is left in the biopsy dish (for the diagnostic laboratory), while the blastocyst is returned to the culture dish prior to vitrification, allowing time for the genetic analysis and potential transfer in a subsequent cycle. (A black and white version of this figure will appear in some formats. For the color version, please refer to the plate section.)

droplets merging together. Any sequential medium yielding a good blastocyst formation rate and blastocyst quality can be used for extended culture. HTF-HEPES is used during the biopsy procedure to keep a constant pH. In contrast to cleavage-stage biopsy, a Ca/Mg-free medium is not used for trophectoderm biopsy. PVP is used to prime (and empty again) the aspiration pipette so as to create a thin and viscous film on the inner wall to avoid sticking of the biopsy pieces.

B. In our laboratory, a blastocyst formation rate of about 40% to 45% per fertilized oocyte is obtained. Of these, 10% to 15% are top-quality blastocysts (at least Gardner stage 3, ICM grade A or B, trophectoderm grade A), and the remaining 30% are good quality (at least Gardner stage 3, ICM grade A or B, trophectoderm grade B) or early blastocysts (BL1, BL2). Day 5 patients are, on average, 32 years of age and present with an average of 12 cumulus-oocyte complexes.

C. Certain laboratories do not take this severe and rather expensive measure but instead rinse the pipette in between blastocysts with HTF-HEPES very carefully and thoroughly.

D. When opening the zona pellucida on day 3 or 4, it may occasionally (<10% of all blastocysts) happen that the ICM is located in the herniating part and thus badly located for further biopsy. Much in contrast to day 3 cleavage-stage biopsy, it is, however, possible to create a second opening and continue trophectoderm biopsy from the other side without any further problem.

E. Our experience with intended trophectoderm biopsy is that, on average, 10% of the started cycles showed insufficient development until day 5 or 6 to allow blastocyst biopsy. On average, 3.9 (SD 2.7) blastocysts were available per biopsy cycle. About 65% of the blastocysts were biopsied on day 5, whereas the other 35% were biopsied on day 6. Patients were, on average, 34.4 (SD 5.1) years of age and presented with an average of 11.6 (SD 6.9) cumulus-oocyte complexes.

F. In cases of fully hatched blastocysts, our experience is that zona-free biopsy is a feasible approach.

G. Settings are very specific per laser system used. Settings used: Saturn 5, 0.594 to 0.649 ms; Octax Laser Shot, 3 to 4 ms; Fertilase, 8 ms.

H. Some laser systems can be used automatically, that is, presetting a straight line as a target where the laser will fire a certain number of pulses of a certain energy. However, it is preferred to fire individual pulses so that each time the operator can anticipate how the blastocyst reacts. The number of pulses needed is difficult to specify and case dependent (on average, three to five pulses or sometimes more) (Note I). Then the biopsy piece can be detached carefully by pulling alone, as such limiting the number of pulses. By stretching, trophectoderm cells become elongated, and one can specifically target the cell tips instead of firing in the middle of the cell. When using a pedal for laser firing (which is an accessory available for the laser system), both hands can be kept on the injectors. As such, full and continuous control of holding and aspiration/pulling is guaranteed.

I. Occasionally, after multiple firing, the trophectoderm can become extremely rigid, rendering all additional pulses inefficient and without further impact. In these cases, mechanical biopsy, by rubbing the created trophectoderm bridge against the holding pipette can be attempted.

References

1. Dokras, A., Sargent, I. L., Ross, C., Gardner, R. L. and Barlow, D. H. Trophectoderm biopsy in human blastocysts. *Hum Reprod* 1990; 5:821–5.

2. Kokkali, G., Vrettou, C., Traeger-Synodinos, J., Jones, G. M., Cram, D. S. et al. Birth of a healthy infant following trophectoderm biopsy from blastocysts for PGD of beta-thalassaemia major. *Hum Reprod* 2005; 20:1855–9.

3. McArthur, S. J., Leigh, D., Marshall, J. T., de Boer, K. A. and Jansen, R. P. Pregnancies and live births after trophectoderm biopsy and preimplantation genetic testing of human embryos. *Fertil Steril* 2005; 84:1628–36.

4. McArthur, S. J., Leigh, D., Marshall, J. T., Gee, A. J., De Boer, K. A. et al. Blastocyst trophectoderm biopsy and preimplantation genetic diagnosis for familial monogenic disorders and chromosomal translocations. *Prenat Diagn* 2008; 28:434–42.

5. Scott, R. T., Upham, K. M., Forman, E. J., Zhao, T. and Treff, N. R. Cleavage-stage biopsy significantly impairs human embryonic implantation potential while blastocyst biopsy does not: a randomized and paired clinical trial. *Fertil Steril* 2013; 100:624–30.

6. Franasiak, J. M., Forman, E. J., Hong, K. H., Werner, M. D., Upham, K. M. et al. The nature of aneuploidy with increasing age of the female partner: a review of 15,169 consecutive trophectoderm biopsies evaluated with comprehensive chromosomal screening. *Fertil Steril* 2014; 101:656–63.

7. Capalbo, A., Rienzi, L., Cimandomo, D., Maggiulli, R., Elliott, T. et al. Correlation between standard blastocyst morphology, euploidy and implantation: an observational study in two centers involving 956 screened blastocysts. *Hum Reprod* 2014; 29:1173–81.

8. Gleicher, N., Kushnir, V. A. and Barad, D. H. Preimplantation genetic screening

(PGS) still in search of a clinical application: a systematic review. *Reprod Biol Endocrinol* 2014; 12:22.

9. Lee, E., Illingworth, P., Wilton, L. and Chambers, G. M. The clinical effectiveness of preimplantation genetic diagnosis for aneuploidy in all 24 chromosomes (PGD-A): systematic review. *Hum Reprod* 2015; 30:473–83.

10. Harper, J. C., Wilton, L., Traeger-Synodinos, J., Goossens, V., Moutou, C. et al. The ESHRE PGD Consortium: 10 years of data collection. *Hum Reprod Update* 2012; 18:234–47.

11. De Rycke, M., Belva, F., Goossens, V., Moutou, C., SenGupta, S. B. et al. ESHRE PGD Consortium data collection XIII: cycles from January to December 2010 with pregnancy follow-up to October 2011. *Hum Reprod* 2015; 30:1763–89.

12. Fragouli, E., Katz-Jaffe, M., Alfarawati, S., Stevens, J., Colls, P. et al. Comprehensive chromosome screening of polar bodies and blastocysts from couples experiencing repeated implantation failure. *Fertil Steril* 2010; 94:875–87.

13. Yang, Z., Liu, J., Collins, G. S., Salem, A. S., Liu, X. et al. Selection of single blastocysts for fresh transfer via standard morphology assessment alone and with array CGH for good prognosis IVF patients: results from a randomized pilot study. *Mol Cytogenet* 2012; 5:24.

14. Gardner, D. K., Lane, M., Stevens, J., Schenkler, T. and Schoolcraft, W. B. Blastocyst score affects implantation and pregnancy outcome: towards a single blastocyst transfer. *Fertil Steril* 2000; 73:1155–8.

15. Van Landuyt, L., Stoop, D., Verheyen, G., Verpoest, W., Camus, M. et al. Outcome of closed blastocyst vitrification in relation to blastocyst quality: evaluation of 759 warming cycles in a single-embryo transfer policy. *Hum Reprod* 2011; 26:527–34.

Chapter 37

Routine Embryo Transfer in the IVF Laboratory

Sangita K. Jindal

37.1 Background

In a very real sense, there is nothing routine about an in vitro fertilization (IVF) embryo transfer. It is the final and critical step in a patient's fertility treatment that has enabled millions of infertile couples to realize their dream of having a child. After completing all steps up to this point as part of their IVF cycle, it is the embryo transfer on which the entire process of bringing a new life into the world depends.

A key to a smooth embryo transfer is an experienced and engaged embryologist. Depending on the laboratory workflow, the embryologist may choose embryos for transfer, move embryos into the transfer dish, load the catheter with embryos and hand off the catheter to the clinician for transfer into the uterine cavity. Every step of the embryo transfer is critical and requires attention to detail and the ability to troubleshoot any issue that may arise.

37.2 Embryologist Experience

The embryologist must be trained and have acquired embryo transfer experience under supervision before performing transfers independently. While each laboratory has its own training regimen, it is important that embryologists observe transfers ($n = 20$), perform transfers under supervision ($n = 20$) and have pregnancy rates within two standard deviations of the mean pregnancy rate for the programme prior to being authorized to do transfers alone. During their training, embryologists should also become aware of how to troubleshoot unforeseen problems such as embryo return, re-loading of embryos and options for difficult transfers.

37.3 Reagent and Supply Inventory

At all times, a supply of catheters and syringes should be available for embryo transfer. There are a number of catheter options available commercially, and often the choice of catheter is clinician specific. Catheters typically come packaged with an outer sheath that contains a longer inner flexible catheter with an open lumen. The outer sheath and the inner catheter can be connected to each other via fitting their hubs together at the top and leaving the inner catheter protruding and visible at the open end. A tuberculin syringe is attached to the catheter collar at the top, and the syringe plunger is manipulated to both aspirate and expel the contents of the inner catheter.

Sometimes difficult transfers require catheters with a malleable stylet that guides the catheter with more stiffness into the uterine cavity. A 'trial of transfer' or mock catheter (without an open lumen) is often used right before the live catheter in order to 'map out' the catheter route into the uterus. Sometimes a pass-through or after-loading technique is used, whereby the catheter's outer sheath is placed into the uterus, and the live inner catheter is fed through the sheath. This transfer technique is helpful when clinicians are being trained to do embryo transfers.[1]

37.4 Guidelines for Transfer

Every embryo transfer requires a signed consent by the patient and, if applicable, the patient's partner. Based on American Society for Reproductive Medicine (ASRM) guidelines, between one and three embryos from normally fertilized oocytes will be transferred to the patient.[2] Following consensus between the clinician and the embryologist, the plan for transfer should be summarized for the patient.[3] The embryologist must confirm patient identity either by patient wristband and/or by verbally confirming the patient's name and date of birth; two unique identifiers should be confirmed. The patient often will have a full bladder in order to provide contrast when visualizing the uterus by ultrasound,[4] so embryo transfers should proceed in a timely fashion. Patients may express concerns or preferences that lead to modifications of the transfer plan at this time.[5] Typically, the patient is asked to attest in writing to her agreement with the plan of embryo transfer.

37.5 Reagents, Supplies and Equipment

The following equipment is required for an intrauterine embryo transfer in the embryology laboratory:

- Stereomicroscope in laminar flow hood at 37°C
- Incubator, trigas or CO_2
- Centre-well transfer dish equilibrated overnight containing 1.5 ml of culture medium with standard protein supplementation. Can also have medium with more than 50% protein supplementation or medium supplemented with hyaluronan.[6] Can place 5 ml of culture oil in outer well of dish to maintain osmolality.
- Stripper pipetter with 290-μm ID tips
- Glass pipette with bulb
- 1-ml tuberculin syringe, individually wrapped or glass Hamilton syringe
- Transfer catheter
- Gloves, sterile and non-latex
- Face mask
- Flask of warmed phosphate-buffered saline (PBS) or HEPES-buffered medium for clinician use

37.6 Quality Control

Universal precautions should be observed at all times. All quality control readings should be noted daily. It is good laboratory practice to record for each patient the lot number and expiration date of medium and protein source used. Only media, reagents and plastic ware that have been cleared for embryo toxicity may be used. No embryos are to be discarded or cryopreserved until the transfer has been completed successfully.

37.7 Transfer Protocol

1. The laminar flow hood is on and cleared for embryo transfer. Begin the transfer by placing a sterile catheter, syringe, gloves and mask in the hood to warm on the 37°C surface. If applicable, gas a bell jar in the warmed laminar flow hood with a blood gas mixture for use during the transfer procedure.

2. Remove the transfer dish and the culture dish containing the patient's embryos from the incubator, and place them in the warmed laminar flow hood.

3. Using the stereomicroscope in the hood, confirm the name and second unique identifier (e.g. date of birth, accession number) on the culture dish as that of the transfer patient. Make sure that a witness such as another embryologist also confirms that the name and second unique identifier on the culture dish are those of the transfer patient.[7] Active witnessing is recommended, whereby the patient's name is stated and spelled out loud. Both the embryologist and the witness must document the witnessing procedure on the embryology worksheet.

4. Evacuate one wash drop in the culture dish using a sterile glass pipette, and replace it with medium from the transfer dish. Keep the transfer dish warmed and gassed for flushing the catheter post-transfer.

5. Once the embryos have been graded and the embryos for transfer have been selected, use the 290-μm stripper to move the embryos to the drop, which now contains transfer medium, for at least 10 minutes, leaving them under the bell jar or in the incubator until time of transfer. At all times the embryos should be kept gassed at 37°C under an oil overlay.

6. The embryologist may be asked to provide the following to the clinician prior to transfer: the live transfer catheter, mock transfer catheter and/or sterile medium to wash the patient's cervix and to remove any mucus.

7. To prepare a catheter for loading, open the catheter packaging but do not remove the catheter. Flush a 1-ml tuberculin syringe one or two times with medium in the transfer dish. Fill the syringe with medium, attach it to the catheter, which is now removed from the packaging, and depress it to flush the catheter with medium. Then discard the medium. The rinsed and fully depressed syringe is attached to the rinsed catheter.

8. Move the patient dish containing the embryos for transfer under the stereomicroscope, and locate the embryos. The stereomicroscope may have a camera that is hooked to a monitor in the transfer room. You can place the patient dish under the microscope and make visible the patient-identifying information on the monitor (e.g. patient's name). The patient is able to see the still image from the microscope with her embryos and her name, enhancing the process for her. Alternatively, you can take a photograph of the embryos with the camera attached to a printer and give it to the patient as she exits.

9. The clinician may request that you load the catheter and hand off the inner and outer catheters to him or her with the catheter hubs loosely connected. Or the clinician may be doing an after-loading technique and requires only the loaded inner catheter be brought in by you and advanced through the outer sheath already in place in the patient's cervix until the catheter hubs can be connected prior to expulsion of the embryos into the uterus. If you are handling only the flexible inner catheter, be very careful to use sterile technique and use both hands to immobilize the catheter during transport.

10. Load the embryos under an oil overlay. Keep a stripper pipette nearby in case manipulation of embryos is required. Figure 37.1 is a diagram of catheter loading. How

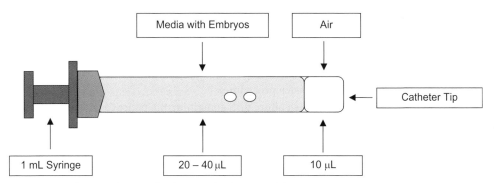

Figure 37.1 Schematic diagram of catheter loading (not to scale).

to draw up embryos into the catheter: 20 to 40 μl of medium column containing embryos + 10 μl of air column.

You will want to aspirate the embryos(s) into the catheter in a column of fluid, typically 20 to 40 μl. This fluid column should be followed by a 10-μl column of air to allow for easier visualization via ultrasound. Transfer volumes of more than 60 μl may result in expulsion of the embryos into the vagina, whereas volumes less than 10 μl may also negatively affect implantation rates.[8]

11. After loading the embryos into the catheter, enter the transfer room, and hand the entire catheter to the physician or thread the live catheter through the outer sheath already placed in the cervix. The patient will be awake during the procedure and will often have her partner in attendance. Patients are rarely medicated at the time of transfer. Before beginning the embryo transfer, call a 'time out' and confirm out loud the following information:

a. Patient's name
b. Planned procedure (embryo transfer or frozen-thawed embryo transfer)
c. Number of embryos to be transferred

The patient should verbally confirm her name. Also be sure to note the time that the catheter was handed to the physician.

12. Once the catheter tip is visualized via ultrasound in the mid-portion or lower mid-portion of the uterus, either the clinician or the embryologist should depress the syringe plunger to expel the embryos. This should be done slowly to protect the embryo(s) from the pressure gradient changes. After injecting the embryos, maintain pressure on the plunger until the catheter is completely withdrawn from the uterus. Be sure to completely retract the outer sheath and remove it simultaneously with the inner catheter to avoid a 'plunger effect'. Withdrawing the catheter slowly will also minimize negative pressure.

13. You will receive the catheter back so that you can return to the laboratory and flush the catheter with media in the transfer dish, to check for any retained embryos. If none are seen, give the 'all clear' call, signalling the successful transfer of all embryos.

14. The embryos should not remain in the catheter for more than two minutes. If the transfer is not successful after approximately 1 minute and 40 seconds, you should verbally remind the physician of this.[9] After two minutes, you will receive the catheter

back so that you can return to the laboratory and flush out the embryos. Be sure to identify all embryos in the culture dish before proceeding with the next transfer attempt.

15. Together you and the physician will make a decision about the next step. The physician may request a different catheter. He or she may also request that a curve be placed into the catheter.

37.8 Final Documentation and Review

At completion of transfer, fill out the necessary information on your embryology work-sheets, and add any comments on the quality of the transfer. You may want to note information such as multiple attempts to enter uterus, multiple catheters, multiple loading of embryos, pain, blood in the catheter, mucus in the catheter, no visualization by ultrasound and so on. Dispose of all transfer catheters, dishes and so on into a non-biohazard receptacle, and clean the laminar flow hood. Begin cryopreservation of any supernumerary embryos as previously determined. Make sure that all paperwork is completed.

37.9 Troubleshooting Notes

Ideally, embryos should not be loaded into the catheter until the clinician confirms that he or she is able to visualize the uterus via ultrasound and is able to map out the path that the catheter will take. In some cases, the clinician is unable to introduce the live catheter loaded with embryos into the uterus. This may be due to a patient's anatomy, an overly full bladder distorting the pathway of the catheter or inexperience on the part of the clinician, who must rely on clinical touch to advance the catheter. If the clinician is having difficulty advancing a catheter into the uterus, you may be asked to provide alternative catheters as needed or to place a curve in a catheter.

Embryos should not remain indefinitely in the catheter during multiple attempts to enter the uterine cavity. The catheter should come back to the laboratory, and the embryos should be unloaded from the catheter back into the culture dish and returned to culture until another transfer attempt is made. There is always a risk of losing embryos during loading and re-loading. Be sure to handle the embryos carefully at the time of transfer, especially if they have been hatched. If any embryo is lost or damaged during the transfer procedure, notify the clinician so that he or she can notify the patient. Another embryo from that patient may have to be transferred in its place.

You must check the catheter once the transfer has been completed. Sometimes not all embryos are expelled into the uterus, and on checking under the microscope, you may see that one or more embryos are still in the catheter. If this happens, calmly inform the clinician and the patient that an embryo has been returned to the laboratory. A new catheter should be prepared, and a second transfer should be performed immediately. Always check the catheter for retained embryos.

If the clinician is unable to visualize clearly the uterus by ultrasound, it may mean that the patient's bladder is overfull. The patient may be able to partially empty her bladder and resume the transfer procedure. Another possibility for better visualization may involve switching from abdominal to vaginal ultrasound.

In rare cases, the transfer cannot be performed. In such cases, the embryos may need to be cryopreserved until a plan of action is devised.

Every successful embryo transfer is the culmination of fertility treatment for the couple but also for the clinician and the laboratory. Routine embryo transfer is carried out every day by trained embryologists who are committed to ensuring success and the fulfilment of dreams for our patients.

References

1. Neithardt, A. B., Segars, J. H., Hennessy, S., James, A. N. and McKeeby, J. L. Embryo afterloading: a refinement in embryo transfer technique that may increase clinical pregnancy. *Fertil Steril* 2005; 83(3):710–4. PMID: 15749502; PMCID: 3444287.

2. SART PCAaPC. Criteria for number of embryos to transfer: a committee opinion. *Fertil Steril* 2013; 99:44–6.

3. Brauer, A. A. and Schattman, G. Embryo transfer. *Methods Mol Biol* 2014; 1154:541–8. PMID: 24782027.

4. Buckett, W. M. A meta-analysis of ultrasound-guided versus clinical touch embryo transfer. *Fertil Steril* 2003; 80(4):1037–41. PMID: 14556830.

5. Healy, M. W., Hill, M. J. and Levens, E. D. Optimal oocyte retrieval and embryo transfer techniques: where we are and how we got here. *Semin Reprod Med* 2015; 33(2):83–91. PMID: 25734346.

6. Loutradi, K. E., Prassas, I., Bili, E., Sanopoulou, T., Bontis, I. et al. Evaluation of a transfer medium containing high concentration of hyaluronan in human in vitro fertilization. *Fertil Steril* 2007; 87(1):48–52. PMID: 17074336.

7. de los Santos, M. J. and Ruiz, A. Protocols for tracking and witnessing samples and patients in assisted reproductive technology. *Fertil Steril* 2013; 100 (6):1499–502. PMID: 24427790.

8. Mains, L. and Van Voorhis, B. J. Optimizing the technique of embryo transfer. *Fertil Steril* 2010; 94(3):785–90. PMID: 20409543.

9. Matorras, R., Mendoza, R., Exposito, A. and Rodriguez-Escudero, F. J. Influence of the time interval between embryo catheter loading and discharging on the success of IVF. *Hum Reprod* 2004; 19(9):2027–30. PMID: 15192071.

Chapter 38

Quality Management in the IVF Laboratory
Witnessing

David H. McCulloh, Patty Ann Labella and
Caroline McCaffrey

Introduction

In our laboratory, we currently perform verification of specimen identity (VSI) by having two laboratory personnel independently check and verify the identity of each patient, gamete specimen and embryo at each step that is susceptible to a mismatch so that we can ensure accurate and complete traceability throughout the processes. Since this is the system currently in place in our laboratory, this method of verification and witnessing is the main focus of discussion in this chapter.

38.1 Purpose

The purpose of VSI is to provide an additional independent verification of the identification of patients (parents) and specimens during the performance of procedures in the in vitro fertilization (IVF) laboratory. Provision of this independent verification ensures laboratory personnel that the embryos were generated using oocytes from the intended specified female and the sperm from the intended specified male. In addition, this same process of VSI is useful in ensuring that each embryo either transferred or cryopreserved is the same embryo that was biopsied and either screened (pre-implantation genetic screening (PGS)) or diagnosed (pre-implantation genetic diagnosis (PGD)) to be of a desired genetic qualities. Rigorous procedures to validate the identification of all oocytes, sperm and embryos also ensure patients that they will receive only the correct embryos (of the expected ploidy, the expected genetic complement and arising from their own gametes). Patients state that one of their greatest anxieties when undertaking IVF treatment is whether the laboratory can maintain accurate identification of their gametes and embryos. It is imperative that the laboratory have a system in place that ensures this essential and critical process.

38.2 Outlining the Procedures for Which VSI Is Necessary

Steps that require VSI include any step during which a specimen is received from a patient, any step in which two specimens must be combined, any step in which gametes or embryos are moved from one container with a label to a different container with a label and/or any step in which a specimen is returned to a patient. The specimens that we use are gametes (oocytes, sperm) and embryos that result from fertilization of an oocyte by sperm. Each of these specimens is so small that it is impractical to label the gametes or embryos directly. Rather, we indirectly label the gametes/embryos by labelling the containers in which we maintain these biological materials. During the course of gamete/embryo culture, the biological material may be transferred from one container to another several times. Since the only means of identifying the specimens is through labelling the containers, it is imperative that the identification be checked and then independently re-checked and verified whenever a specimen is moved from one container to another. This means that there must be a clear chain of custody documented and verified whereby the gametes and embryos can be tracked starting with receipt of specimens from the patient through to final disposition of gametes or embryos. These transfer-of-custody steps include

Receipt of specimens from patients. Every time a specimen is accepted from a patient, it is important to accurately establish and maintain identity of that specimen as belonging to that patient. Therefore, both the patient's identity and the identification label must be confirmed and matched on the container into which the specimen will be placed.

> For oocytes, this means (1) identifying the patient while the patient is still awake and prior to administering anaesthesia and (2) verifying the identification labels on the dishes or tubes into which the patient's oocytes will be placed. The patient's identity must match the identification on the culture dishes.

> For sperm, this means (1) identifying the patient prior to accepting his semen or tissue specimens and following his affirmation that it is his specimen and (2) verifying the identification labels on all the vessels into which the specimen will be moved during sperm processing. The patient's identity must match the identification on the processing vessels (centrifuge or culture tubes).

Insemination (combining two specimens). Immediately prior to the mixing of sperm and oocytes (insemination procedure, regardless of the method), identification of the sperm specimen and identification of the oocyte specimen must be verified. Insemination of the oocytes must only occur when there is confirmation that the gametes are correctly matched to each other.

Specimen moved from one container to another container. Gamete and embryo specimens are moved from vessel to vessel during their culture and treatment in the embryology laboratory. At each transition from one container to another container, the identification on the container from which the gametes/embryos will be taken must match the identification on the container into which the gametes/embryos will be placed. Without this verified matching process, the gametes/embryos must not be moved. Examples of the switch in vessel include steps in semen processing as well as steps in oocyte/embryo handling:

- Vessel changes for semen/sperm processing
- Vessel changes for oocytes and embryos and for embryo biopsies

Return of specimen to patients. When the female patient is ready to have an embryo(s) placed into her reproductive tract to attempt to achieve pregnancy, it is imperative that the patient's identity and the embryos' identities are verified and match. No transfer of embryos to a patient should occur unless the identity of the embryos can be verified to match the patient and can be verified throughout every step of the embryos' processing/treatment from gametes obtained through embryo placed in the catheter.

38.3 Equipment, Reagents, Standards and Controls

- Performance and witnessing identification sheet (Figure 38.1)
- Witness with qualifications for personnel who perform VSI

Figure 38.1 Performance and Witnessing Identification Sheet.

	Last name	First name	Middle name	Medical record no.	Procedure no.
Female					
Male					

Procedure: Inscription of your initials under ID#1 or ID#2 indicates that you have viewed the identification on the materials listed below and have found that the identification on the materials matches between the materials and with the Identification on this form	ID #1	ID #2
Oocyte retrieval (patient and dishes)		
Oocyte thaw (tank location, cryo vessel, dishes)		
Sperm collection (patient, specimen cup and tubes)		
Sperm processing (specimen cup and tubes)		
Removal of cumulus/corona prior to ICSI (including move to new dish) (dishes before and after)		
Insemination/ICSI (including move to new dish) (oocyte dishes, sperm tube, insemination dish)		
Fertilization check (dish)		
Embryo thaw (embryo ID, tank location, cryo vessel, dishes)		
Day 2 check (dish)		
Day 3 check (and transfer to new dishes) (dishes before and after)		
Day 4 check (dish)		
Day 5 check (dish)		
Day 7 check (dish)		
Embryo transfer (patient ID and dish)		
Embryo biopsy (dish, embryo ID, biopsy dish, biopsy tube)		
Embryo cryopreservation (dish, embryo ID, cryo vessel)		

A person who provides VSI must be qualified to provide this important function. Qualification should include the ability to read names and numerals used to identify the patients and specimens; the ability to distinguish between single-letter or single-digit differences in names and numerals used to identify patients and specimens; and a knowledge of the workflow within the embryology laboratory so that the individual is available when needed and is not causing distractions when not needed. Most technical staff within a medical facility are trained to identify patients, and clinical staff are generally aware of the importance of what can and cannot be touched within the embryology laboratory. It is not necessary that the person who provides VSI be an embryologist. In fact, individuals with much less training and experience can function as providers of VSI. In some cases, we permit observers, designated by the patient, to observe the procedures within the laboratory. Although these observers provide comfort and assurance to the patient, they should not serve as witnesses. We rely on our own internal system of VSI because we are responsible for the identifications; therefore, all witnesses are paid employees of our facility.

38.4 Sample Required

1. **Oocyte retrieval.** Female patient arm band (after the arm band has been placed on the patient's arm following an identification step (check of the patient's name and identification), it must match identifiers on the dishes to receive the oocytes.
2. **Sperm collection.** Male patient's name and identification (state-provided identification card) must match the identification on the specimen cup and preparation tubes.
3. **Insemination:**
   a. Female patient's name and unique identifier(s) must match the identifiers on the oocyte dish.
   b. Male patient's name and unique identifier(s) must match the identifiers on the sperm tube.
   c. Female patient's identifiers must match the male patient's identifiers, and both must match those expected for the patient couple.
4. **Move specimens from one container to another.** Patient's name and unique identifier(s) must match on the first container and the next container.
5. **Biopsy.** Patient's name and unique embryo identifier(s) for the culture dish must match the identifiers on the biopsy receptacle (vial or tube).
6. **Cryopreservation.** Patient's name and unique embryo identifier(s) on culture dish must match the identifiers on the cryo container.
7. **Embryo transfer.** Patient's name and unique identifier(s) must match the identifiers on the culture dish.
8. **Embryo thaw.** Patient's name and unique embryo identifier(s) on the orders must match the identifiers on the cryo container and the dishes for culture.

38.5 Preliminary Steps

Prior to verification of identity, the facility must decide what type of identification is necessary to uniquely identify each patient in the programme. The use of unique identifiers is crucial to ensure that two patients with the same name are not mistakenly considered to be the same person. Since patients occasionally have the same names or the same dates of birth, these two identifiers are not effective unique identifiers. Many programmes have unique patient identifiers (medical record number) or unique procedure numbers (accession numbers) that may be useful in uniquely identifying samples for either or both partners in a couple.

Further, we must now consider the use of unique identifiers for multiple specimens for the same patient or patient couple. Two examples could be (1) two sperm specimens that may be used in one IVF procedure and (2) multiple oocytes/embryos, especially when we wish to link the results of specific embryo testing (PGS, PGD, morphokinetics, mitochondrial activity) to a particular embryo belonging to a patient couple. Therefore, methods of identification must now be able to uniquely identify more than just the patient or the patient couple. This raises the difficulty and highlights the precision needed by an order of magnitude in the laboratory. Careful thought must be exercised in planning how unique identifiers will be designed and implemented in the assisted reproductive technologies (ART) laboratory. This becomes even more difficult because the complexity of identification tends to require more and more characters (digits), and the tools onto which we must affix unique identifiers (for cryopreservation of individual embryos) are becoming smaller and smaller.

Next, it is necessary to decide how patients will be identified when they present in your programme. Will you require that they show identification with each visit (or at least during application of patient ID arm bands)? Will you provide patients with identification cards? Will you rely on newer digital fingerprint, palm print or retinal scan technology? Will you consider patients' memory of identifying numbers as sufficient (reciting name, telephone number, date of birth, Social Security Number)? Or will you rely on visual recognition of patients by staff. All these have their advantages and disadvantages, and your decision should be a match to the volume, complexity and your desire to avoid misidentification in your programme.

38.6 Step-by-Step Instructions

1. The first step in identity verification is to determine the identity of the individual(s) for whom the verification is to be performed. Who is the person that you expect? Who are the partners that you expect? Generally, several identifiers are required to be certain of a patient's identity. These would include the patient's first and last names (one identifier) plus the patient's medical record number at your facility (a unique identifier), the patient's procedure number (a unique identifier – several may be associated with the same patient/couple) or the patient's date of birth (a not-so-unique identifier). The identifiers should be written or printed legibly on paperwork (performance and witnessing identification sheet) and on dishes, tubes, vials and cryo containers. The person performing the procedure must ensure that the paperwork indicating the identifiers to be verified has been prepared.

2. Now that the expected identifiers are legibly inscribed, the labelling used to identify the sample must match the expected identifiers. Sample identifiers that must be matched are different depending on the type of sample being identified (please see Section 38.4).

3. The person performing the procedure must alert the witness and ensure that the witness is present before beginning the procedure. The witness must be available to perform VSI when the person performing the procedure is ready to perform the procedure.

4. The witness must review the paperwork indicating the identification to be verified during the procedure. The person performing the procedure must permit the witness to view all the crucial identifying labels prior to the initiation of the procedure. For the double-checking method to be valid and not suffer from either detrimental automaticity or lack of independence, the person performing the procedure must honestly assess the identity of the specimens and patients or containers without deferring to the person performing the VSI. Only when the person performing the procedure and the witness perform identity verification independently is the double-check system valid. Unfortunately, since we do not wish to expose gametes or embryos to conditions outside the incubator for excessive periods, we try to limit their time on the bench to a minimum, and this tends to lead to a rushed identification procedure by both parties verifying identification simultaneously. If, at any time, the identification does not match

the expected identification, the procedure must be halted. All material must be returned to a safe location (incubator, freezer). In this situation, it is imperative that the reason for the lack of match be determined and resolved prior to proceeding. Consult a supervisor or the laboratory director prior to proceeding.

5. Once the procedure and witnessing are complete, both the person performing the procedure and the VSI must indicate their identities on the paperwork for verification. This paperwork provides documentation of the steps that were verified and the personnel who verified them.

38.7 Calculations

None

38.8 Frequency and Tolerance of Controls

There are no controls per se. However, please note that the matching of identification is always performed by comparing one set of names and identifiers to a second (reference or control) set of names and identifiers. Whenever these do not match exactly, the matching is considered out of tolerance, and all procedural steps must be halted, and gametes and embryos should be returned to their safe locations (back in the incubator if they came from the incubator or back in the cryotank if they came from the cryotank.)

38.9 Expected Values

It is expected that all names and identifiers match whenever they are compared.

38.10 Procedural Notes

38.10.1 Limitations

We use a witnessing system[1] to reduce the incidence of identification errors. Personnel performing witnessing should be aware of the faults with this system,[2–4] including involuntary automaticity,[5,6] lack of independence of witnesses and interruption of personnel performing other critical procedures.[7] We believe that when witnessing is acknowledged as an important step in procedures and when its performance receives appropriate personnel attention, it reduces errors.

Only when the person performing the procedure and the witness perform identity verification independently is the double-check valid. Unfortunately, since we do not wish to expose gametes or embryos to conditions outside the incubator for excessive periods, we try to limit their time on the bench to a minimum, and this tends to lead to a rushed identification procedure by both parties verifying identification simultaneously.

38.10.2 Alternative Methods to the Use of a Second Laboratory Person

Future advances include direct bar coding of oocytes/embryos using avidin/biotin reaction to affix chemical bar codes directly to the zona pellucida of oocytes/embryos.[8] This application (presently at the research stage) may provide useful methods of unique identification in the future. This method may be more appropriate in the case of identifying individual embryos prior to, during and following embryo biopsy procedures.

The electronic systems commercially available provide an effective alternative to the two-person witnessing[3] and are in use in laboratories around the world. Use of these methods relies on electronic equipment to perform the witnessing steps described earlier. These systems include the use of bar codes (Matcher, IMT International, Chester, UK) and radiofrequency identifiers or RFID tags (Witness, Research Instruments, Cornwall, UK) that can be read by identity readers placed at workstations within the laboratory. Both of these systems address the limitations of the two-person witness system by removing errors of automaticity, improving traceability and eliminating the need to call other laboratory personnel away from their duties. In this way, it is argued that both systems make more efficient use of time and personnel and ensure independent unbiased verification if implemented properly.

References

1. Brison, D. R., Hooper, M., Critchlow, J. D., Hunter, H. R., Arnesen, R. et al. Reducing risk in the IVF laboratory: implementation of a double witnessing system. *Clin Risk* 2004; **10**:176–80.

2. Jarman, H., Jacobs, E. and Zielinski, V. Medication study supports registered nurses' competence for single checking. *Int J Nurs Pract* 2002; **8**:330–5.

3. Rienzi, L., Bariani, F., Dalla Zorza, M., Romano, S., Scarica, C. et al. Failure mode and effects analysis of witnessing protocols for ensuring traceability during IVF. *Reprod Biomed Online* 2015; **31**:516–22.

4. Thornhill, A. R., Orriols Brunetti, X. and Bird, S. Measuring human error in the IVF laboratory using an electronic witnessing system. In *Proceedings of the 17th World Congress on Controversies in Obstetrics, Gynecology & Infertility* (COGI '13) (pp. 101–6) (Lisbon, Portugal: Monduzzi Editoriale, 2013).

5. Toft, B. and Mascie-Taylor, H. Involuntary automaticity: a work-system induced risk to safe health care. *Health Serv Manag Res* 2005; **18**:211–16.

6. Armitage, G. Double-checking medicines: defense against error or contributory factor? *J Eval Clin Pract* 2007; **14**:513–19.

7. Biron, A. D., Loiselle, C. G. and Lavoie-Tremblay, M. Work interruptions and their contribution to medication administration errors: an evidence review. *Worldviews Evidence-Based Nursing* 2009; **6**(2):70–86.

8. Novo, S., Nogues, C., Penon, O., Barios, L., Santalo, J. et al. Barcode tagging of human oocytes and embryos to prevent mix-ups in assisted reproduction technologies. *Hum Reprod* Hum Reprod 2013; **29**(1):18–28.

9. www.alphaconference.org/media/London_2012/Presentations_Speakers/17_15_Orriols_Xavier.pdf (accessed 17 July 2015).

10. www.slideshare.net/RIUKROB/embryology-id-systems-i-steve-fleming-sydney (accessed 31 August 2015).

Chapter

39

Quality Management in the IVF Laboratory

Quality Improvement, Document and Process Control and Adverse Events

Rebecca Holmes and C. Brent Barrett

Introduction

Over the last 35 years, in vitro fertilization (IVF) has transformed the treatment of infertility. Concurrently, IVF has become more complex due to the adoption of highly technological laboratory procedures, including cryopreservation of eggs and embryos, micromanipulation and pre-implantation genetic screening. In addition, the patient population being treated has broadened and often includes not only the intended parents but also gamete donors or gestational surrogates. It is critical therefore for IVF laboratories to implement and maintain the highest standards of quality, and this chapter has been written to guide laboratory directors and embryologists in this endeavour.

Quality can be an elusive concept and is often in the eye of the beholder. In an IVF laboratory it is frequently defined by a clinic's success rates or the results of inspections by regulatory agencies such as the College of American Pathologists (CAP) or a laboratory's ability to offer the latest technology. While these attributes are very important and a vital part of a high-quality laboratory, quality comprises many other elements that are often overlooked.

According to one definition, 'quality' is, 'the totality of features and characteristics of a product or service that bear on its ability to satisfy stated or implied needs'. In the case of an IVF laboratory, the stated and implied needs are primarily those of our patients and physicians and include proper identification (ID) and chain of custody, appropriate care of gametes and embryos, clear and accurate communication, transparency and use of procedures and techniques that are consistent with satisfactory outcomes. How these needs are fulfilled relates to the features and characteristics of the service that the IVF laboratory provides. Among many things, this involves training and on-going assessment of laboratory personnel, use of appropriate and quality-controlled equipment and supplies, accurate and complete records and documentation, protocols that are clear and accurate, robust procedures for identification and correction of errors and problems and a system for ensuring that laboratory quality is continually being reviewed and improved.

Every organization has a unique system for ensuring that quality is maintained. However, there are basic principles that apply to all quality management systems (QMS) no matter what industry, company or laboratory. This chapter discusses these foundational concepts and applies them to IVF laboratories with the intention of providing a resource that can be used to create or strengthen a QMS.

39.1 Management

39.1.1 Responsibility and Authority

Generally, the laboratory director is empowered and given the necessary financial and human resources by the business owners and/or physicians in order to create and maintain a functional and effective laboratory QMS. In larger clinics, a laboratory manager or supervisor might oversee the quality of specific areas, such as embryology, cryopreservation or andrology. In situations where there is an offsite director, a laboratory manager is often in charge of day-to-day work and quality.

39.1.2 Communication

The laboratory director must have an established and effective means of communicating quality issues to laboratory personnel. This could be in the form of regular laboratory meetings, posted bulletins and/or emails. Equally important as communication within the laboratory is communication between the laboratory and the other departments of the clinic. Clear delineation of responsibilities and understanding of interactions between departments is vital. Flowcharts can be a very effective means for describing these interactions (see section on documents below).

39.1.3 Goal-Setting

The QMS should contain measurable goals that the director oversees and reviews periodically. These goals will be different from laboratory to laboratory but might include statistical measurements of quality, accuracy of data entry (determined by random checks of records), quality control (QC) and Proficiency testing (PT) success, non-conformance report reviews, document reviews and so on.

39.1.4 Compliance with Regulations

Each country has a different set of governmental or regulatory bodies that has oversight of IVF laboratories. Understanding and complying with all the applicable regulations is an important aspect of a high-quality laboratory. For example, in the United States, laboratories must comply with regulations from many or all of the following: Food and Drug Administration (FDA), College of American Pathologists (CAP), Clinical Laboratory Improvement Amendments (CLIA), Occupational Safety and Health Administration (OSHA), Joint Commission on Accreditation of Healthcare Organizations (JCAHO), Health Insurance Portability and Accountability Act of 1996 (HIPAA) and state regulations.

In addition, there are international organizations such as the International Standards Organization (ISO) which have created quality standards that apply universally to companies in every industry. Some IVF clinics, particularly in Europe, have chosen to use the ISO 9001:2008 quality standard and have based their QMS on its requirements. Certified clinics are inspected at least annually to ensure their continued compliance with the standard.

39.2 Document and Record Control

'Document control' refers to who has control of the documents; how they are written, updated, managed, reviewed and distributed; and their form of storage and accessibility. There are many companies that provide excellent online document control, and this will be the best choice for many laboratories that do not want to develop their own system. Other laboratories may choose to develop an in-house document control system. Whether a laboratory uses an external or internal document control system, it is critical that everyone in the laboratory or clinic understand the basic concepts of document control, as described below.

39.2.1 Types of Documents

There are many different documents that must be controlled, including

- Flowcharts (process maps)
- Procedures and protocols
- Work instructions (short one-page 'cheat' sheets)
- Forms
- Administrative records (laboratory bulletins and meeting minutes)
- Organizational charts
- External documents that are used in the laboratory (equipment manuals, validation reports and QC certificates)

Most documents are created and stored as electronic copies, and these electronic versions must be controlled as well as the hardcopy versions. It is very helpful to create a list of documents, who controls them and the current version.

While editing privileges are given only to the person who controls the document, everyone should be able to read the document. If documents are printed, revision numbers must be clearly visible, and careful attention must be paid to ensuring that only the current version is available.

39.2.2 Assigning Control of Documents

An important step in document control is deciding who is authorized to make changes in a document. Usually, there is one person who is designated as controlling a document; for example, the laboratory director may control all laboratory procedures and be the only one who can make changes. If a physician would like to change a procedure, the change must first be approved by the laboratory director.

39.2.3 Templates and Document ID

Creating a template for documents is essential. While templates can take many forms, they should contain the following information (see example below):

- Type of document
- Name of the document or procedure
- Name or title of person who controls document
- A unique ID
- A revision number

Example template for a laboratory procedure (the company logo can be inserted in the left box):

	PROCEDURE *Semen Analysis*	*Approved by:* *Lab Director*	P-AE-1000 Revision : 17 Page 1 of 18

39.2.4 Document Revision

A procedure for updating and changing documents should be established. As noted earlier, only authorized personnel may make changes, and those changes must be communicated to all appropriate employees. Minor changes may be communicated by email or verbally, but personnel should sign off on significant changes to show that they have understood the changes. There are many different ways to achieve this, but one example is to use a 'laboratory bulletin' that is posted and must be initialled by all appropriate staff.

Documents should be updated as needed, but many regulatory bodies require that all protocols be reviewed at least annually. In addition, it is particularly important to review and update all documents at the time of a change in management, such as a new laboratory director.

Tracking changes in documents is important, and there are many ways to achieve this. One method is to use a table that identifies who created the document and approved any revisions and the dates of the changes. This form could be a cover page or a back page:

Review and revision history

Revision number	Authorized signature(s)	Date	Description of changes (If no changes, write N/A)
0		2/1/03	N/A
1		11/11/03	Rpm changed to 1100
2		2/24/04	Verbal orders verified, spill clean up

39.2.4.1 Example: Creating a New Document

You have decided to start to vitrify embryos instead of using a slow-freezing technique. Since this is a significant protocol change, you have decided to create a new procedure and discontinue the old procedure. The steps to complete this include

1. Identify the appropriate document template for creating a new procedure.
2. Write the procedure.
3. Assign the unique code.
4. If the laboratory has a list of current documents, add this to the list.
5. As director, sign off on the procedure and have all laboratory members read and sign off on it.
6. Move the electronic copy of the old slow-freeze method into the discontinued procedure folder.
7. Remove any hard copies of the old slow-freeze procedure from workstations and replace with the new vitrification procedure.

39.2.5 Flowcharts

Otherwise known as 'process maps', flowcharts are extremely helpful when creating, modifying or troubleshooting a procedure. Because each step in a process and each decision point must be clearly defined, flowcharts can reveal inconsistencies or potential problems in a process and can aid in ensuring that everyone completely understands all the steps in a process. Flowcharts can be easily created using software such as Microsoft Visio.

Below is an example flowchart consisting of the first steps in andrology processing:

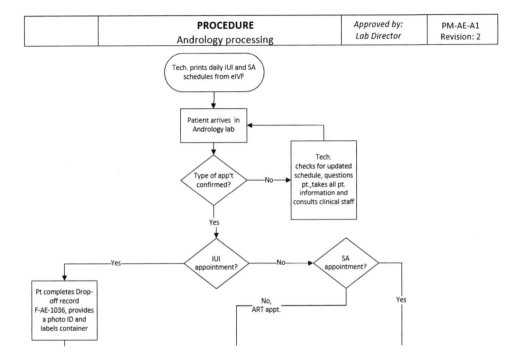

| | PROCEDURE | Approved by: | PM-AE-A1 |
| | Andrology processing | *Lab Director* | Revision: 2 |

39.2.6 Control of Records

Records are generally completed forms and will be both electronic, as with an electronic medical record, and paper. The form itself will be created and controlled by an authorized person, and changes to the form can only be made by this person. Critical records, such as embryology and frozen egg, sperm and embryo information, should be reviewed prior to filing to ensure that the record is accurate. Once stored, the records must be appropriately stored and accessible as needed. The amount of time records need to be stored varies but is generally at least two years and in the case of critical records will be indefinitely.

39.3 Human Resources

39.3.1 Qualifications

In the United States, the CLIA'88 and CAP regulations specify the minimum qualifications in regard to educational level and experience for technical, supervisory and director-level laboratory personnel. With a few exceptions, directors are required to have a PhD and be certified by an agency such as the American Board of Bioanalysis. Off-site directors must visit the laboratory at least once every three months to review all critical aspects of laboratory functions. It is also recommended that supervisory embryologists be certified in either andrology or embryology. Continuing education is required to maintain these certifications.

There are numerous other criteria that are important when hiring embryologists and technicians, including

- Technical skill
- Dependability
- Attention to detail
- Teamwork
- Communication and interpersonal skills
- Organizational ability
- Judgement
- Initiative

39.3.2 Training

Training embryologists, especially those without experience in the human field, is critically important. Generally, training occurs in four phases, and each phase should be documented and reviewed and approved by the director or designee before the next phase is begun:

1. An introduction to the procedure and, as needed, practice in basic skills such as pipetting or micro-injection using animal or discarded material (often there is a specified number of repetitions that must be documented).
2. Performing a procedure clinically under the direct supervision of a trained embryologist in conjunction with monitoring of success rates and, again, completion of a specified number of repetitions. At this stage, new embryologists must become fully competent with laboratory documents, be able to maintain and troubleshoot the equipment required for the procedure and understand the role and importance of patient ID and chain of custody.
3. Working independently with a supervisor available as needed.
4. Ability to work completely independently with no requirement for supervision.

39.3.3 Competency Assessment

All laboratory personnel who perform practical applications in the laboratory must be monitored for performance. There are many different ways for assessing performance, including:

- Direct observation by a director or supervisor who is present in the laboratory and performing procedures can provide invaluable information that cannot be gained in any other way about the performance of individuals as well as any deviations from established procedures (protocol drift) or improvements that could be made.
- Some procedures, such as intracytoplasmic sperm injection (ICSI) fertilization rates and thaw survival rates, can be statistically tracked, and these rates should be monitored for all embryologists who perform them.
- Competency in all procedures should also be formally assessed and documented at least annually and more often if there have been any problems.

Table 39.1 Number of embryologists in relation to cycle numbers

Number of cycles	ASRM minimum no.	High-performing laboratorys
250	3	2
500	4	4
1000	6	8
1500	9	12
2000	11	16
3000	16	24

39.3.4 Number of Embryologists

The laboratory director has to determine the appropriate number of embryologists, andrologists and technicians to employ. This depends on a number of factors, including

- Volume and timing (whether the laboratory batches or not) of cases
- Experience level of the embryologists
- Amount of other, non-technical work (embryo transports, data entry, etc.) assigned to each employee
- Budgetary considerations

As the number of more complex procedures, such as PGS and embryo vitrification and thawing, increases, the number of embryologists required will concomitantly increase, and staffing levels should be carefully monitored.

The American Society for Reproductive Medicine (ASRM) does have published guidelines on the minimum number of embryologists depending on the number of cycles a clinic performs a year[1] (summarized in Table 39.1). Also, Van Voorhis et al.[2] looked at the number of embryologists in 10 high-performing laboratories in the United States and found that these high-performing laboratories generally have more embryologists than the ASRM guidelines.

39.4 Space and Infrastructure

Ideally, IVF laboratories have an adequate amount of space for the number of procedures performed; in practice, however, the space is often less than ideal. It is the responsibility of the director to ensure that the space and infrastructure (i.e. electrical outlets, sinks and eye washes, lighting, air quality)

- Are safe for employees
- Minimize the risk of a mistake
- Are able to produce acceptable results

39.5 Control of Supplies, Equipment and Processes

An IVF laboratory must control all the processes that occur within the laboratory and all the supplies and equipment. This comprises all the steps from scheduling, cycle initiation and specimen arrival to the final review of data.

39.5.1 Purchasing and Control of Supplies

All vendors should be approved by the laboratory director, and it is helpful to maintain a current list of approved vendors, contact information and supplies ordered. Many products purchased for use in an IVF laboratory are validated by the vendor, often by using a mouse embryo assay (MEA). Products that come into contact with gametes or embryos that are not validated by the vendor should be validated by the laboratory using an MEA test or a human sperm survival assay. Upon arrival, supplies should be checked for proper shipping conditions (e.g. ice packs are still cold with products that must be shipped cold). Some supplies, particularly plastic ware, should be allowed to off-gas prior to use. The dates of use must be tracked for each lot of medium or supplies, and expired supplies discarded. Use of a database to record such information is highly desirable. A searchable database should include the name and brand of product, when it was received, the lot number, expiration date, transport conditions, type of QC and dates in use and discarded.

39.5.2 Validation of Equipment

Much of the equipment in an IVF or endocrine laboratory must be validated before put into use. Typically, blood analyzers are validated by the manufacturer, and many instruments come with a validation certificate from the manufacturer. In the embryology laboratory, particular attention must be paid to the incubators – temperature, humidity and gas concentrations should be checked, and they should also be validated using MEA or another biological assay.

39.5.3 Quality Control of Equipment

All equipment must be monitored on a regular basis to ensure proper function. In an IVF laboratory, this often involves checking temperature for incubators and warming plates, humidity and gas concentrations for incubators, volume for pipettors and rpms for centrifuges. All devices used to monitor the equipment such as thermometers, gas analyzers and so on must be calibrated on a regular basis with a calibration device that is certified to be accurate. Blood analyzers used in endocrine testing are controlled using QC samples with known concentrations and by comparison with other laboratories. Many types of equipment require preventive maintenance or calibration on a regular basis, and it is helpful to have a calendar to keep track of these events.

39.5.4 HVAC Systems

Modern IVF laboratories generally have specialized heating, ventilation and air-conditioning (HVAC) filters to control particulates and volatile organic compounds (VOCs) that may negatively affect embryo development in the laboratory.[4] This equipment needs to be validated prior to opening the laboratory by analysis of particles and VOCs in the air, and they must be maintained and filters changed on a regular basis. Air quality should be monitored periodically to ensure that the equipment is functioning properly.

39.5.5 Control of Processes

Processes in an IVF laboratory are controlled by observation and data collection and analysis. Daily observation by the director or a supervisor of egg quality, fertilization rates and embryo development is essential to ensure that there are no hidden problems such as unseen contamination in an incubator, oil or medium. Embryologists must be supervised as protocol drift is a constant possibility.

There are a number of processes that are especially critical in an IVF laboratory and should be closely monitored: (1) accurate identification and a clearly documented chain of custody for gametes and embryos, (2) procedures for ensuring that current and valid consents are in place and (3) in the United States, documentation that FDA screening and results have been performed within the proper time period for all gamete and embryo donations. Each of these processes must be tightly controlled and should be reviewed periodically. Process mapping and/or FMEA analysis (see Section 39.6.1) can be very helpful in identifying steps in these processes that may be weak. Also, embryologists and andrologists should be fully trained and instructed on how to handle discrepancies from protocol.

Data collection and analysis are important in order to identify any trends in the data that may not be easily seen on a daily basis. Laboratories choose different parameters, statistical methods and time points to track and analyze their data based on their own experience. Important parameters that are often monitored include fertilization rates (both IVF and ICSI), cleavage and blastocyst development, thaw survival rates, implantation, pregnancy and delivery rates and volume of different procedures. Many other parameters can be tracked, and it is advisable to carefully track the results of new procedures. Acceptable ranges for each parameter should be established, and values outside these ranges should be carefully reviewed and corrective action taken if needed (see Section 39.6.1). Graphical presentations such Levy-Jennings charts or p-charts can be helpful in identifying and monitoring trends.[5]

39.5.6 Implementation of New Procedures

All IVF laboratories implement new procedures or introduce new equipment from time to time. A procedure that has been established commercially or is functional in another laboratory still requires testing, validation and quality control in the testing laboratory. Proper training and documentation of validation should be completed before rolling out the new test/procedure.

39.6 Errors and Corrective and Preventive Action

The opening sentence in the ASRM guideline on disclosure of medical errors involving gametes and embryos[7] states: 'Clinics have an ethical obligation to disclose errors out of respect for patient autonomy and in fairness to patients.' All human beings make mistakes, and the IVF laboratory is no exception. It is the medical and laboratory director's responsibility to foster a culture of truth-telling so that when a mistake is made, it is not hidden but brought forward to the appropriate managerial personnel. Not only is this an ethical duty, but it also brings problems to light and allows improvements to be made. For a brief discussion on error rates in an IVF laboratory, see Sakkas et al.[8]

Errors, or non-conformances, in an IVF laboratory can range from benign in the case of an easily correctable misspelling on a dish to catastrophic if incorrect gametes are mixed or the wrong embryo is transferred. Minimizing errors in the laboratory has always been an integral part of a high-quality laboratory and has become an even higher priority as the complexity in IVF procedures has increased.

39.6.1 Non-Conformances and Corrective Action

A 'non-conformance' is any problem, error or deviation from protocol, and non-conformances must be resolved, documented (preferably in an electronic database) and reviewed for possible corrective action and/or trends. Often non-conformances are resolved quickly, either by the employee alone or with the help of a supervisor, and this resolution must be documented as well. Once the immediate problem or error is resolved, the director or quality manager should review the incident to determine whether the root cause of the problem has been identified. A process called 'root cause analysis'[6] can aid in determining why the problem happened and how to prevent it from happening again. The overall process of identifying the root cause and fixing it is often termed 'corrective action'. In addition to reviewing individual non-conformances as they occur, they should also be reviewed together periodically to spot any trends that may be present.

For example, a document from a physician's nurse states that a patient wants to thaw two embryos, but when the laboratory reviews the patient's frozen embryo inventory, it finds that the patient only has one embryo. This is corrected by discussing the problem with the nurse, and the nurse calls the patient to inform her that she only has one embryo. The embryologist documents the error and the resolution and submits it to the director. Upon review, the director finds that the root cause of the problem was that the nurse used an old database to determine how many embryos the patient had. The director initiates corrective action by removing the database from the server and documenting this correction.

39.6.2 Preventive Action

It is equally important to provide a mechanism for identifying areas of concern before a problem occurs. This is often called 'preventive action', and it involves examining a procedure or set of procedures to determine where problems might be likely to occur. Several tools that can be very useful in this process are 'flowcharts' (also known as 'process mapping') and a process known as 'failure mode and effects analysis' (FEMA).[6] Flowcharts are extremely helpful in mapping each step in a process and identifying steps that may vary from person to person or which may need to be reinforced, and FEMA can help to identify areas where the greatest risk lies.

39.7 Conclusions

Due to the nature of IVF laboratories and the regulatory agencies that oversee them, many laboratories have strengths in certain areas, such as equipment maintenance and QC, setting statistical goals and tracking trends in outcomes, keeping up-to-date protocols and procedures, record keeping and so on. However, there are many aspects of a QMS that are not regulated, and these are frequently weaker areas that can be improved upon.

As our IVF clinics and laboratories expand and become more complex, we need to strengthen and improve the QMS structures in place in those laboratories as well as, ideally, putting a strong QMS in place throughout the clinic. There are many resources available to aid clinics and laboratories in improving their QMS. Notably, ISO is recognized throughout the world for quality standards; certification to a standard such as ISO 9001:2015 or ISO 15189:2012 (which is designed specifically for medical laboratories) will ensure a strong and dynamic QMS.

References

1. Practice Committee of the Society for Assisted Reproductive Technology, Practice Committee of the American Society for Reproductive Medicine. Revised minimum standards for practices offering assisted reproductive technologies. *Fertil Steril* 2006; 86:S53–6. doi: http://dx.doi.org/10.1016/j.fertnstert.2006.07.1484

2. Van Voorhis, B., Thomas, M., Surrey, E. and Sparks A. What do consistently high-performing in vitro fertilization programs in the U.S. do? *Fertil Steril* 2010; 94:1346–9. doi: http://dx.doi.org/10.1016/j.fertnstert.2010.06.048

3. CLIA Law and Regulations, available at www.n.cdc.gov/clia/Regulatory/ (accessed October 2015).

4. Morbeck, J. Air quality in the assisted reproduction laboratory: a mini-review. *Assist Reprod Genet* 2015; 32:1019–24.

5. Carey, R. *Improving Healthcare with Control Charts* (New York: ASQ Quality Press, 2003).

6. Mortimer, S. T. and Mortimer, D. *Quality and Risk Management in the IVF Laboratory* (2nd edn.) (Cambridge University Press, 2015).

7. Ethics Committee of the American Society for Reproductive Medicine. Disclosure of medical errors involving gametes and embryos. *Fertil Steril* 2011; 96:1312–14.

8. Sakkas, D., Pool, T. B. and Barrett, C. B. Analyzing IVF laboratory error rates: highlight or hide? *Reprod Biomed Online* 2015; 31.

Chapter 40

Troubleshooting in the IVF Laboratory

Kathryn J. Go and Thomas B. Pool

40.1 Background

A fully equipped laboratory with state-of-the-art air handling and climate control; meticulously calibrated and maintained incubators and microscopes; culture media and medium supplements scrupulously selected after stringent after-market assays; validated, efficient and effective laboratory protocols and techniques; skilled, experienced, knowledgeable embryologists; and board-certified reproductive endocrinologists. What could go wrong? Why and how could there *ever* be a poor outcome, such as failure of fertilization, oocyte degeneration, arrested development of embryos or low blastocyst formation rate, poor survival of embryos after cryopreservation or low embryo implantation rates?

Every laboratory and clinic must be prepared to encounter one, some or all of these undesired events and set out on a systematic analysis of the entire process to identify and address 'the problem'. The tendency to react with a toxic mix of assigning blame and panic will only result in a squandering of energy and the loss of opportunity to conduct a timely objective investigation into all candidate factors that are disrupting or negatively affecting the process.

In this chapter, some suggested strategies and tools for an effective investigation and focused troubleshooting are presented. These are designed to assist the embryologist, as well as the entire clinical team, to embark on a structured evaluation of each factor that may underlie, cause and/or contribute to a failure or a sub-optimal outcome. Indeed, the engagement of the *team* is encouraged, providing not only support but also valuable perspective in a time when one must resist the temptation to ascribe poor performance in in vitro fertilization (IVF) solely to the laboratory.

40.2 The Overview

A divide-and-conquer strategy is frequently effective when applied to many situations, and troubleshooting in assisted reproductive technology (ART) is no exception. Identifying the individual but interdependent compartments of the ART laboratory provides a map by which one can navigate the experience of the gametes and embryos. These categories may be defined as

1. Environment
2. Instruments
3. Culture system
4. Equipment and materials
5. Technical execution

In a world of simplistic solutions without challenges, one would hope, for instance, to quickly find 'bad' medium and simply open a new bottle of a new lot number or discover a negative nuance in technique and immediately adjust the method, but this is rarely the case. ART is the assistance to a biological process, not an industrial one, so one is denied the easy troubleshooting experience of punching through a list of scenarios to land on the omission or defect (example from the troubleshooting section of the user's manual for many electrical appliances: 'Is the unit plugged in?').

Troubleshooting in ART must be a thoughtful process by which one considers each component and step in the context of gamete and embryo function. *How* might the egg, sperm or embryo be negatively affected? And how will that negative impact be revealed? Looking at the factors in each of the broader categories listed earlier can be both incisive and revealing, providing information on deviations or, conversely, reassurance, that the set point or performance expectation is being met. The process of elimination allows the investigative process to advance through the list of factors with opportunity for adjustment and fine-tuning of the entire system.

Some categories lend themselves to study by a root cause analysis; others, by checklist-driven protocols or by decision trees. In this chapter, examples of each will be provided, allowing the reader to select the approach that best fits his or her individual style of investigation or the object of the investigation.

40.3 Environment of the Laboratory

The embryology laboratory must be a clean room or suite with filtered air and temperature and humidity set to achieve constant and comfortable levels. In considering how to study the laboratory's climate, a checklist accounting for and addressing each environmental factor may be helpful and may include the following:

40.3.1 Checklist for Evaluation of Laboratory Environment

- Temperature range achieved?
- Humidity range achieved?
- Air handling system functioning?
- Filters maintained/changed on schedule?
- Is environment free of and protected against volatile organic compounds (VOCs)?
  - No new, un-tested, non-approved cleaning agents or materials in the laboratory
  - No solvents
  - No painting or construction
  - No adhesives or caulks
  - No new cabinetry or fixtures

- Are there restrictions on access, and have they been observed?
- Do staff and patients observe prohibitions on colognes and scented cosmetics?
- Has there been painting or construction in or around the laboratory or operating/procedure room?
- Are there any potential sources of deviation in or disruption of the laboratory's ambient air quality?

Because conservation of an optimal environment in the laboratory is central to its work, running through a checklist of factors such as these can be useful. Protection of the gamete and embryos cultures from deviations in temperature or exposure to potential toxins in the air is critical as both represent opportunities for negative effects. Even transient drops in temperature in the cultures may affect, for instance, meiotic spindle formation or micro-tubular organization.[1] For instance, a too-cold temperature in the laboratory presents a steep temperature gradient to culture plates removed from incubators for microscopic examination or transfer or gametes or embryos from culture vessel to culture vessel.

The negative effects of VOCs on the outcomes of IVF have been described and well recognized for many years.[2,3] The checklist also highlights that the rooms and spaces surrounding the laboratory or operating/procedure room are vulnerable to environmental contaminants or disruptors such as paints, adhesives, carpeting and so on, so any sources in adjoining rooms or corridors must also be considered.[4]

40.4 Instruments

As ART has expanded to include cryopreservation and thawing of gametes and embryos, micro-manipulation for intracytoplasmic sperm injection (ICSI), assisted hatching and embryo biopsy and extended embryo culture, the catalogue of instruments installed and maintained in the laboratory has correspondingly increased.

While the earliest laboratories were minimally outfitted with a laminar flow hood, dissecting and inverted microscopes, a centrifuge and a couple of incubators, the twenty-first-century laboratory will typically house multiple incubators and laminar flow worksta-tions with integrated microscopes, potentially two or more inverted microscopes with micro-manipulators and a laser, centrifuges, and possibly programmable cell freezers and micro-tool fabricating machines such as pipette pullers, micro-forges and grinders in laboratories maintaining these skills. There are likely also several appliances such as refrigerators, water baths, sonicators, autoclaves, drying ovens and the instrumentation required to evaluate routine operational parameters such as thermometers, pH meters, hygrometers and carbon dioxide analyzers.

All these instruments demand maintenance and confirmation that they are operating correctly, integral as they are to providing the correct culture or procedural environment to gametes and embryos directly or indirectly.

Creating a systematic query for the operation of each instrument can be a useful exercise in ruling out deviations or sub-optimal function. Examples for three types of instrument – an incubator, microscope and micro-manipulators, and centrifuges – are provided in Figure 40.1.

This model can complement a checklist to consider an array of possible conditions that characterize an instrument, from complex (micro-manipulators) to simple (pipetters) and can be integrated into a routine quality control programme for the laboratory. Indeed, a rigorous quality control programme is a valuable ally during troubleshooting.[5]

40.5 Culture System

Far and away the most common response to poor or failed embryonic growth is to blame the culture medium, even though embryo culture media are, perhaps, the most heavily tested and scrutinized component of an IVF cycle, including the ovulatory and triggering medications as well as other clinical factors. It is crucial to realize that culture medium is

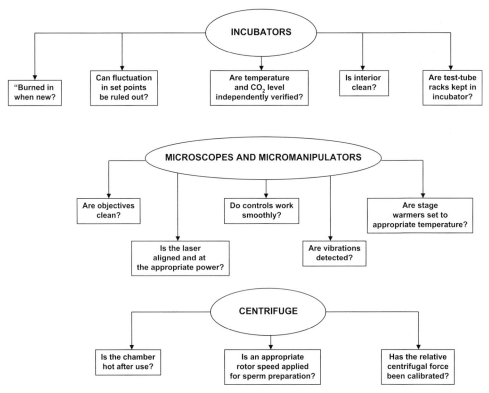

Figure 40.1 Factors to consider while troubleshooting processes in the IVF laboratory.

only one component of an entire embryo culture system that also encompasses medium protein supplements, oil overlay and culture plastic ware plus the physical environment provided by the incubator to include temperature, humidity and gas phase.[6] Additionally, poor performance manifest during embryo culture may well have roots in the retrieval and insemination/injection phases of the IVF cycle. Issues in embryo culture that appear with time, such as declining growth rates and reduced blastocyst conversions, should be addressed in a different manner than issues that arise catastrophically. One of the very best tools for troubleshooting performance that declines with time is to compare the performance and results of fresh cycles to frozen embryo transfer cycles. In this way, factors resident in the culture system can be dissected from those whose cause is associated with the events of embryo transfer and/or even luteal support as embryo production and transfer are separated in time with frozen cycles.

For performance failures that appear abruptly, the laboratory is charged not only with troubleshooting the immediate situation but also with simultaneously attempting to rescue the ongoing case. One effective way to do this is to formulate a process diagram prospectively that can be activated and followed should culture issues arise cataclysmically. Such a diagram is illustrated in Figure 40.2. In this example, it is assumed that daily quality control measures of incubator performance (temperature, oxygen and CO_2 concentrations, pH) are within defined limits. The detail one may extract from this troubleshooting activity will be

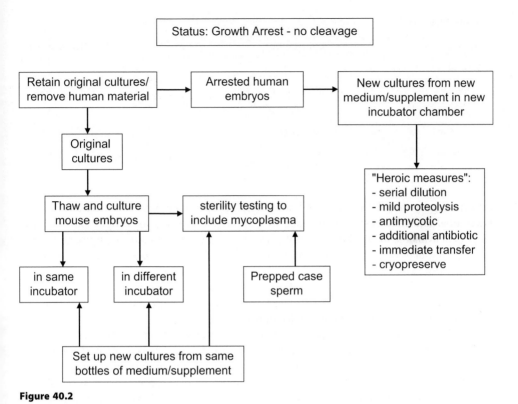

Figure 40.2

largely dependent on culture volumes used for embryo growth. If sufficient volumes are available, this process diagram will address and separate incubation environmental factors from medium and medium supplement issues. It also addresses the insemination phase of the cycle while suggesting some 'heroic' measures for saving the ongoing IVF cycle. Most importantly, it provides a template that can be revised and adapted to the specific approach taken by individual laboratories regarding embryo culture. The power of process diagrams is derived from their prospective design; troubleshooting can be initiated immediately with a thoughtful, comprehensive approach.

40.6 Equipment and Materials

Meticulous quality control, performed daily or at least once in each eight-hour shift for larger laboratories, is a key activity in augmenting effective troubleshooting. The commercial availability of data logging and alarm devices can provide 24-hour surveillance that can detect instrument malfunctions in precise moments that can be correlated in time with other troubleshooting data. Catastrophic equipment failures are rare with effective preventive maintenance programmes but do occur, and one must be prepared to troubleshoot equipment failures along with compromised procedural outcomes. For example, with microscopes, performance issues must be quickly triaged into electrical versus optical causes. Extra bulbs and fuses must be on hand, and the capacity for checking electrical

Table 40.1 Current Contact Materials in the Laboratory, Week of 21 September 2015

Item	Lot number	Lot OK	Date in use
Gas cyliners:			
CO_2, inc. 1/2	XG01T234A	Y	9/9/2015
CO_2, inc. 5/6	XG00U093A		16/9/2015
CO_2, inc. C/D	XG0IU009A	Y	2/*/2015
CO_2, inc. D b/u	XD04UT09A	Y	5/6/21015

circuit integrity must be available. A knowledge of proper alignment of optical components is essential and may best be embedded in a sequential checklist of proper chronological alignment available to all laboratory staff. Ancillary failure of associated equipment, such as micro-manipulators or lasers, must also be considered and contingencies made available. Having partial zona dissection (PZD) needles in the laboratory may save a case of embryo biopsy while laser malfunction is thoroughly evaluated for software or hardware causes. Again, checklists are excellent tools, used in conjunction with quality control data, in effective troubleshooting of equipment failures.

The IVF laboratory uses a wide variety of contact materials in the form of chemicals, gasses and laboratory ware. A systematic way to catalogue the date of first use and lot numbers of these items in a fashion that can be queried is imperative. First, only materials that have passed appropriate toxicity assays (mouse embryo assay, sperm survival test) should be allowed into the IVF laboratory. When introduced into usage, a simple table in a spreadsheet such as Excel can be updated on a weekly basis. An example of such a table is shown in Table 40.1. In this example, specific lots of compressed carbon dioxide in use with specific incubators are listed, along with the date when their use was initiated. The most important column is labelled 'Lot OK'. A 'Y' (yes) in the column means that since introduction into use, this particular lot of the item has been associated with results consistent with key performance indicators (KPIs) or outcomes for the laboratory. Thus, when laboratory performance falters, a rapid query of all items that have been placed into use but not yet evaluated against KPIs or routine outcomes can be quickly identified for further evaluation. This can greatly accelerate the troubleshooting process, often steering it into more productive pathways once it is clear that no new contact materials are the likely culprit.

Note that a quick visual inspection of the table shows that the cylinder in use for incubators 5 and 6 has not yet been associated with standard laboratory performance and, thus, would be suspect should performance be subpar. This examples illustrates how a strong quality control programme is a valuable ally in effective troubleshooting.

40.7 Technical Execution

There is a strong technical component to every activity performed in the IVF laboratory, and technical execution must always be evaluated in comprehensive troubleshooting activities. This begins with embryologists being forthright when mistakes occur, but often they go undetected without further analysis. In essence, one must determine whether the event involved deviation in the technical execution of a given procedure and, if so, were the roots

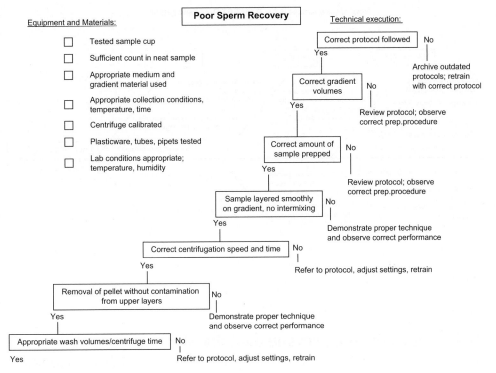

Figure 40.3

of it due to following an improper protocol, to incorrect technique, to improper or inadequate training or a combination of these. Checklists and a decision tree are effective tools in making these determinations, an example of which is given in Figure 40.3. In this example, the laboratory supervisor has noticed that the recovery of highly motile, morphologically normal sperm from neat samples has declined and has employed a decision tree, in conjunction with a checklist, to troubleshoot the procedure. Evaluation of the equipment and materials checklist eliminates those as a cause; thus, the decision tree is followed for technical execution beginning with the protocol. Was the proper protocol followed, and if not, why not? At each node of the tree, successive steps of a procedure are evaluated with remedial actions suggested when the answer is 'No'. Decision trees such as this are not only fundamental tools for troubleshooting but are also instrumental in ensuring that technical deviations are not repeated in the future.

Another tool for investigating outcomes in which suboptimal technique is suspected is a root cause analysis. An example is presented for poor results in an embryo freezing and thawing programme using an Ishikawa diagram[7] (also known as a 'fishbone diagram') depicted in Figure 40.4. This method provides another way of taking stock of all the factors that could influence the technique under consideration, including those outside the laboratory's influence, such as whether the patient's cycle is natural or hormonally programmed. Again, the encouragement is offered to consider *all* potential factors, not only those that originate in the laboratory, to provide an all-encompassing analysis.

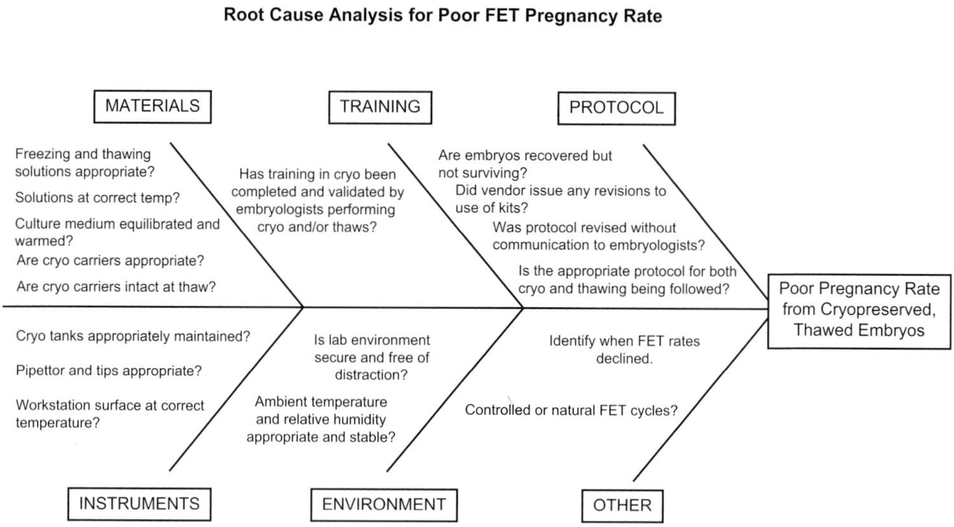

Root Cause Analysis for Poor FET Pregnancy Rate

Figure 40.4

40.8 Troubleshooting beyond the Laboratory

The same quest for meticulous quality control pursued in the embryology laboratory should be a tenet of the clinical procedures. A metric approach can be taken by tracking the clinical outcomes for each physician (e.g. pregnancy rate per treatment cycle, per embryo transfer performed), thereby ensuring that these phases of the treatment process receive the same scrutiny for consistency and optimal performance.

Taking stock of clinician-driven procedures should also be part of an effective troubleshooting effort. Agonist versus antagonist for suppression, new approaches to stimulation, endometrial thickness, new physicians, new transfer catheters, new ultrasonographers, new imaging, even the scrub technicians or operative assistants who handle the follicular aspirates at retrieval all merit some consideration in the investigation.

Finally, the patient introduces a number of factors that may elude all control: female age, response to gonadotrophin stimulation, ovarian reserve, body weight and mass, severity of male factor and ejaculated versus testicular sperm. Some consideration of how the clinical and medical factors may influence outcomes is a fair part of troubleshooting beyond the confines of the laboratory. An excellent culture environment can conserve the developmental potential of 'good' eggs, but it cannot induce an egg grown in a poor follicular environment, for instance, to improve its prospects for implantation.

In this context, a cooperative and collaborative spirit should ideally permeate the troubleshooting process. Assumptions that the laboratory, clinician or patient is individually to *blame* for poor outcomes will not serve the purpose of achieving best practice. Working together to thoughtfully address the problem and conduct the investigation is a chance for each member to learn more about the global process and attain the insight that may catalyze the problem solving at the heart of troubleshooting.[8]

40.9 Effective Troubleshooting Is an All-Inclusive Activity

Envision this scenario: you have noticed that the percentage of metaphase II oocytes has dropped and that the fertilization rate is reduced as well as the percentage of fertilized oocytes that cleave. There are few centres that would not be scrutinizing the laboratory environment and performance as the culprit, but in this case these were all attributed to the use of a short GnRH agonist protocol as opposed to a long one.[9] There are myriad examples of effects seen in the ART laboratory that are caused by factors outside the laboratory, not the least of which may be clinical characteristics of the patient, including compliance with treatment or medication instructions.

In many respects, the methods and expendable supplies used in the laboratory are the most heavily scrutinized factors involved in an ART procedure, given requirements for laboratory accreditation (educational and experience requirements of testing personnel, patient test management, proficiency testing, quality control, quality management) and bioassay of contact materials. In contrast, there are no recurring requirements for competency examinations or proficiency testing of clinical personnel. It is assumed, for example, that all ovarian follicles are identified and measured with little to no inter-observer variability. Further, cataloguing the gonadotrophins used in ovulation induction by source, lot number, storage conditions and so on is a challenging, maybe impossible task, but that does not exclude them as a potential root cause of downstream effects manifest in the laboratory.

What can and should be recorded are specific dates of changes made to clinical protocols (ovulation induction agents and strategies, trigger criteria and agents, luteal-phase support medications, duration, delivery systems) as well as any deviations in patient compliance. The physical properties of the retrieval room (temperature, humidity) should be recorded for each procedure as well as equipment performance characteristics such as the temperature of warming blocks, surfaces and chambers and vacuum values for aspiration pumps. Cleaning agents and procedures for the retrieval room, instruments and the clinical space must be proven initially to be compatible with gamete and embryo viability and must be documented at each use. Events outside the centre, such as the use of pesticides and fumigants, or activities that generate significant amounts of VOCs, such as the application of coatings to parking lots, must be noted as well.

Effective troubleshooting can only be achieved when investigations into unacceptable laboratory performance are initiated centre-wide. Any of the tools employed within the laboratory for troubleshooting are applicable to extra-laboratory evaluations, and the quickest way to perform this task is to have a template for a checklist, process map or cause/effect analysis (RCA) ready at all times. Archived documentation of QC measures can then be rapidly queried and applied to the template as an adjunct to laboratory investigations. It is also catalytic to the process to determine when and by whom a centre-wide troubleshooting activity will be activated and evaluated.

40.10 Conclusion

Troubleshooting is a demanding enterprise, and because it is triggered by negative or poor outcomes, it is carried out frequently in an environment of duress, consternation, disappointment and impatience, none of which is conducive to a measured pace. Typically, a solution to the problem is expected to be found in short order, followed by design and implementation of an immediate corrective action. Alas, there is no on-board computer in an embryology laboratory or ART clinic to run multiple diagnostic tests in a closed system to produce the meaning behind an error message. Troubleshooting is the resolute look into multiple systems and processes for a dual purpose: confirm that operations are sound and detect the deviation or fault. Through its requirement for analysis of processes and the role it fulfils in assessing compliance with protocols, troubleshooting is intertwined with the vital activities of quality control and risk management.[10]

To fulfil the mission of expediently correcting a 'fault' and returning to optimal operation, several methods for conducting an organized investigation into each part of an ART laboratory and clinic have been described. Each affords a systematic and comprehensive look into a physical object such as an instrument or an activity such as a laboratory technique where one hopes to validate correct operation or to detect a flaw, the correction of which will vanquish the problem and prevent recurrence.

As well as prescribing a methodology for troubleshooting, a philosophy and attitude of global thinking and team-oriented approaches to problem solving are strongly encouraged. While troubleshooting may be required and launched by a negative event or trend, its effective completion can yield insight into all the processes of IVF treatment and reveal ART as an ecosystem of professionals, the tools they deploy and the patients whom they treat.

References

1. Wang, W.-H., Meng, L., Hackett, R. J., Odenbourg, R. and Keefe D. L. Limited recovery of meiotic spindles in living human oocytes after cooling-rewarming using polarized light microscopy. *Hum Reprod* 2001; **16**:2374–8.

2. Cohen, J., Gilligan A., Esposito W. and Schimmel T. Ambient air and its potential effects on conception *in vitro*. *Hum Reprod* 1997; **12**:1742–9.

3. Hall, J., Gillian, A., Schimmel, T., Cecchi, M. and Cohen, J. The origin, effects and control of air pollution in laboratories used for human embryo culture. *Hum Reprod* 1998; **13**(Suppl. 4):146–55.

4. Sparks, L. E., Guo, Z., Chang, J. C. and Tichenor, B. A. Volatile organic compound emissions from latex paint: 1. Chamber experiment and source, model development. *Indoor Air.* 1999; **9**:10–7.

5. Elder, K., Van den Bergh, M. and Woodward, B. *Troubleshooting and Problem-Solving in the IVF Laboratory* (Cambridge University Press, 2015).

6. Gardner, D. K. and Lane, M. Culture systems for the human embryo. In *Textbook of Assisted Reproductive Techniques, Laboratory and Clinical Perspectives*, ed. D. K. Gardner, A. Weissman, C. M. Howles and Z. Shoham (2nd edn., pp. 211–34) (London: Taylor & Francis).

7. Ishikawa, K. *Guide to Quality Control* (Tokyo: JUSE, 1968).

8. Go, K. J., Patel, J. C. and Dietz, R. Troubleshooting in the clinical embryology laboratory: the art of problem-solving in ART. In *Practical Manual of In Vitro Fertilization. Advanced Methods and Novel Devices*, ed. Z. P. Nagy, A. C. Varghese and A. Agarwal (pp. 631–7) (New York: Springer, 2012).

9. Greenblatt, E. M., Meriano, J. S. and Casper, R. F. Type of stimulation protocol affects oocyte maturity, fertilization rate, and cleavage rate after intracytoplasmic sperm injection. *Fertil Steril* 1995; **64**:557–63.

10. Mortimer, D. and Mortimer, S. T. What's gone wrong? Troubleshooting. In *Quality and Risk Management in the IVF Laboratory* (pp. 135–44) (Cambridge University Press, 2005).

Index